Practical Case Studies in Dentistry

Practical Case Studies in Dentistry

Editor: Lailah Stewart

AMERICAN
MEDICAL PUBLISHERS
www.americanmedicalpublishers.com

AMERICAN
MEDICAL PUBLISHERS
www.americanmedicalpublishers.com

Cataloging-in-Publication Data

Practical case studies in dentistry / edited by Lailah Stewart.
p. cm.
Includes bibliographical references and index.
ISBN 979-8-88740-654-1
1. Dentistry. 2. Clinical medicine. I. Stewart, Lailah.
RK51 .C55 2023
617.6--dc23

American Medical Publishers,
41 Flatbush Avenue,
1st Floor, New York,
NY 11217, USA

ISBN 979-8-88740-654-1 (Hardback)

Contents

Preface

This book aims to highlight the current researches and provides a platform to further the scope of innovations in this area. This book is a product of the combined efforts of many researchers and scientists, after going through thorough studies and analysis from different parts of the world. The objective of this book is to provide the readers with the latest information of the field.

Dentistry is an important branch of healthcare that focuses on the diagnosis, prevention and treatment of issues related to oral health. One of the primary aspects of dentistry is preventive care. Regular dental check-ups, cleanings, and oral examinations help in detecting early signs of dental problems such as tooth decay, gum disease and oral cancer. Restorative dentistry is another fundamental aspect of the field. It involves repairing and restoring damaged or missing teeth. Dental fillings, crowns, bridges, and dentures are some of the common restorative treatments which are offered within dentistry. It also encompasses specialized fields such as orthodontics, which corrects misaligned teeth and bite irregularities, and endodontics, which involves root canal treatments to save infected teeth. This book contains some path-breaking studies in the field of dentistry. It will serve as a reference to a broad spectrum of readers.

I would like to express my sincere thanks to the authors for their dedicated efforts in the completion of this book. I acknowledge the efforts of the publisher for providing constant support. Lastly, I would like to thank my family for their support in all academic endeavors.

Editor

1

Detachable Lip and Cheek Plumper for Rehabilitation of Facial Disfigurement

Nada Fathalla Abdelbagi,[1] **Ibrahim Ahmed Ismail**,[1] **Fadia Awadalkreem**,[1] **and Mohammed Nasser Alhajj**[1,2]

[1]*Department of Oral Rehabilitation, Faculty of Dentistry, University of Khartoum, Khartoum, Sudan*
[2]*Department of Prosthodontics, Faculty of Dentistry, Thamar University, Dhamar, Yemen*

Correspondence should be addressed to Mohammed Nasser Alhajj; m.n.alhajj@hotmail.com

Academic Editor: Konstantinos Michalakis

Background. Hemimaxillectomy of acquired palatal defects may predispose the patient to hypernasal speech, leakage of fluids into the nasal cavity, impaired masticatory function, and swallowing difficulties leading to a detrimental impact on the quality of life. Sequentially, it can also affect individual character and trust in social life, leading to social phobia and anxiety. This article presents prosthodontic management of a young male patient with deformation of the entire right half of the face due to surgical removal of odontogenic myxoma. It describes a method where the clinician utilized a simple, noninvasive, and cost-effective technique to cut the weight of the obturator and to attain aesthetics, utilizing a detachable lip and cheek plumper. *Case Presentation.* A 19-year-old male attended the Prosthodontic Clinics at Faculty of Dentistry, the University of Khartoum, eight months after the surgical removal of a tumor. The chief complaint was difficulty eating or drinking. Furthermore, he dropped out of school because of his facial deformity and his indistinct voice. Medical and dental history revealed surgical resection of the entire right half of the maxillary alveolar bone due to myxoma. Intraoral examination revealed a well-healed surgical defect in the maxillary right buccal vestibule creating an oroantral communication. A treatment plan was formulated, keeping the patient's demand in mind. The decision was made to treat the patient with a maxillary obturator that would gain its support from the remaining teeth and tissues with a detachable cheek and lip plumper. The use of dental magnets as a means of attachment was elected. *Conclusion.* This article has described a simple, noninvasive, and cost-effective method to improve facial appearance in patients with hollow faces. The plumper prosthesis successfully improved the patient's appearance to the extent that comfort and function would permit and encourage self-esteem.

1. Background

The face is a significant constituent of body image; and those with facial disfigurement, self-worth, and self-concept are tightly entangled. It carries on how one is perceived and judged by others, guiding their impressions and behavior [1]. Most body deformities can be obscured from sight, but those of the face are open for all to view [2]. A young person might hold exterior looks to be very important; contrary to our thought, disfigurement to females is equally distressing to male patients; and it causes severe dislocation in their lives [2]. Hemimaxillectomy of acquired palatal defects may predispose the patient to hypernasal speech, leakage of fluids into the nasal cavity, impaired masticatory function, and swallowing difficulties leading to a detrimental impact on the quality of life [3, 4]. Sequentially, it can also affect individual character and trust in social life, leading to social phobia and anxiety [3, 5]. This tends to occur more often in patients with a maxillofacial defect than those with other defects of other organs of the body [3]. Cheeks impart greatly to facial aesthetics. Slumped or hollow cheeks can add years to a person's age. At times, the flanges of the prosthesis can be enough to provide fullness to the cheeks and lips, but sometimes, this is not entirely satisfactory [6].

Prosthodontic rehabilitation of a patient is no longer confined to the replacement of missing teeth alone. The

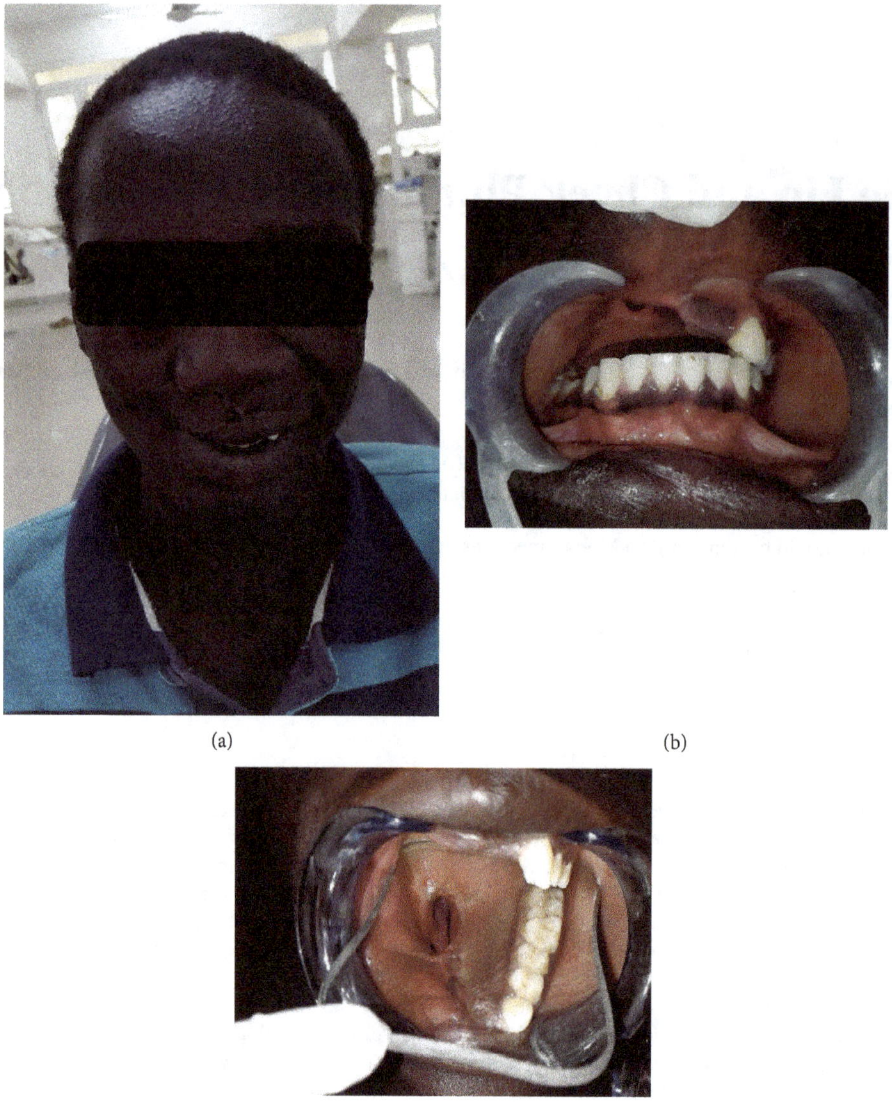

(a) (b)

(c)

Figure 1: (a) Extra oral view showing facial deformation of the right side; (b) maxillary and mandibular arch occlusion; (c) intraoral view of the maxilla showing defect.

importance of facial aesthetics has become an indispensable piece of dental treatment, and patients are increasingly calling for an improvement in aesthetics. A prosthodontist plays an integral part in restoring the losses in the patient with sunken faces. Sometimes, conventional dentures can fulfill these demands. But, in some instances, extra support to the dentures could be supplied. This can be achieved by using cheek plumpers or cheek lifting appliances [7]. The use of plumper prosthesis in maxillofacial prosthodontics is also well documented [8]. Cheek plumper or cheek lifting appliance is a prosthesis for supporting and lifting the cheek to provide required aesthetics that will increase the self-esteem of the patient [6]. A cheek plumper can be of two types: detachable or undetachable. Undetachable cheek plumpers are conventional single-unit prostheses with extensions on either side of the polished buccal surfaces of the denture. Detachable cheek plumpers are those which can be detached from the denture. This can be achieved by magnets or customized attachments [8].

This article presents prosthodontic management of a young male patient with deformation of the entire right half of the face due to surgical removal of odontogenic myxoma. It describes a method where the clinician utilized a simple, noninvasive, and cost-effective technique to cut the weight of the obturator and to attain aesthetics, utilizing a detachable lip and cheek plumper.

2. Case Presentation

A 19-year-old male attended the Prosthodontic Clinics at Faculty of Dentistry, the University of Khartoum, eight months after the surgical removal of a tumor. The chief complaint was difficulty eating or drinking. Furthermore, he dropped out of school because of his facial deformity and his indistinct voice. Medical and dental history revealed surgical resection of the entire right half of the maxillary alveolar bone due to myxoma. Extra oral examination revealed an

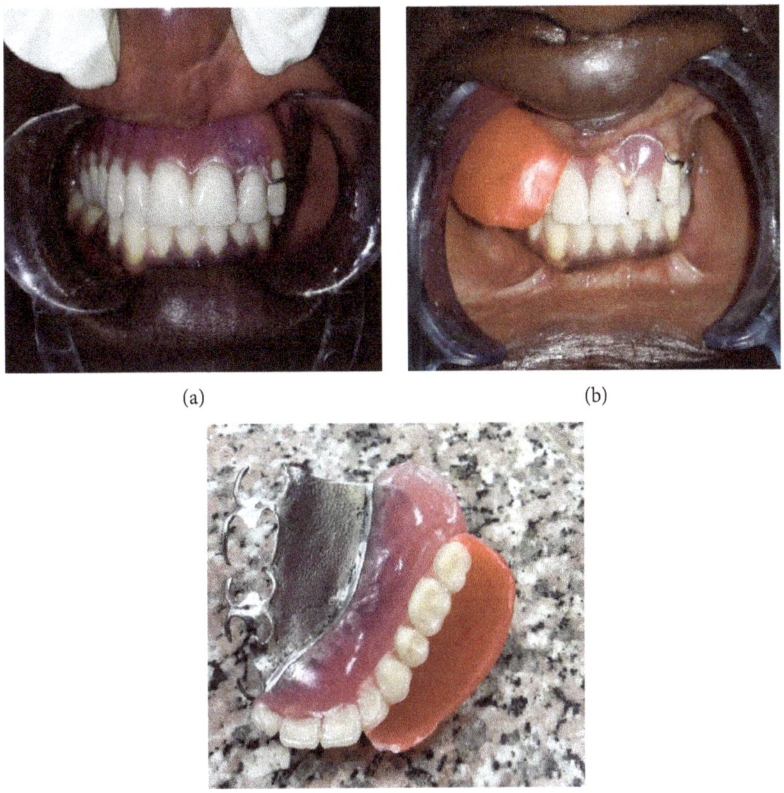

(a) (b) (c)

FIGURE 2: (a) Definitive obturator in maximum intercuspal position; (b) intraoral wax try-in of the plumper; (c) plumper impression hallowed.

asymmetrical face with the loss of lip support and sunken right cheek, depression of the right nasolabial fold, and ptosis on the right eye with many wrinkles around it (Figure 1(a)).

Intraoral examination revealed a well-healed surgical defect in the maxillary right buccal vestibule creating an oroantral communication. The missing teeth were 11, 12, 21, 22, 23, 24, 25, 26, and 27. All the remaining maxillary teeth and complete mandibular dentition were examined clinically as well as radiographically and found to be caries-free with no significant gingival/periodontal problems. Masticatory and phonetic functions of the patient were severely affected due to missing maxillary structures. The panoramic radiograph showed a large radiolucency in the right maxillary region. The defect area extended from the right side, reaching the premaxilla on the left side, crossing the midline, and the patient was classified as class IV according to Aramany's classification of acquired hard palatal defects. The patient had not used an interim obturator (Figures 1(b) and 1(c)).

It was noted that the patient was socially demoralized due to poor aesthetics. He was conscious of his sunken cheek and lip and desired a prosthesis which would make his face look fuller and healthier. A treatment plan was formulated, keeping the patient's demand in mind. The decision was made to treat the patient with a maxillary obturator that would gain its support from the remaining teeth and tissues with a detachable cheek and lip plumper. The use of dental magnets as a means of attachment was elected.

2.1. Treatment Procedures. Preliminary impressions of both maxillary and mandibular arches were made using irreversible hydrocolloid material (Alginate, Dentsply) for the maxillary and mandibular arches and then poured with type III dental stone. The maxillary study cast was surveyed, and undercut areas were blocked, and an interim obturator was constructed (®DPI Heat Cure) with no teeth incorporation, and wire clasps for retention were attached to it around two selected teeth. The interim obturator was worn by the patient while the definitive obturator was in process. On that study cast, the framework was designed and drawn, and then, a custom tray was constructed using an autocure acrylic resin. Necessary mouth preparations were carried out, and the rest seats were prepared on 12, 13, 14, 15, 16, and 17. Border molding was performed using a high fusing compound (Hiflex Tracing Sticks) for the borders and a low fusing compound (Hiflex impression compound) for the defect area. The final impression was recorded using light-body addition silicone material (Aquasil, Dentsply). This impression was poured with die stone (type IV). After preparation, the master cast was duplicated in refractory material (Whip Mix Beauty-Cast Investment/Gypsum-Bonded) and the partial framework of the cast was fabricated with the help of appropriate wax patterns. The framework was invested and casted using cobalt-chromium alloy (Remanium® GM 380+), and try-in was done with the help of pressure indicator paste (PIP, Mizzy Inc. USA) to affirm the accuracy of fit of the framework. An occlusal bite block was constructed on the

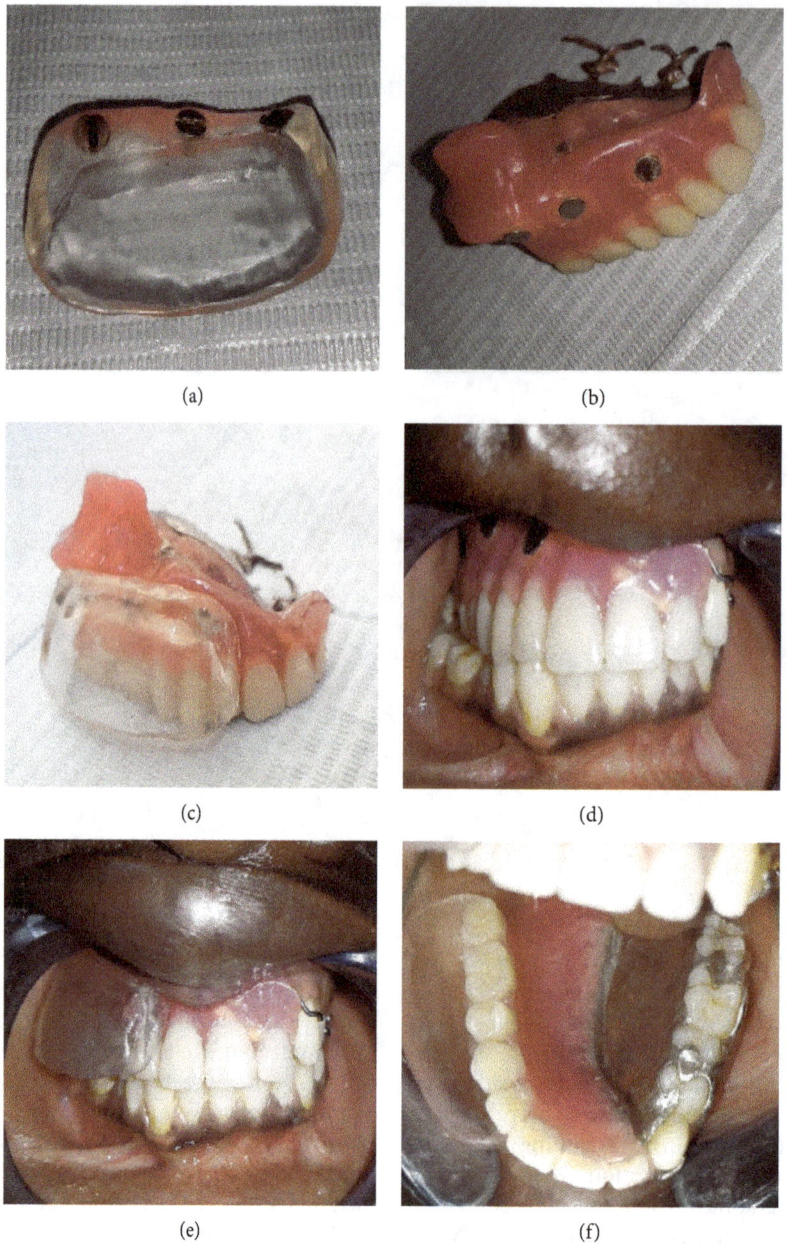

Figure 3: (a) Magnets attached to the removable part of the plumper; (b) magnets attached to the definitive obturator; (c) definitive obturator with plumper parts attached together, (d) intraoral view showing magnets attached to the definitive obturator; (e) intraoral view of the plumper; (f) occlusal view of the view of the plumper.

framework, and jaw relation was recorded. The casts were mounted; tooth arrangement and a try-in were done. The prosthesis was cured with heat-cured acrylic resin and adequately finished and polished (Figure 2(a)). A pressure indicator paste (PIP) was used to check and eliminate any pressure areas at the insertion appointment. The patient was educated regarding oral hygiene and the future care of the prosthetic device. A recall system for follow-ups was established.

One month later, the patient was recalled for the construction of a cheek and lip plumper to give him a fuller upper lip and cheek and asymmetrical facial appearance. Wax was added on the buccal side of the maxillary obturator (Figure 2(b)), and border movements were done until the wax was well adapted. Movements were repeated till the cheek and lip gained the required fullness, and the facial contour was restored, and the patient approved a pleasing appearance. The waxed-up plumper was sent to the dental laboratory which was kept in its position by an index of an addition silicone (Panasil Putty Soft, Kettenbach GmbH & Co. KG, Eschenburg, Germany). The plumper was hollowed (Figure 2(c)), and only a thin border was held back. The waxed-up plumper was separated from the obturator, and three holes were made on the right obturator flange and also on the corresponding area on the plumper. Flasking and dewaxing of the plumper with both parts of the magnets

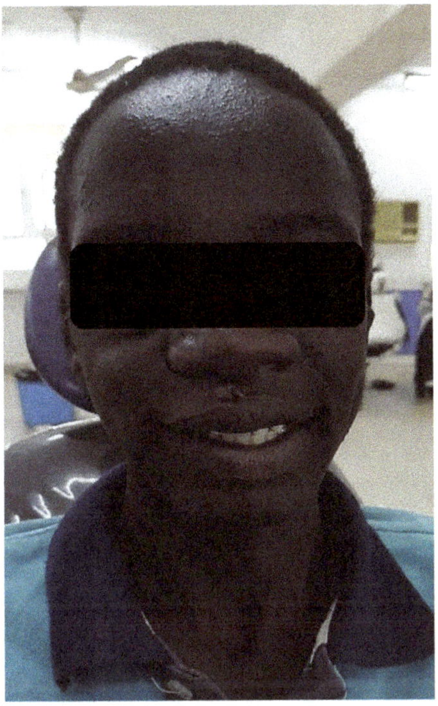

FIGURE 4: Postoperative frontal view of the patient wearing the lip and cheek plumper having and having better fullness.

(cobalt-samarium, Ambika Corporation) attached were done (Figure 3(a)). The resultant mold space was then packed with a clear heat-activated denture base resin, and curing procedures were completed (Figure 3(b)). After curing, the magnets of the obturator were attached (Figure 3(c)). Trimming, finishing, and polishing procedures were performed (Figures 3(d)–3(f)). The patient was given instructions on the use of the plumper and was encouraged to make efforts to learn to adapt to it. Within one week, the patient expressed satisfaction in his aesthetic (Figure 4) and even signed up for school.

3. Discussion and Conclusion

Facial aesthetics plays a vital role in shaping the psychology of patients. The primary function of a maxillofacial prosthesis is to restore the masticatory function, speech, mastication, and aesthetics. Maxillofacial disfigurement can be congenital, developmental, traumatic, or because of ablative surgery. Such defects compromise appearance and function and render an individual incapable of leading a relatively healthy life and affect his\her psyche. As the patient's quality of life gets worse, social integration becomes difficult, and the expectation of returning to "normalcy" collapses. The prognosis for a successful treatment result depends on getting a correct diagnosis and anticipating issues beyond the land of dentistry alone [9].

The established method of treating a sunken cheek is placing via an additional row of teeth to achieve the fullness of the face [10]. However, this can affect both the retention and stability of the obturator and also cause muscle fatigue. Cheek plumper is a prosthetic device used to support and flesh out the severely sunken cheeks [6]. They were previously used as intraoral splints in patients with Bell's palsy [11]. Such prosthesis is indicated in patients with maxillofacial defects or for restoring aesthetics in patients with hollow or sunken cheeks [12]. Although there are various attachments available for the fabrication of detachable cheek plumpers such as magnets, push buttons, and orthodontic separators, each has its pros and cons [10]. Dental magnets have been used in this case, and they have the benefit of being small and easy to insert because of their magnetic forces and are comfortable to remove and clean. Nevertheless, over a point of time, the magnets used intraorally require replacement due to a lack of long-term durability in oral conditions. The patient was informed about the limitations, and he was put in a six-month recall for a regular checkup and to replace the magnets if required. Conventional cheek plumpers, when used, append to the weightiness of the prosthesis, which can cause muscle fatigue and denture instability [13].

This case report described a secure method to restore facial form by fabrication of detachable plumper and the use of dental magnets to improve the facial aesthetics in a patient with extremely sunken cheeks and lips without affecting the retention of the obturator. In this case, extra lightweight plumper was used for compensation of severely slumped cheeks and lips, with minimal additional weight to the obturator, despite the massive level of compensation required. Assessing the tolerable width for the plumper using scientific and physiological knowledge has not been reported until now. The magnet-retained plumper prosthesis successfully restored the contour of the cheek and improved the aesthetics and the psychological well-being of the patient, and his lost smile was given back. Management of a patient with a maxillary defect should not be confined to the restoration of oral functions only but should equally include the identification of the patient psychological needs and appearance concerns.

This article has described a simple, noninvasive, and cost-effective method to improve facial appearance in patients with hollow faces. An effort was made to improve a patient's appearance by providing better support. The plumper prosthesis successfully improved the patient's appearance to the extent that comfort and function would permit and encourage self-esteem.

Authors' Contributions

NFA performed dental treatment and drafted the manuscript. IAI and MNA suggested the treatment method and drafted the manuscript. FA provided comprehensive judgment and assisted in editing the final version of the manuscript. All authors read and approved the final version of the manuscript before submission.

Acknowledgments

The authors would like to thank Dr. Magdi Gilada, Mr. Mahir Mousad, Dr. Rufida Mohammed, and all dental staff at the Department of Prosthodontics in Khartoum Dental Teaching Hospital and University of Khartoum for their appreciated assistance during the treatment of this case.

References

[1] W. J. Rifkin, R. S. Kantar, S. Ali-Khan et al., "Facial disfigurement and identity: a review of the literature and implications for facial transplantation," *AMA Journal of Ethics*, vol. 20, no. 4, pp. 309–323, 2018.

[2] A. Deshpande and R. Ghooi, "Narrative: the fear of disfigurement in cancer patients," *Indian Journal of Palliative Care*, vol. 23, no. 3, pp. 347–349, 2017.

[3] M. N. Alhajj, I. A. Ismail, and N. Khalifa, "Maxillary obturator prosthesis for a hemimaxillectomy patient: a clinical case report," *Saudi J Dent Res.*, vol. 7, no. 2, pp. 153–159, 2016.

[4] M. Singh, A. Bhushan, N. Kumar, and S. Chand, "Obturator prosthesis for hemimaxillectomy patients," *Natl J Maxillofac Surg.*, vol. 4, no. 1, pp. 117–120, 2013.

[5] D. Arunachalam, A. Thirumoorthy, and S. Devi, "Quality of life in cancer patients with disfigurement due to cancer and its treatments," *Indian Journal of Palliative Care*, vol. 17, no. 3, pp. 184–190, 2011.

[6] A. Wangoo, M. Kaur, S. Kaur, and A. Singh, "Facial lift in geriatric patient: the prosthodontic way," *Journal of Advanced Medical and Dental Sciences Research*, vol. 5, no. 11, pp. 76–78, 2017.

[7] S. Poovani and G. Shetty, "Complete dentures with detachable cheek plumper-a case report," *International Journal of Scientific Research.*, vol. 8, no. 12, pp. 44–46, 2020.

[8] S. S. Deepthi and S. Sudeep, "Detachable cheek plumpers: an innovative approach for rehabilitating smiles," *Intl J Sci Res*, vol. 9, no. 7, pp. 71-72, 2020.

[9] A. D. Gupta, A. Verma, T. Dubey, and S. Thakur, "Maxillofacial prosthetics part-1: a review," *International Journal of Advanced Research*, vol. 5, no. 9, pp. 31–40, 2017.

[10] S. R. Venkatachalapathy, G. N. Chander, and P. Gnanam, "A magnetically retained cheek plumper in a maxillary single complete denture: a clinical report," *Journal of Interdisciplinary Dentistry.*, vol. 9, no. 1, p. 25, 2019.

[11] J. B. Lazzari, "Intraoral splint for support of the lip in Bell's palsy," *The Journal of Prosthetic Dentistry*, vol. 5, no. 4, pp. 579–581, 1955.

[12] A. Shah, S. Latoo, A. Malik et al., "Odontogenic myxoma of the maxilla: a report of a rare case and review on histogenetic and diagnostic concepts," *Natl J Maxillofac Surg.*, vol. 2, no. 2, pp. 189–195, 2011.

[13] P. Bhushan, M. A. Aras, I. Coutinho, P. Rajagopal, A. R. Mysore, and S. Kumar, "Customized cheek plumper with friction lock attachment for a completely edentulous patient to enhance esthetics: a clinical report," *Journal of Prosthodontics*, vol. 28, no. 1, pp. e1–e5, 2019.

2

Verrucous Carcinoma of Buccal Mucosa in Female: A Rare Case Report of Traumatic Tooth Origin

V. Keerthi Narayan

Department of Oral Pathology and Microbiology, Thai Moogambigai Dental College and Hospital, Dr. MGR Educational and Research Institute, 600107, Chennai, Tamil Nadu, India

Correspondence should be addressed to V. Keerthi Narayan; narayankrth55@gmail.com

Academic Editor: Giovanni Mergoni

Verrucous carcinoma or Ackermann's tumor is considered a low-grade variant of squamous cell carcinoma frequently presenting at the oral mucosa and skin. Oral verrucous carcinoma clinically presents as a proliferative or cauliflower-like lesion or as ulceroproliferative lesion on the buccal mucosa followed by other sites such as the gingiva, tongue, and hard palate. Tobacco in both smoking and smokeless form, alcohol, and opportunist viral infections are the most associated etiologies in most of the reported literature cases. Here, in this paper, we discuss a rare case scenario of a 52-year-old female diagnosed with verrucous carcinoma of the left buccal mucosa with constant traumatic irritation caused by tooth as etiology for the occurrence of lesion, though verrucous carcinoma is described as a benign lesion with minimum aggressive potential but long-standing cases have shown transformation into squamous cell carcinoma. Therefore, early diagnosis and surgical excision of the lesion are the most appropriate treatment modality of verrucous carcinoma.

1. Introduction

Cancer of the head and neck region is of significant public health importance in India. Most often, it is diagnosed at advanced or late stages resulting in extremely low and poor treatment outcomes with considerable financial constrain [1]. Oral cancer often manifests itself in about 45%-48% of cases as ulcers or ulcerated tumors. Owing to its wide range of causative factors and unpredictable presenting features, the diagnosis of oral ulcerative lesions might be quite challenging. In initial cases, these carcinomatous ulcers can be confused with other pathological entities and often misdiagnosed as nonneoplastic ulcerative lesion. Such lesions lasting for two weeks or longer often create a dilemma due to its chronicity and unresponsive behaviour to various treatments prescribed [2].

In order to arrive at a definitive diagnosis, earlier detection of oral cancer followed by laboratory tests and additional investigations to narrow the diagnosis offers the best chance for long term survival and has the potential to improve treatment outcomes and make healthcare services affordable [3–5]. In this paper, we discussed an unusual presentation of verrucous carcinoma (VC) of the buccal mucosa in a female patient with rapid progression of the disease even after the removal of etiological agent suggesting a new variation in a disease process. In addition to this unfamiliar etiological factor and course of the disease, these findings could shed new light on the possible pathogenesis of verrucous carcinoma.

2. Case Report

2.1. About the Case. A 52-year-old female patient visited the Outpatient Department of Our Dental College and Hospital with a chief complaint of a nonhealing ulcerated tissue on the left lower back tooth region for the past 6 months, associated with pain and burning sensation during intake of spicy or hot food items occasionally. She developed continuous severe burning sensation accompanied by pain since 1 week in the same region. No relevant past medical, dental, occupational, and habit history was observed in relation with the chief complaint.

2.2. On Intraoral Examination

2.2.1. Visit 1. On soft tissue examination, a solitary, firm, ulcerative tissue measuring 2 × 2 centimetres was found on the alveolar mucosa near premolar region separated from it by clinically healthy mucosa. On stretching the cheek mucosa, a tooth root was found extruding from the socket impinging on the soft tissue counterpart surrounding areas (Figures 1 and 2). No other lesions were observed on either side of the oral mucosa. After comprehensive intraoral examination followed by analysis of the past dental and relevant history, an interim diagnosis of traumatic ulcer was given in association with the tooth as the source of origin. Patient consent was obtained before proceeding with the treatment. Extraction of the tooth root was performed under local anaesthesia (Figure 3). The procedure was uneventful, and postoperative instructions were given for the same. The patient was normal and freed of complaints during postoperative follow-up made after 15days.

2.2.2. Visit 2. The patient reported again to the outpatient department with similar complaints of pain and severe burning sensation after 3 months in the same region. On intraoral examination, nodular proliferous ulcerative growth measuring 3 × 2 centimetres was found on the alveolar mucosa near the premolar-molar region with focal areas of white spots (Figure 4). She was referred immediately to our oral pathology department followed by prescription of topical application of antiviral drugs (2% acyclovir) for a week. As the lesion did not show signs of regression, routine blood investigations were carried out to rule out complications following biopsy and were found to be normal. An incisional biopsy was advised for the same with differential diagnosis of focal epithelial hyperplasia; traumatic fibroma, verruciform leukoplakia, verruca vulgaris, verrucous carcinoma, and ulcerative squamous cell carcinoma were suggested.

2.3. Histopathological Analysis. Histopathological analysis showed a broad bulbous rete pegs with pushing margins in many areas along with features of mild dysplasia and few areas of parakeratin plugging. There were also few areas of severe dysplasia without significant break in the basement membrane and malignant cells infiltrating into the subjacent minimal connective tissue stroma with inflammatory cells which led to a provisional diagnosis of verrucous carcinoma of buccal mucosa.

2.4. Differential Diagnosis and Its Consideration. Verrucous carcinoma has particular clinical and histopathological features that agree its diagnosis to be obtained, which was an uncharacteristic observation in the present case. First, the clinical reasons for rejection were considered followed by the histological ones for each diagnosis, to obtain a final diagnosis thus clearly separating from others. Oral traumatic fibroma was ruled out since it presents as a firm smooth papule in the mouth, usually the same colour as the rest of the mouth lining, but is sometimes paler or, if it has bled, may look a dark colour. The surface may be ulcerated due to trauma or become rough and scaly. It is usually dome-shaped but may be on a short stalk like a polyp or pedunculated [6]. It should be noted no histological dysplastic features and other observations are not present and fibromas

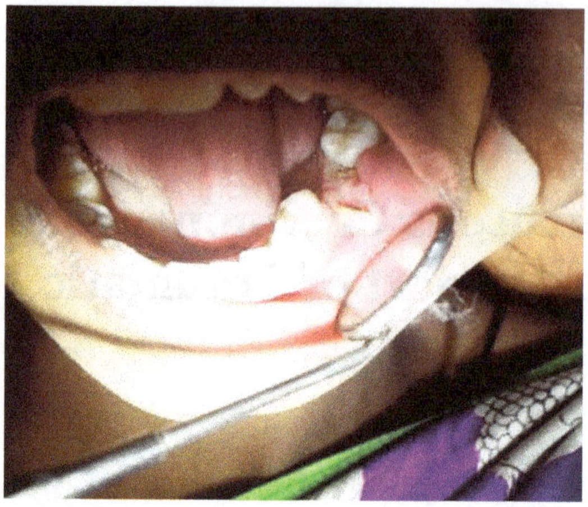

Figure 1: Clinical photograph showing a solitary, firm, ulcerative tissue measuring 2 × 2 centimetres on the alveolar mucosa near the premolar region.

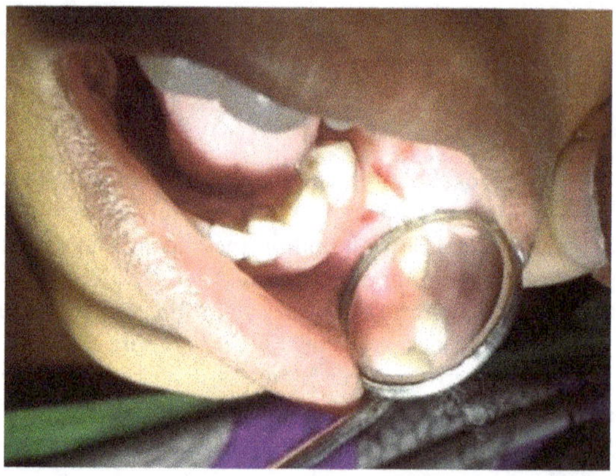

Figure 2: Clinical photograph showing the stretching of the cheek mucosa a tooth root found extruding from the socket impinging on the soft tissue counterpart surrounding areas.

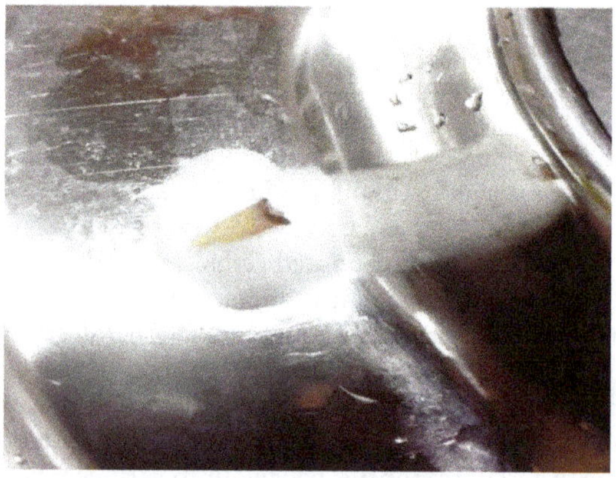

Figure 3: Clinical photograph showing a completely removed tooth under local anaesthesia.

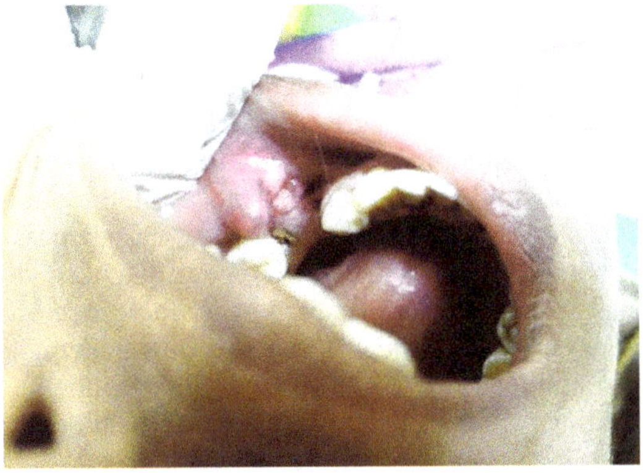

FIGURE 4: Clinical photograph showing nodular proliferous ulcerative growth measuring 3 × 2 centimetres on the alveolar mucosa.

never develop into oral cancer, similarly verrucous hyperplasia (VH) are often associated with papillomas or arise as a de novo lesion. VH (verrucous hyperplasia) and PVL (Proliferative Verrucous Leukoplakia) are irreversible clinicopathologic lesions with considerable potential for evolving into verrucous or squamous cell carcinoma. PVL is a disease of the oral cavity in which VH is a part of its developmental spectrum. Human papillomavirus, as a cofactor, may play an important role in some of these lesions [7, 8]; however, no signs suggestive of HPV infection were observed in the present histopathology section.

2.5. Treatment and Follow-Up. In the present case, as no other findings like nodal involvement or metastasis were observed, clinical staging of T2N0M0 was given. A wide local surgical excision was planned and performed under local anaesthesia (Figure 5). To ensure complete removal of the lesion with clear margins, further examination of the complete surgical specimen was sent for histopathological investigation and also to rule out infiltrating squamous cell carcinoma. The procedure was uneventful, and postoperative instructions were given. A postoperative follow-up was performed at an interval of every 15 days over a period of 3 months. No further complaints were observed.

2.6. Final Diagnosis. In this instance, though varied clinical course of the disease was noted, the histological result of the complete surgical specimen showed features of verrucous carcinoma similar to the reports obtained during the incisional biopsy thus ruling out squamous cell carcinoma evolved from a verrucous carcinoma (Figure 6). Thus, on complete evaluation of clinical and histological findings, a conclusive diagnosis of verrucous carcinoma (VC) was given.

3. Discussion

Verrucous carcinoma (VC) is a rare, low-grade, well-differentiated SCC of the skin or mucosa presenting with a verrucoid or cauliflower-like presence. It shows in the vicinity aggressive behaviour and has low metastatic potential, a low grade of dysplasia, and a good prognosis. It is a tumor that tends to erode more than infiltrate with predominantly

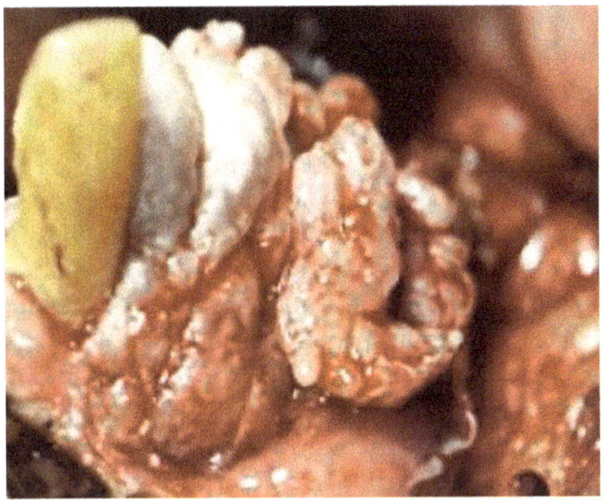

FIGURE 5: Clinical image showing a wide local surgical excision performed under local anaesthesia.

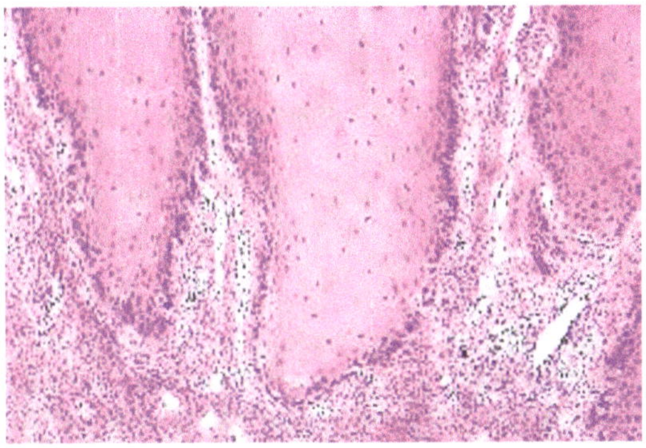

FIGURE 6: Histopathology of completely excised specimen showed verrucous configuration with a broad bulbous rete pegs with pushing margins in many areas along with features of mild dysplasia and few areas of parakeratin plugging (H&E, original magnification: ×40).

horizontal growth and does not present with distant metastasis. It has been presented with various names such as Ackerman tumor and carcinoma cuniculatum which are correlated to specific anatomic sites [9, 10].

In the oral cavity, verrucous carcinoma constitutes 2% to 4.5% of all forms of SCC seen mainly in men older than 50 years and also is associated with a high incidence (37.7%) of a second primary tumor mainly in the oral mucosa (e.g., tongue, lips, palate, and salivary gland) [11]. Kalsotra et al. reported a male to female ratio of 3.6 to 1 in patients with verrucous carcinoma, with a mean age of 53.9 years. In the present report of a case, it is seen with female older than 50 years though it is thought to predominantly affect elderly men [12]. The etiology of VC is related to various local and systemic sources such as Human Papilloma virus and chemicals from cigarettes (smoking) or physical source such as constant trauma and irritation [13, 14]. In this case, the patient did not present with most common factors like tobacco, alcohol consumption, or any occupational factors but presented with history of irritation to the buccal mucosa by tooth.

However, epidemiological studies generally analyse the relationship between chronic traumas of the oral mucosa originated by dentures and cancer, but mostly, they do not include other traumatic factors such as defective teeth or parafunctional habits, and they do not analyse the relationship between dental factors and oral potentially malignant disorders (OPMD). Although faulty restorations, sharp teeth, and ill-fitting dentures have been implicated in a few epidemiological studies, it is not clear whether confounding factors like tobacco and alcohol have been addressed in these studies [15, 16].

Valente et al. [17], Tornes et al. [18], and Rahali et al. [19] reported few cases of squamous cell carcinoma misdiagnosed as a denture-related traumatic ulcer. Meanwhile, de Sant'Ana dos Santos et al. reported misdiagnosis of lip SCC as actinic cheilitis [20]. A case of gingival SCC masquerading as an aphthous ulcer was also reported by Kumari et al. This time elapse might jeopardize patients' overall prognosis; therefore, attempts should be done for timely diagnosis by more logical routes such as decision trees rather than test-and-error methods [6]. The present case scenario admits the fact that other traumatic factors such as sharp teeth or defective teeth are a possible agent for arising of lesion but the primary etiology of trauma as a true etiological factor has to be analysed further by investigation on a larger scale by reporting of various cases across the world.

Histopathologically, VC frequently presents with a hyperplastic epithelium with abundant keratin superficially projecting as exophytic church-spire keratosis with bulbous well-oriented rete ridges shows an endophytic growth pattern with pushing borders. Rapid transition from a normal epithelium to endophytic ingrowth is taken as a significant feature to differentiate it from benign verrucous growths [21]. A classic case of VC shows minimal or no pleomorphism of cells, and no mitotic activity above the basal and suprabasal layers of the epithelium and lymphoplasmacytic inflammatory host reaction are marked, especially in cases where keratin has plunged deep into the connective tissue inducing foreign body granuloma formation as not seen or appreciated in the present case. Insufficient depth of the section, the absence of adjacent normal epithelium, presence of dysplastic features, and evidence of micro invasion create a dilemma for the pathologist. To avoid such scenario, deeper sections were taken and conclusive evidences were considered as it becomes mandatory to rule out SCC [22, 23].

Among various therapeutic approaches, surgical intervention is the primary therapeutic mode to treat verrucous carcinoma. Surgical excision with adequate margins has been proven to be effective in the management of these tumors, and radiotherapy has generally been recommended in the presence of adverse risk factors in the histopathology report such as metastatic lymph node positivity and invasion to the deeper vital structures like nerves and blood vessels [24, 25]. In the present case as no other findings like nodal involvement or metastasis was observed, clinical stating of T2N0M0 was given. Only surgical intervention for complete removal of tumor by intraoral approach was recommended since it may not be effective as in the case of larger area extension of the carcinogenic lesion.

4. Conclusion

In the present case, an unexpected or unusual demonstration of verrucous carcinoma caused by local irritation in the form of tooth, with rapid progression of the disease lesser than the usual demonstration even after removal of the etiological agent, suggests a new variation in a disease process. VC should be considered in the differential diagnosis of slow growing ulcerative lesion though not characteristic as noted in the present case considering the evolving epidemiological and etiopathological trends and in addition to the fact that these findings could shed new light on the possible pathogenesis of verrucous carcinoma. In this case, proper diagnosis was made as early as possible to avoid further complication and was appropriately treated. Thus, both clinicians and pathologists must be cautious about chronic traumatic ulcers or ulcerative lesions of the oral cavity and propose diagnostic alternatives to ensure the most appropriate treatment to be given at the right time.

Acknowledgments

The study was self-funded by the author.

References

[1] M. W. Finkelstein, "A guide to the clinical differential diagnoses of oral mucosal lesions," in *CrestOral-Bat dentalcare.com*, vol. 1, pp. 1–41, Continuing Education Course, 2010.

[2] H. Mortazavi, Y. Safi, M. Baharvand, and S. Rahmani, "Diagnostic features of common oral ulcerative lesions: an updated decision tree," *International journal of dentistry*, vol. 2016, no. 1, pp. 1–14, 2016.

[3] M. Muñoz-Corcuera, G. Esparza-Gómez, M. A. González-Moles, and A. Bascones-Martínez, "Oral ulcers: clinical aspects. A tool for dermatologists. Part I. Acute ulcers," *Clinical and Experimental Dermatology*, vol. 34, no. 3, pp. 289–294, 2009.

[4] A. J. Bruce, T. S. Dabade, and N. M. Burkemper, "Diagnosing oral ulcers," *Journal of the American Academy of Physician Assistants*, vol. 28, no. 2, pp. 1–10, 2015.

[5] P. S. Khandekar, P. S. Bagdey, and R. R. Tiwari, "Oral cancer and some epidemiological factors: a hospital based study," *Indian Journal of Community Medicine*, vol. 31, no. 3, pp. 157–159, 2006.

[6] P. S. Kumari, G. P. Kumar, Y. D. Bai, and E. Y. Reddy, "Gingival squamous cell carcinoma masquerading as an aphthous ulcer," *Journal of Indian Society of Periodontology*, vol. 17, no. 4, pp. 523–526, 2013.

[7] W. C. Gonsalves, A. A. Chi, and B. W. Neville, "Common oral lesions: part II. Masses and neoplasia," *American family physician*, vol. 75, no. 4, pp. 509–512, 2007.

[8] D. A. Lederman and M. L. Fornatora, *Oral fibromas and fibromatoses*, Medscape Reference, 2002.

[9] E. T. Stoopler and F. Alawi, "Clinicopathologic challenge: a solitary submucosal mass of the oral cavity," *International Journal of Dermatology*, vol. 47, no. 4, pp. 329–331, 2008.

[10] M. Zanini, C. Wulkan, F. M. Paschoal, M. H. M. Maciel, and C. D.′. A. S. Machado Filho, "Carcinoma verrucoso: uma variante clínico-histopatológica do carcinoma espinocelular,"

Anais Brasileiros de Dermatologia, vol. 79, no. 5, pp. 619–621, 2004.

[11] S. Chaudhary, C. Bansal, and U. Ranga, "Verrucous carcinoma of the buccal mucosa with extension to the cheek," *Cutis*, vol. 99, no. 2, pp. E16–E18, 2017.

[12] P. Kalsotra, M. Manhas, and R. Sood, "Verrucous carcinoma of hard palate," *JK Science*, vol. 2, pp. 52–54, 2000.

[13] Q. Peng, Y. Wang, H. Quan, Y. Li, and Z. Tang, "Oral verrucous carcinoma: from multifactorial etiology to diverse treatment regimens (review)," *International journal of oncology*, vol. 49, no. 1, pp. 59–73, 2016.

[14] V. V. Kamath, R. R. Varma, D. R. Gadewar, and M. Muralidhar, "Oral verrucous carcinoma: an analysis of 37 cases," *Journal of Cranio-Maxillofacial Surgery*, vol. 17, no. 7, pp. 309–314, 1989.

[15] B. L. Chen, C. C. Lin, and C. H. Chen, "Oral verrucous carcinoma: an analysis of 73 cases," *Clinical Journal of Oral and Maxillofacial Surgery*, vol. 11, pp. 11–17, 2000.

[16] S. Warnakulasuriya, "Causes of oral cancer - an appraisal of controversies," *British Dental Journal*, vol. 207, no. 10, pp. 471–475, 2009.

[17] V. B. Valente, A. S. Takamiya, L. L. Ferreira et al., "Oral squamous cell carcinoma misdiagnosed as a denture-related traumatic ulcer: a clinical report," *The Journal of Prosthetic Dentistry*, vol. 115, no. 3, pp. 259–262, 2016.

[18] K. Tornes, G. Bang, H. S. Koppang, and K. N. Pedersen, "Oral verrucous carcinoma," *International Journal of Oral Surgery*, vol. 14, no. 6, pp. 485–492, 1985.

[19] L. Rahali, Y. Omor, K. Mouden et al., "Oral verrucous carcinoma complicating a repetitive injury by the dental prosthesis: a case report," *The Pan African Medical Journal*, vol. 20, p. 297, 2015.

[20] F. D. dos Santos, M. A. Isper, J. P. Novo-Neto, A. C. Marqueti, C. P. Pereira, and F. G. Isper, "Misdiagnosis of lip squamous cell carcinoma," *RSBO Revista Sul-Brasileira de Odontologia*, vol. 9, pp. 114–118, 2012.

[21] E. D. Piemonte, P. J. Lazos, and M. Brunotto, "Relationship between chronic trauma of the oral mucosa, oral potentially malignant disorders and oral cancer," *Journal of Oral Pathology & Medicine*, vol. 39, pp. 513–517, 2010.

[22] A. K. Shergill, M. C. Solomon, S. Carnelio, A. T. Kamath, C. Aramanadka, and G. S. Shergill, "Verrucous carcinoma of the oral cavity: current concepts," *International Journal of Scientific Study*, vol. 3, no. 3, pp. 114–118, 2015.

[23] S. Varshney, J. Singh, R. K. Saxena, A. Kaushal, and V. P. Pathak, "Verrucous carcinoma of larynx," *Indian Journal of Otolaryngology and Head and Neck Surgery*, vol. 56, pp. 54–56, 2004.

[24] D. L. McClure, P. J. Gullane, R. P. Slinger, and G. P. Wysocki, "Verrucous carcinoma-changing concepts in management," *The Journal of Otolaryngology*, vol. 13, no. 1, pp. 7–12, 1984.

[25] M. L. Asha, K. Vini, I. Chatterjee, and P. Patil, "Verrucous carcinoma of buccal mucosa: a case report," *International Journal of Health Sciences*, vol. 1, no. 4, pp. 19–23, 2014.

3

"Orofacial Dystonia—A Silent Killer": Mandibular Fractures with Orofacial Dystonia, A Report of a Case and Review

Anand deep Shukla, G. Srikanth, A. Chitra, Anupam Singh, and Sunil Nayak

Department of Oral and Maxillofacial Surgery, MCODS, Manipal, India

Correspondence should be addressed to Anand deep Shukla; drandymanipal@gmail.com

Academic Editor: Leandro Napier de Souza

Mandibular parasymphysis fracture is very commonly observed especially in old age when there is resorptions of the alveolar ridges. In cervical dystonia, there is centrally mediated disease in which there is uncontrolled and spasmodic contraction of the facial and the masticatory muscles. Due to the application of this sudden and uncontrolled force, there is a tendency of the bone to unfavourably remodel and weaken. The case presented here is of a geriatric patient who presented to us with a fracture at the right parasymphysis and left dentoalveolar region of the mandible and was suffering from cervical dystonia. Management of this case posed a challenge in every step, and it needed a resurgery where the fracture was managed by the placement of reconstruction plate. Not many cases in the literature have been reported where dystonic movements have resulted in the fracture of the mandible.

1. Introduction

Orofacial dystonia is a neuromuscular disorder of central origin which causes involuntary, spasmodic, and periodic movements of the muscles of the orofacial, masticatory, and lingual region [1].

Most of the cases are idiopathic (63%), other causes include drug induced (22.8), peripheral induced (9.3), post anoxic (2.55%), neurodegenerative disorder associated (1.8%), and head injury associated (0.8%) [2]. The triggering factors for this basically include physical or emotional stress, depression, or orofacial surgical procedures [3]. There is no clear-cut outline for the diagnosis and the management of this condition. The options mentioned in the literature for the management of dystonia include chemodenervation [4], medical management, and CNS procedures [5]. In the case that is presented, we came across a case of dystonia of long-term duration, which used to increase and decrease in intensity. The chronic dystonia led to the weakening of the mandible which resulted in the fracture of the parasymphysis region ultimately. There was also loosening of the teeth because of the dystonic movements. The case presented with challenge at each step.

2. Case Report

This is a case of 56 years old male, who presented to us with the complaint of pain in the lower jaw since last one month ago (Figures 1 and 2). On thorough clinical and radiological examination, the patient was diagnosed with infected right mandibular parasymphysis and left dentoalveolar fracture (Figures 3, 4, and 5) and was admitted under our unit for the management of the same. The patient was also suffering from dystonia for the past one year. After clearances from the concerned units, the patient was taken up for surgery, where it was decided to do a thorough debridement of the infected area, send the bone for biopsy, and perform an open reduction and internal fixation of the fractured mandible.

During the surgery, the mandibular parasymphysis and the dentoalveolar fracture were approached intraorally by giving a vestibular incision and performing layered dissection, after approaching the mandibular parasymphysis

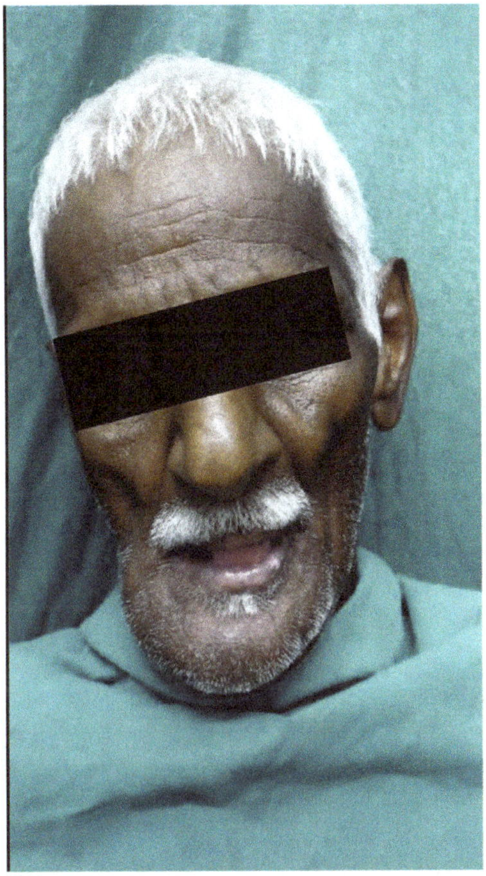

FIGURE 1: Preop photograph.

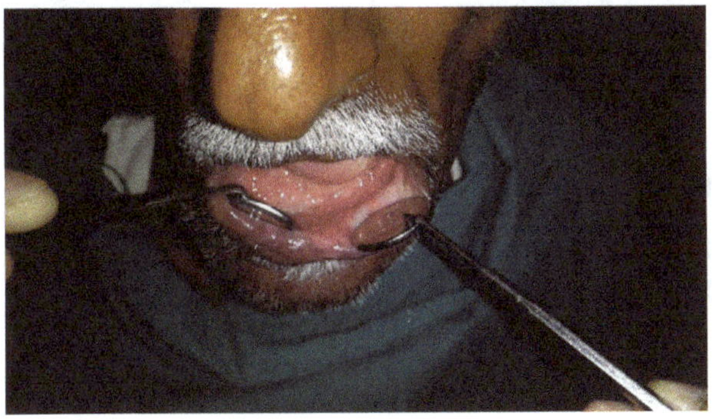

FIGURE 2: Intraoral view presop.

region, thorough debridement was done and the infected chunks of bone were removed. Following this, the fractures were fixed using two miniplates. Following the fixation, the incision site was thoroughly debrided and closed in layers (Figures 6 and 7).

Following the surgery, the patient was shifted to postop ICU and then to the ward.

On postop day one, the patient was having persistent cough in view of which blood and sputum culture was taken which revealed E. Faecalis sensitive to Linezolid and K. Pneumonia sensitive to Gentamycin. The patient was given IV Ampicillin, IV Gentamycin, and Tab Linezolid as advised

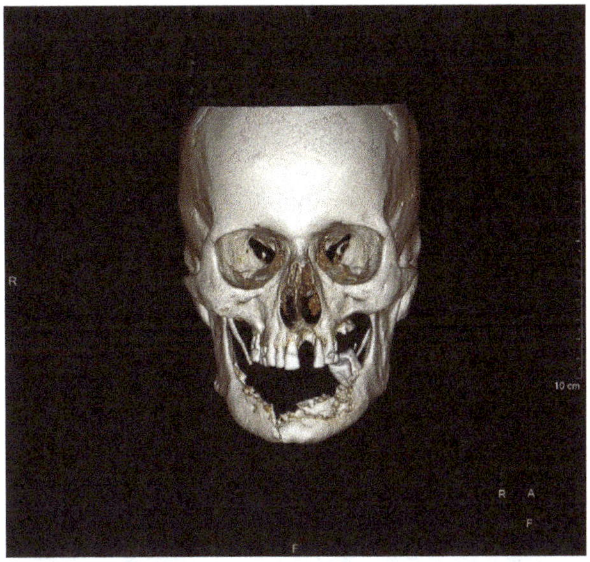

FIGURE 3: Preop CT scan showing right parasymphysis and dentoalveolar factures.

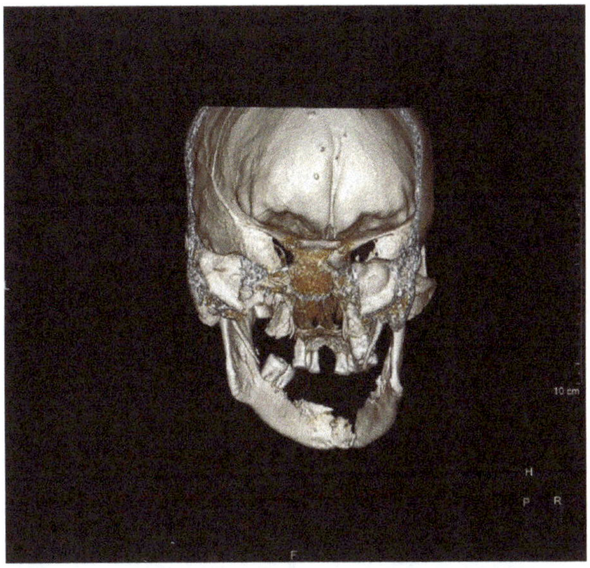

FIGURE 4: Lingual view of the same CT scan.

by the medicine department. Neurology was consulted, and the same medication was continued. ENT consultation was sought in view of difficulty in speech for which conservative management was advised, and the patient recovered well post surgery. Malignancy and osteomyelitis were ruled out by histopathology report, and the fracture was attributed to the constant occlusal trauma due to cervical dystonia. Following this, the patient was discharged.

Following this surgery, the patient again reported to our outpatient department after three months with similar complaints of pain in the anterior region of the mandible. On examination, there was slight opening in the mucosa on the right parasymphysis region and segmental mobility over the right parasymphysis region. Clinical and radiological examination confirmed hardware failure to be the cause of pain and

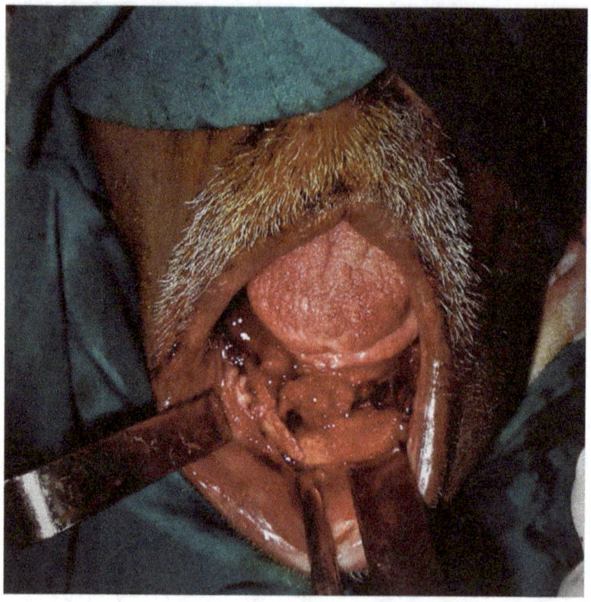

Figure 5: Coronal CT image.

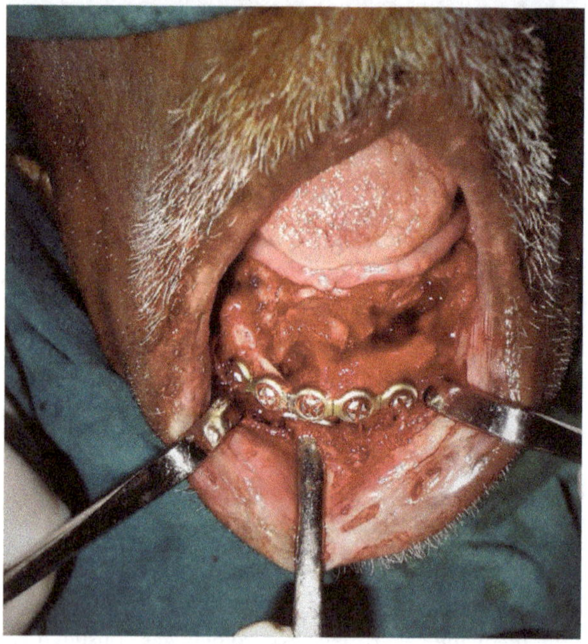

Figure 6: On-table exposure of the fracture site (first surgery).

mobility over the right mandibular parasymphysis region (Figures 8 and 9).

The patient was again taken up for the surgical intervention where after securing adequate anesthesia, extraoral incision from the right body region of the mandible to the left body region of the mandible was given. After layered dissection, the right mandibular parasymphysis region was exposed. On exposure, a dumbbell plate was found attached to the soft tissues with its two screws, which was subsequently retrieved (Figures 10 and 11). The superior 6-holed plate and 5 screws were also retrieved. Following this, the infected bone

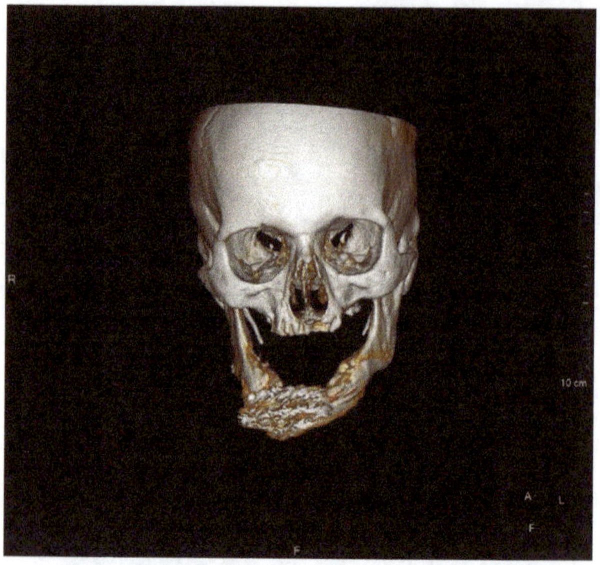

Figure 7: Plates in situ 9 (first surgery).

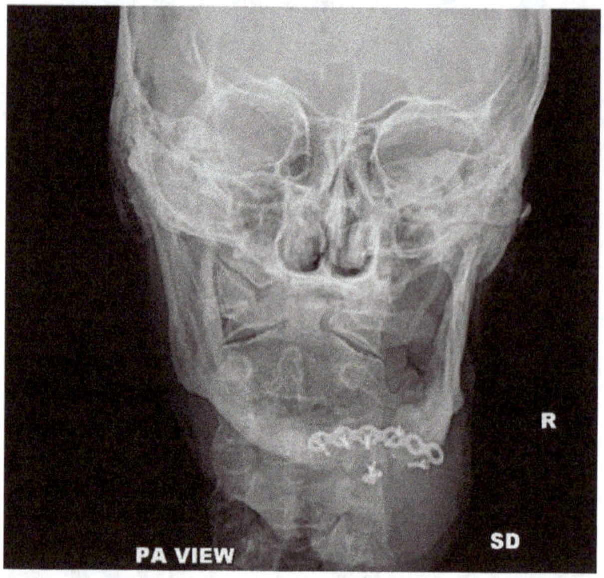

Figure 8: CT scan after hardware failure.

chunks were curetted out, and the mandible was fixed using a 15-hole 2.5 mm reconstruction cut plate and 8 (2×14 mm) locking screws (Figures 12 and 13). Homeostasis was achieved, and the wound was closed in layers.

The patient recovered well post surgery and was subsequently discharged after a week (Figure 14).

3. Discussion

Meige was the first person to describe orofacial dystonia in detail [6].This condition is also known by the name of Meige syndrome when it occurs in conjunction with blepharospasm [7]. This disease still poses a dilemma as far as its understanding is concerned. This condition may affect the muscles on one side or both the sides of the face, hence causing a

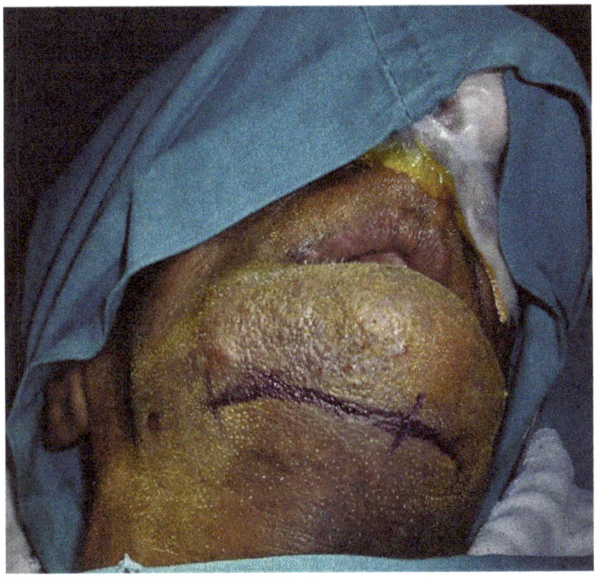

FIGURE 9: PA view of the mandible taken at the same time.

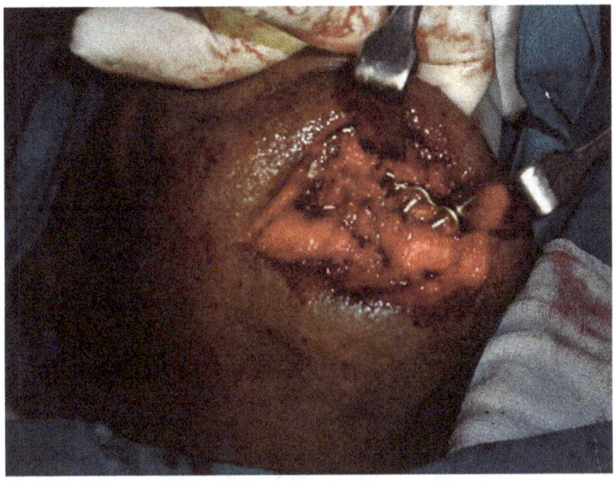

FIGURE 10: Extraoral markings for incision (second surgery).

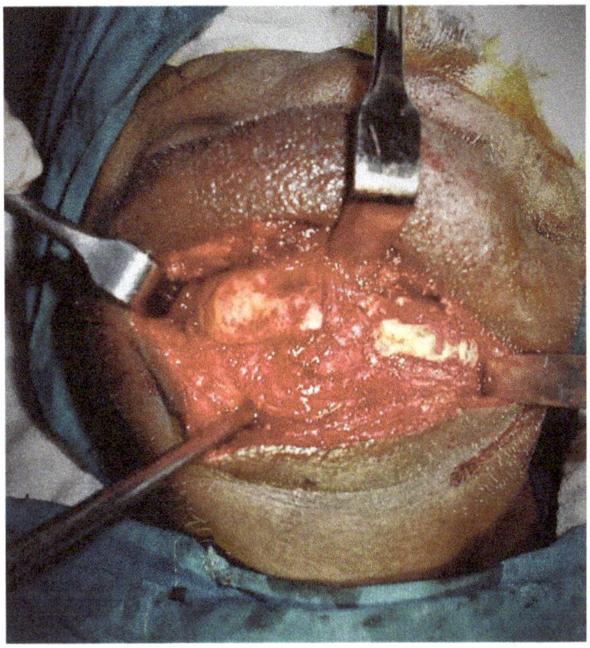

FIGURE 11: Exposure of the site, revealing a loose hardware.

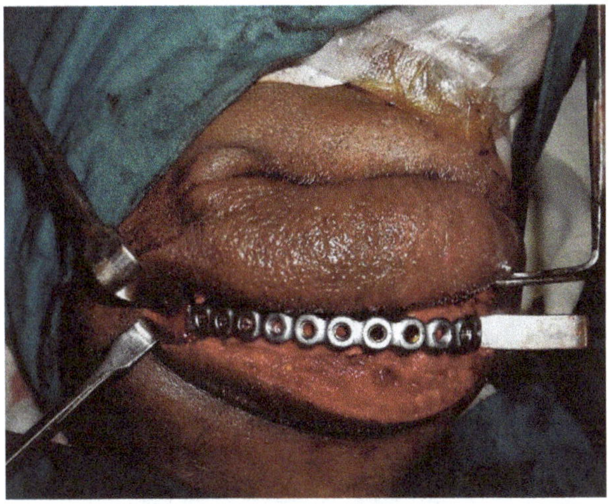

FIGURE 12: After the removal of the hardware and necrotic bone.

different clinical presentation. All the jaw movements that include protrusion, retrusion, and side-to-side movements may be affected. When the muscles of facial expression and lingual musculature are affected, there may be spasmodic contraction; there are a number of features like twitching of the face, abnormal lip movements, nasal contractions, clenching/grinding of teeth, retractions of oral commissures, and/or abnormal movements of tongue [8].

There may be involvement of platysma also resulting in contractions of the neck. Involvement of laryngeal muscles has also been reported resulting in difficulty in breathing, dysphagia, dysphonia, and dysarthria [9].

Slowly, these uncontrolled spasms result in accumulation of products of anaerobic metabolism in the muscles and thus results in myalgia [10].

The pain further involves the antagonist muscles. On the other hand, spasms consistently lead to further damage to the soft tissue envelope. If the condition is not managed promptly, the condition becomes very serious resulting in intolerable pain and discomfort [11].

Stimulating factors for this episode are stress, depression, or any kind of activity involving the orofacial musculature. Even trauma has also been associated with the triggering of the episode of dystonia [12].

Over a period of time, the patient learns to live with the condition and they tend to deal with it by engaging in more pleasurable activities. The contraction of facial musculature gradually results in bruxism, clenching of the teeth, wearing away and loosening of the teeth, and even dislocation of the condyles [13]. In a few instances, it has also resulted in the fracture of the mandible due to excessive masticatory force generated, as was the presentation in our case.

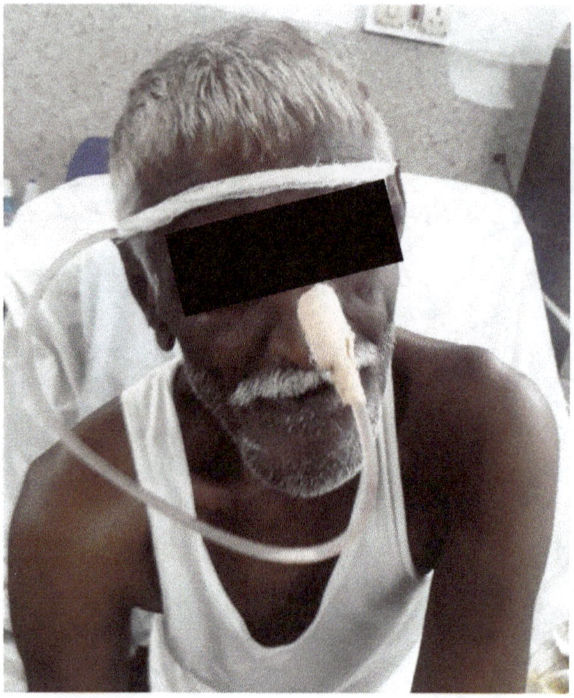

Figure 13: Plates in situ.

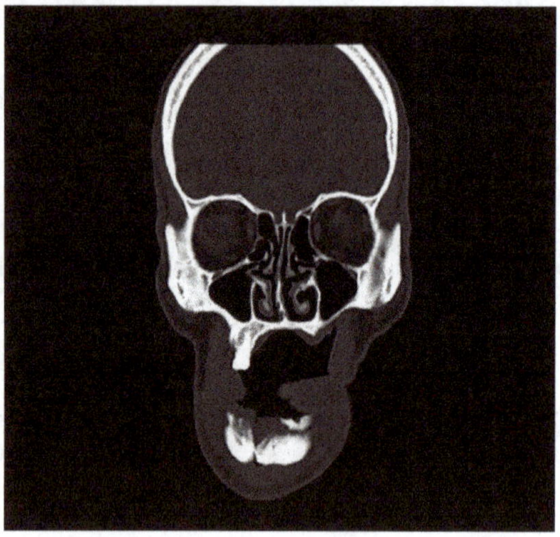

Figure 14: Postop photograph after second surgery.

Currently, there is no standard cure for dystonia, although various treatments have been documented. Treatment options for dystonia are as follows.

(1) *Medical Management.* This includes administration of pharmacological agents like anticholinergics, anticonvulsants, antiparkinsonians, benzodiazepines, carbamezipine, lithium, and gabapentin, which are very effective in this condition [14]

(2) *Chemodenervation.* It implies injections of botulinum neurotoxin in the form of Botulinum toxin A and B in focal dystonia

(3) *Surgical Management including Peripheral/Central Nervous System Procedures.* This is used as the last retort when nothing is helping. Peripheral procedures include TMJ arthroscopy and surgery, myotomies, rhizectomies, and ramisectomies. CNS procedures involve deep brain stimulation or identification and ablation of a desired nucleus in the brain. Thalamotomy and pallidotomy are also reported to provide relief in some cases [15]

In our case, the patient was a 56-year-old male who was suffering from dystonia for the past 1.5 years. The patient came from a very low socioeconomic background and was not undergoing any treatment for cervical dystonia. The patient showed signs of twisting of the head and chin towards the side which was involuntary. He had difficulty in coordinating the movements of his jaw muscles. He was partially edentulous and was not using any dental prosthesis. When the patient presented to us, his chief complaint was the pain and tenderness over the right mandibular parasymphysis region; on examination and radiological examination, a diagnosis of fracture of the right mandibular parasymphysis region was made. There was no history of any trauma on that region. In all likelihood, the fracture had occurred some time back since there were obvious signs of infection evident. Since there was no history of trauma which was confirmed by the history taken from the patient as well as the relatives accompanying the patient, the most obvious cause of the fracture can be the occlusal forces due to dystonia resulting in the fracture of the mandibular parasymphysis. The patient also showed signs of bruxism which was confirmed by the presence of occlusal facets on the remainder of teeth. There were only two lower molar present which may have caused improper distribution of occlusal forces resulting in the fracture of the mandibular region. The patient and the patient's party gave the history that the dystonia that the patient was suffering from was idiopathic. He was also partially edentulous with loss of few anterior teeth and did not used a denture. Due to these factors, the occlusal load on the anterior mandible would have been increased multiple times leading to the eventual weakening of the region and leading to fracture of the anterior mandible. The primary surgery was aimed at thorough debridement of the infected bone, curettage, biopsy to know if it was a pathological fracture, and fixation of the mandible. The fixation that was done using two miniplates which were load sharing.

The biopsy report ruled out any pathological involvement in the form of malignancy or osteomyelitis. When the patient reported to us again, he had a hardware failure most probably due to dystonia and excessive masticatory forces. He was then taken up for surgery again, and the loosened hardware were removed, followed by fixation with a reconstruction plate, which is a load-bearing plate. The use of a heavy-load-bearing plate gives additional strength to the mandible and hence bears the excessive forces of mastication in dystonia patients. The patient recovered well after the surgery and had shown good improvement on his follow-up visits.

4. Conclusion

Orofacial dystonia is a very distressing condition which causes a lot of problems to the person concerned. Some general recommendations to be followed in these patients are as follows:

(1) Periodic dental visits to look for health of the teeth and the surrounding structures

(2) Periodic X-rays to be taken of the maxillofacial region, to rule out facial fractures or pathology caused due to dystonia

(3) Good maintenance of oral hygiene

(4) Proper administration of the medications for orofacial dystonia

If all these measures are undertaken and a periodic check-up, any problem arising can be diagnosed early and patients suffering can be reduced considerably.

References

[1] E. S. Tolosa, "Clinical features of Meige's disease (idiopathic orofacial dystonia). A report of 17 cases," *Archives of Neurology*, vol. 38, no. 3, pp. 147–151, 1981.

[2] E. K. Tan and J. Jankovic, "Botulinum toxin A in patients with oromandibular dystonia: Long-term follow-up," *Neurology*, vol. 53, no. 9, pp. 2102–2107, 1999.

[3] B. L. Scott, "Evaluation and treatment of dystonia," *Southern Medical Journal*, vol. 93, no. 8, pp. 746–751, 2000.

[4] R. Tintner and J. Jankovic, *Botulinum toxin type A in the management of oromandibular dystonia and bruxism. Scientific and therapeutic aspects of Botulinum toxin*, PA: Lippincott Williams & Wilkins, Philadelphia, 2002.

[5] K. H. Lee, "Oromandibular dystonia," *Oral Surgery, Oral Medicine, Oral Pathology, Oral Radiology, and Endodontology*, vol. 104, no. 4, pp. 491–496, 2007.

[6] E. S. Tolosa, "Clinical features of Meige's disease (idiopathic orofacial Dystonia)," *Archives of Neurology*, vol. 38, no. 3, pp. 147–151, 1981.

[7] E. Tolosa and M. J. Marti, "Blepharospasm-oromandibular dystonia syndrome (Meige's syndrome): clinical aspects," *Advances in Neurology*, vol. 49, pp. 73–84, 1988.

[8] J. Jankovic, "Etiology and differential diagnosis of blepharospasm and oromandibular dystonia," *Advances in Neurology*, vol. 49, pp. 103–116, 1988.

[9] E. K. Tan and J. Jankovic, "Botulinum toxin As in patients with oromandibular dystonia: long-term follow-up," *Neurology*, vol. 53, no. 9, pp. 2102–2107, 1999.

[10] M. Hallett, "Is dystonia a sensory disorder?," *Annals of Neurology*, vol. 38, no. 2, pp. 139-140, 1995.

[11] E. K. Tan, L. L. Chan, and M. C. Wong, "Levodopa-induced oromandibular dystonia in progressive supranuclear palsy," *Clinical Neurology and Neurosurgery*, vol. 105, no. 2, pp. 132–134, 2003.

[12] A. E. Lang, "Psychogenic dystonia: a review of 18 cases," *The Canadian Journal of Neurological Sciences*, vol. 22, no. 2, pp. 136–143, 1995.

[13] P. J. Blanchet, O. Abdillahi, C. Beauvais, P. H. Rompre, and G. J. Lavigne, "Prevalence of spontaneous oral dyskinesia in the elderly: a reappraisal," *Movement Disorders*, vol. 19, no. 8, pp. 892–896, 2004.

[14] J. Jankovic, S. Leder, D. Warner, and K. Schwartz, "Cervical dystonia: clinical findings and associated movement disorders," *Neurology*, vol. 41, no. 7, pp. 1088–1091, 1991.

[15] I. S. Cooper, "20-year follow-up study of the neurosurgical treatment of dystonia musculorum deformans," *Advances in Neurology*, vol. 14, pp. 423–452, 1976.

4

Erythema Multiforme Attributable to Herpes Simplex Virus: Clinical Aspects and Treatment

Aya Mtiri,[1] Ghada Bouslama,[1] Nour-sayda Ben Messouad,[1] Iyadh Abidi,[1] Souha Ben Youssef,[1] and Badreddine Sriha[2]

[1]*Department of Oral Surgery, University Hospital Farhat Hached Sousse, University of Monastir, Tunisia*
[2]*Department of Histopathology, University Hospital Farhat Hached, Sousse, Tunisia*

Correspondence should be addressed to Aya Mtiri; aya.mtiri1@gmail.com

Academic Editor: Alberto Delbem

Erythema multiforme is an acute mucocutaneous hypersensitivity reaction with various etiological factors, including herpes simplex virus, medications, autoimmune diseases, and malignancies, but the most common cause is infection by herpes simplex virus. The most characteristic feature is the presence of "target lesions." There are no specific diagnostic tests for EM, and the diagnosis is based on clinical signs and symptoms and biopsy if required. We report a case of recurrent herpes-associated erythema multiforme managed with prophylactic acyclovir for 6 months: a 17-year-old boy had recurrent cutaneous lesions as well as lesions in the oral cavity and lips. Positive serology for herpes simplex virus and histopathological examination confirmed the diagnosis.

1. Introduction

Erythema multiforme (EM) is a reactive mucocutaneous disorder that is characterized by acute cutaneous and mucous bullous lesions. It usually affects adolescents and apparently healthy young adults but may occur at any age, and several reports suggest that males are affected more than females [1].

The detachment of the skin affects less than 10% of the body surface area (BSA), and localized typical and/or raised atypical targets are present.

2. Case Report

A 17-year-old male patient was referred from the internal medicine department to the dental surgery unit of University Hospital Farhat Hached, Tunisia. The patient was complaining about recurrent intraoral ulcers, diagnosed with recurrent aphthous stomatitis. He was treated with colchicine for two months without any improvement.

Our patient was afebrile with all vital signs within normal limits, and his medical history was noncontributory.

Extraoral examination at this point revealed nonspecific 3 to 4 purplish red cutaneous lesions on the forearms. Only some itching was reported. However, intraoral examination revealed diffuse and painful irregular erythematous lesions and postbullous ulcerations on the palate (Figure 1) and all buccal mucosae. Moreover, poor oral hygiene was noticed as the patient was unable to brush his teeth regularly.

Based on the clinical examination, the diagnosis of recurrent aphthous stomatitis was excluded. Yet a bullous disease was suspected such as bullous pemphigoid, lichen planus, or even a drug reaction related to the use of colchicine. Aimed at confirming our diagnosis, a histological exam with a biopsy in the left buccal mucosa was performed.

The patient was told to stop all medications and start using corticosteroids: Solupred (20 mg) 1 tablet *3 per day for 20 days and a topical steroid for the cutaneous lesions in order to relieve him and enable him to eat and speak conveniently.

One week later, the patient showed a clear improvement of mucosal lesions as well as pain relief. The histopathological analysis showed a prominent dermal inflammatory reaction with vasodilation and oedema. A dermal inflammatory

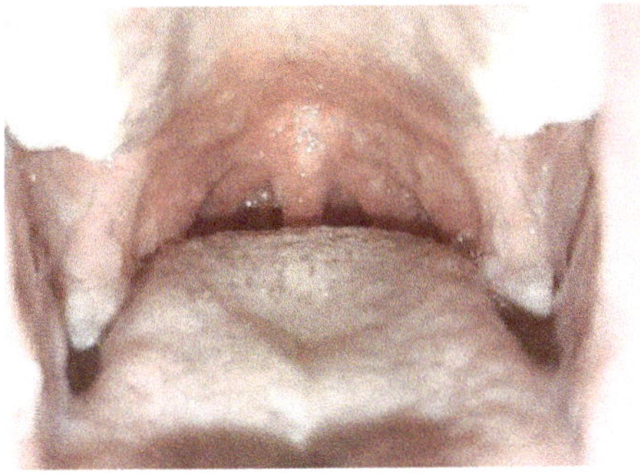

Figure 1: Mucosal involvement of the palate.

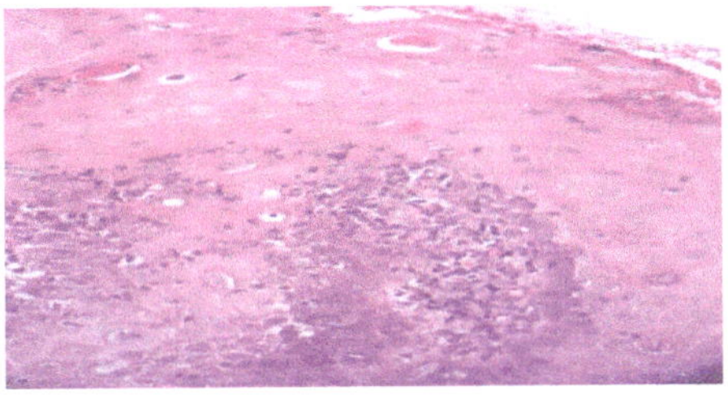

Figure 2: Histopathology of EM minor. A dermal inflammatory infiltrate consisting of lymphocytes, histiocytes, and necrotic epidermal cells.

infiltrate consisting of lymphocytes and histiocytes was identified as well as some necrotic epidermal cells (Figure 2). Thus, the diagnosis of erythema multiforme was retained.

Unfortunately, one month later, the patient reported complaints about more severe postbullous lesions on buccal, gingival, and labial mucosae (Figure 3). The lesions were diffuse, multiple, irregularly mixed, red and white, surrounded by erythematous margins, and covered with white slough in addition to postvesicular heme-crusted polycyclic erosions of vermillion lips and philtrum.

Furthermore, numerous targetoid erythematous lesions over the back of hands, fingers, arms, and back were noticed (Figure 4).

Considering the presence of a herpes lesion and the recurrence in a short period of time, a correlation between herpes simplex infection and erythema multiforme was suspected. Therefore, serology tests were indicated. The patient was negative for human immunodeficiency virus (HIV) while positive for herpes simplex virus (HSV) pinpointing a chronic infection (IgM: negative; IgG: positive).

Clinical evidences, positive serology tests, and pathological findings were in accordance with diagnostic features of HAEM.

The patient was treated with prednisolone 60 mg a day for 10 days, antiseptic, analgesic, and anesthetic mouthwash, topical steroid ointment, and valaciclovir 500 mg a day for 6 months to prevent the recurrence.

The patient when recalled after 2 months showed marked improvement in his condition with no signs of recurrence.

3. Discussion

The diagnosis of EM is based on the clinical appearance supported if necessary by biopsy.

EM patterns can be classified into EM with and without mucosal involvement: the oral cavity and the genital, ocular, laryngeal, and esophageal mucosae may be affected.

EM has been subdivided by some authors [2] into EM minus (involvement of ≤ 1 mucosal site) and EM majus (involvement of ≥ 2 mucosal sites).

Typical targets are defined as lesions less than 3 cm in diameter and characterized by three different concentric zones with predominant acral localization usually symmetrical. Raised atypical targets may occur containing only two zones. In typical and raised atypical targets, the center zone might show bulla formation as a sign of epidermal involvement [2, 3].

Oral involvement may precede lesions on other sites or may arise in isolation [1]. It is usually presented by lesions progressing through diffuse macules to blisters and ulceration, lips becoming swollen, bleeding, and crusted and intraoral lesions typically on the nonkeratinized mucosae and most pronounced in the anterior parts of the mouth.

Infections are the most common cause. Herpes simplex virus (HSV) infection is the most commonly identified cause of EM. Assier et al. identified HSV infection in 17 of 28 patients with recurrent EM. 23% of patients were found to have associated HSV infection [2, 4]. EM typically follows a lesion of recurrent herpes simplex within 1 to 3 weeks. The interval usually is about 10 days; one study found that the lip was the most common site of preceding HSV infection in recurrent EM implicating HSV-1 [1] just like our case. Nonetheless, many causative factors have been implicated including bacterial, viral, and fungal infections, drugs, radiation therapy, and emotional stress [5].

A characteristic histopathological finding of EM is necrosis of some keratinocytes and epidermal damage in the form of basal cells. This is particularly notable in the center of the target lesions of EM [5, 6]. In more severe bullous cases, necrosis of the whole dermis is noted [7, 8].

Direct immunofluorescence is performed to confirm the diagnosis as well as to rule out other diseases with diagnostic immunofluorescence findings such as autoimmune mucocutaneous diseases, in particular pemphigus vulgaris and paraneoplastic pemphigus, mucosal bullous pemphigoid, and linear IgA dermatosis.

There are significant differences in severity and clinical expression between EM and Stevens-Johnson syndrome (SJS) that cause widespread lesions and epithelial detachment involving less than 10% of the body surface and toxic epidermal necrolysis (Lyell's disease, TEN) characterized by extensive detachment of the full-thickness epithelium usually induced by drugs [1, 9]. During clinical investigations, primary herpetic infection, hand-foot-and-mouth disease, urticaria, lupus erythematosus, erosive lichen planus, fixed drug eruption, cutaneous vasculitis, and some neutrophilic dermatoses have to be considered in the differential diagnosis of EM [2, 5, 10, 11].

The treatment of EM depends on the severity of the disease manifestation, the causes, and its acute or chronic course.

In most cases, EM is minor and regresses spontaneously in 2 to 4 weeks. Therapy is similar for EM minor and major

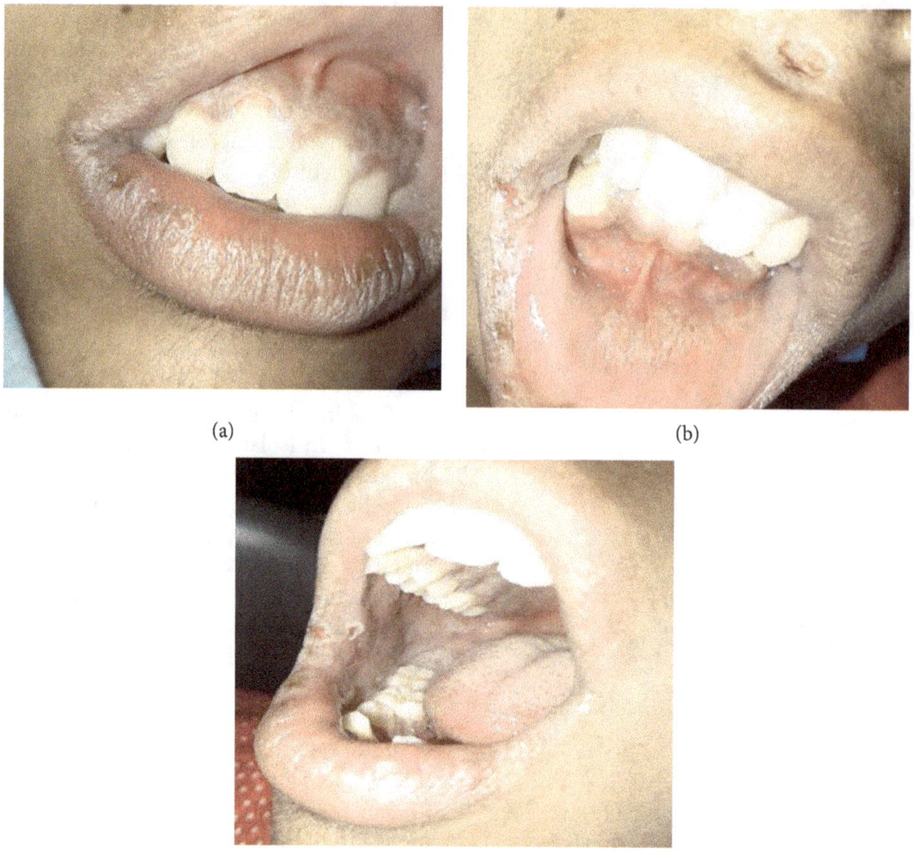

(a) (b)

(c)

Figure 3: Oral lesions of oral erythema multiforme. The oral lesions involve (a) the gingival, (b) labial, and (c) buccal mucosae and vermilion of the lips.

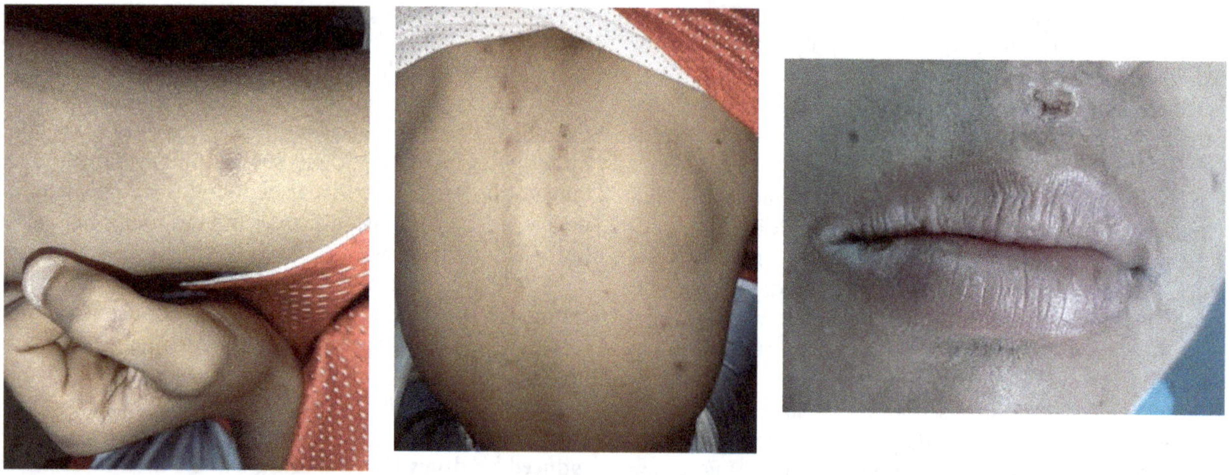

(a) (b) (c)

Figure 4: Clinical presentation of EM: (a) target lesions on the right arm and left thumb; (b) target lesions on the back; (c) crusty blister.

with the addition of oral care for oral EM. When the manifestations are not severe, only symptomatic, conservative care is usually indicated. This may include topical analgesics and oral care which consist mainly of soothing mouth rinses, like viscous lidocaine rinse; topical anesthetics, such as gel benzocaine in Orabase Bland or lidocaine gel; soft liquid diet; and avoidance of spicy and acidic food. Adequate nutrition with high-calorie and high-protein diet is essential.

Systemic treatment may also be used such as systemic analgesics, as well as antibiotic treatment if the lesions are secondarily infected.

Some authors believe that the use of systemic glucocorticoids is unnecessary [10] in this case, and it may worsen the condition [8]. Contrary to acute EM, treatment with systemic corticosteroids and prednisone has been recommended [12], although controlled studies are missing.

In cases with a high suspicion of drug-induced EM, the first measure is to stop the drug or exposure to drugs with a potential for crossreactivity due to similar chemical structures [2].

In patients with recurrent episodes, especially with a history of HSV infection, antiviral therapy is recommended and may be beneficial in preventing recurrences. Tatnall et al. performed a 6-month double-blind placebo-controlled study with 20 patients with recurrent EM, whereof 15 had a proven HSV association, with acyclovir 400 mg twice daily [13]. The study showed significant superiority of acyclovir compared to placebo treatment with regard to the prevention of further EM episodes. Furthermore, after discontinuation of acyclovir, a fraction of patients remained in clinical remission, whereas all patients treated with placebo showed recurrence [2].

In patients with HSV-associated EM resistant to antiviral therapy, oral cyclosporine, thalidomide with its known TNF-α modulating mode of action despite its teratogenic effect [2], and corticosteroid-sparing drugs, such as dapsone, azathioprine, methotrexate, and mycophenolate mofetil, may also be considered for these challenging patients [5].

4. Conclusion

Due to its typical clinical and histological features, its frequent association with HSV, and its potentially recurrent course, EM represents a distinct entity [2]. As there remain no specific diagnostic tests, early clinical recognition of disease remains essential to promptly initiate appropriate treatment [14] and improve life quality.

Thus, in the above case, prompt diagnosis and immediate treatment given to the patient not only cured him but also prevented any recurrence, thereby saving the patient from major discomfort and pain [15].

References

[1] P. Farthing, J. V. Bagan, and C. Scully, "Number IV erythema multiforme," *Oral Diseases*, vol. 11, no. 5, pp. 61-267, 2005.

[2] M. Lerch, C. Mainetti, B. T. Beretta-Piccoli, and T. Harr, "Current perspectives on erythema multiforme," *Clinical Reviews in Allergy & Immunology*, vol. 54, no. 1, pp. 177–184, 2018.

[3] S. Bastuji-Garin, B. Rzany, R. S. Stern, N. H. Shear, L. Naldi, and J. C. Roujeau, "Clinical classification of cases of toxic epidermal necrolysis, Stevens-Johnson syndrome, and erythema multiforme," *Archives of Dermatology*, vol. 129, no. 1, pp. 92–96, 1993.

[4] D. A. Wetter and M. D. Davis, "Recurrent erythema multiforme: clinical characteristics, etiologic associations, and treatment in a series of 48 patients at Mayo Clinic, 2000 to 2007," *Journal of the American Academy of Dermatology*, vol. 62, no. 1, pp. 45–53, 2010.

[5] L. Ayangco and R. S. Rogers 3rd, "Oral manifestations of erythema multiforme," *Dermatologic Clinics*, vol. 21, no. 1, pp. 195–205, 2003.

[6] J. C. Huff, W. L. Weston, and M. G. Tonnesen, "Erythema multiforme: a critical review of characteristics, diagnostic criteria, and causes," *Journal of the American Academy of Dermatology*, vol. 8, no. 6, pp. 763–775, 1983.

[7] A. Buchner, F. Lozada, and S. Silverman Jr., "Histopathologic spectrum of oral erythema multiforme," *Oral Surgery, Oral Medicine, Oral Pathology*, vol. 49, no. 3, pp. 221–228, 1980.

[8] P. M. Dowd and R. H. Champion, "Erythema multiforme," in *Rook/Wilkinson/Ebling Textbook of Dermatology, vol. 4*, J. L. Burton, D. A. Burns, and S. M. Breathnach, Eds., pp. 2081–2087, Blackwell Science, Oxford, UK, 6th edition, 1998.

[9] A. Auquier-Dunant, M. Mockenhaupt, L. Naldi, O. Correia, W. Schröder, and J.-C. Roujeau, "Correlations between clinical patterns and causes of erythema multiforme majus, Stevens-Johnson syndrome and toxic epidermal necrolysis: results of an international prospective study," *Archives of Dermatology*, vol. 138, no. 8, pp. 1019–1024, 2002.

[10] P. O. Fritsch and R. R. Maldonado, "Erythema multiforme," in *Dermatology in General Medicine, vol. 2*, T. B. Fitzpatrick, A. Z. Eisen, K. Wolff, I. M. Freedberg, and K. F. Austen, Eds., pp. 636–643, McGraw-Hill, New York, NY, USA, 4th edition, 1993.

[11] S. D. Helander and R. S. Rogers III, "The sensitivity and specificity of direct immunofluorescence testing in disorders of mucous membranes," *Journal of the American Academy of Dermatology*, vol. 30, no. 1, pp. 65–75, 1994.

[12] F. Drago, A. Parodi, and A. Rebora, "Persistent erythema multiforme: report of two new cases and review of literature," *Journal of the American Academy of Dermatology*, vol. 33, no. 2, pp. 366–369, 1995.

[13] F. M. Tatnall, J. K. Schofield, and I. M. Leigh, "A double-blind, placebo-controlled trial of continuous acyclovir therapy in recurrent erythema multiforme," *The British Journal of Dermatology*, vol. 132, no. 2, pp. 267–270, 1995.

[14] T. Bashir, S. Arti, G. Jyoti, Y. Monu, K. Vijay, and A. Naeem, "Erythema multiforme: a case report," *International Journal of Scientific Study*, vol. 2, no. 7, pp. 249–251, 2014.

[15] H. Kaur and M. Kaur, "Drug induced erythema multiforme: a case report," *International Journal of Oral Health Dentistry*, vol. 4, no. 3, pp. 175–179, 2018.

5

Reconstruction of the Occipital and Parietal Congenital Defect with 3D Custom-Made Titanium Prosthesis: A Case Report with Four and a Half Years of Follow-Up and a Brief Review of Literature

Farnoush Mohammadi,[1] **Abbas Azari**,[2] **Nariman Nikparto**,[1] **and Heliya Ziaei**[3]

[1]*Department of Oral and Maxillofacial Surgery, School of Dentistry, Tehran University of Medical Sciences, 1439955991, Kargar North St., Tehran, Iran*
[2]*Department of Prosthodontics, School of Dentistry, Tehran University of Medical Sciences, 1439955991, Kargar North St., Tehran, Iran*
[3]*School of Dentistry, Tehran University of Medical Sciences, 1439955991, Kargar North St., Tehran, Iran*

Correspondence should be addressed to Nariman Nikparto; n-nikparto@razi.tums.ac.ir

Academic Editor: Consuelo Amantini

Management of patients with congenital skull defects requires a multidisciplinary approach. Considering the defect's location and size, brain protection, and the cosmetic outcome makes such reconstructions challenging. Due to limited resemblance to skull contour and donor site morbidity of autogenous bone grafts, alloplastic materials are widely used for skull reconstructions. Titanium alloys have proper strength values, low infection rates, favorable osseointegration property, and excellent marginal adaptability when manufactured by computer-aided design (CAD) and computer-aided manufacturing (CAM). A 13-year-old female patient presented with congenital defects at the superior third of occipital bone and posterior thirds of the bilateral parietal bones. On CT scan, the exact size and shape of the defect were determined. Using CAD/CAM, a 3D virtual model of the prosthesis was designed and then printed with titanium alloy (TiAl6V4) via additive manufacturing method. The prosthesis was placed on the defect in a total surgery time of only 90 minutes. On 4.5 years of follow-up, the contour of the skull was ideal and the skin over the defect and neurologic status was intact. Due to their biocompatibility and rigidity, custom-made titanium prostheses are promising options for reconstructing complex skull defects.

1. Introduction

Skull defects are mainly due to congenital deformities, trauma, infection, or malignancy. Considering the location and size of the defect, along with brain protection and the cosmetic outcome, it makes such reconstructions challenging [1].

Autogenous bone grafts are assumed to be the gold standard for osseous reconstructions due to their immunocompatibility and low infection rates; however, donor site morbidity and lack of resemblance to skull contour are important drawbacks that limit their usage for the reconstruction of complex skull defects [2].

Due to these limitations, alloplastic materials that are biocompatible, inert, sterilizable, lightweight, noncarcinogenic, and cost-effective can be the option of choice for these reconstructions [3].

Whether prefabricated or custom-made, alloplastic materials are mainly made from titanium or polymathic methacrylate (PMMA) [3]. PMMA is economically affordable [3, 4]; however, it is not as strong as titanium [5]. Moreover, PMMA prostheses are more prone to infection, local

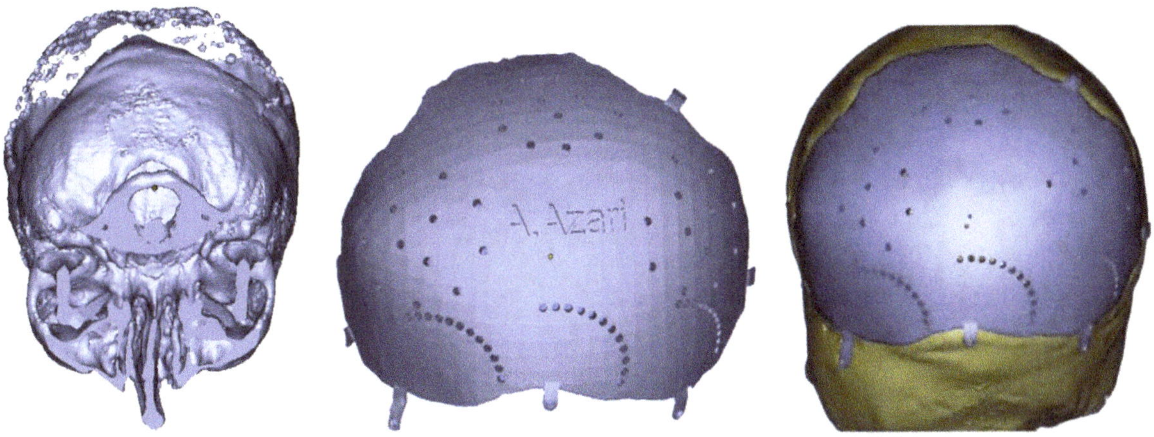

(a) (b) (c)

FIGURE 1: 3D analysis. (a) CT scan shows the exact size and shape of the congenital defect. (b) The 3D virtual model of the prosthesis. (c) The 3D virtual model of the prosthesis adapted into the defect.

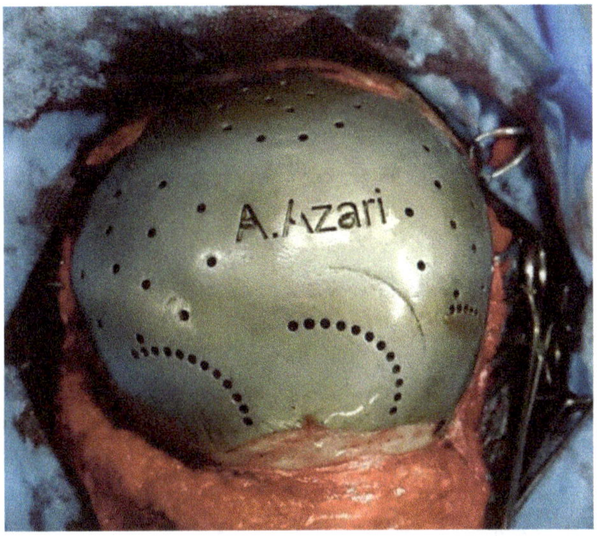

FIGURE 2: Intraoperative photograph showing the prosthesis fitness to the defect.

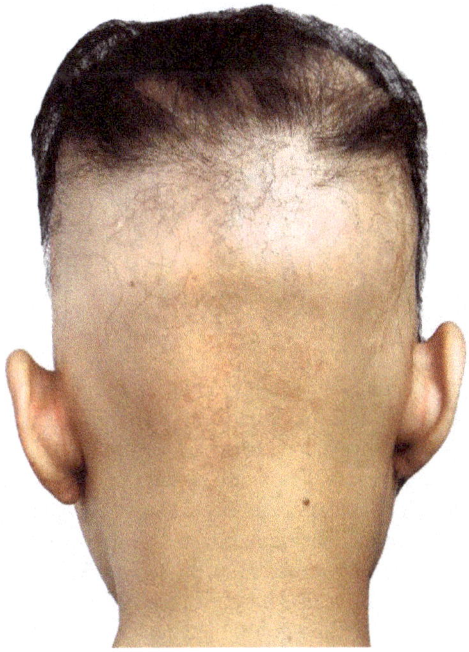

FIGURE 3: Four and a half years of follow-up. Note the perfect contour and healthy intact soft tissue at the age of 17.

irritation, foreign body reaction, and thermal damage during polymerization in the case being used as a cement for prosthesis adaptation. Furthermore, due to the native tissue ingrowth, prosthesis removal may be challenging [6].

Titanium alloys are amongst the most popular metals used in reconstructive procedures due to their high strength, biocompatibility, excellent contour, rigidity, low infection rate, favorable osseointegration property [7, 8], and excellent marginal adaptability, which can precisely fit into the complex geometry of skull defects, especially when 3D printed with CAD/CAM. These 3D-printed prostheses also have fewer radiographic artifacts in comparison to titanium meshes [9]. However, they are more expensive to design and manufacture [10].

Hence, the authors present a case of congenital skull defect with a history of several unsuccessful surgical treatments aimed at restoring the contour of skull. She was successfully treated with a 3D custom-made CAD/CAM titanium implant. For this reconstruction, the total surgery time was 90 minutes, which is 70% less than that of conventional cranioplasty procedures. Moreover, on 4.5 years of follow-up, excellent contour and the aesthetic outcome were evident.

2. Presentation of Case

The patient was a 13-year-old female with congenital skull defects at the superior third of occipital bone along with the posterior thirds of the bilateral parietal bones. Upon physical examination, the neurologic status was intact, and she did not have growth retardation. The genetic analysis showed no hereditary syndromes. She had her first

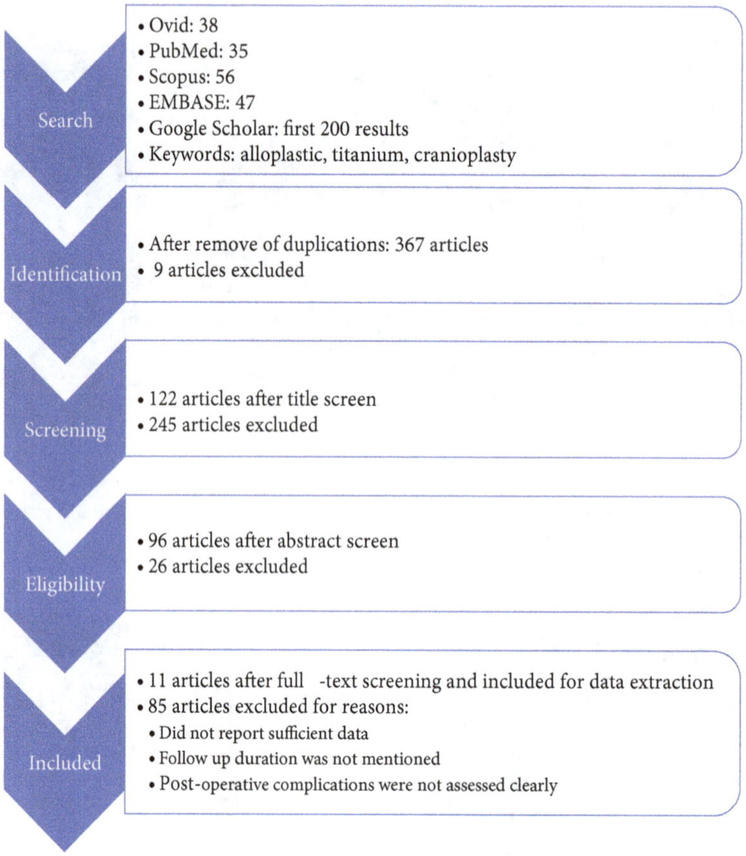

Figure 4: PRISMA flowchart. The details on selection process are reported.

reconstructive surgery in May 2008, at the age of 4 years, when the defect was bridged with a titanium mesh plate. Ever since that surgical treatment, she developed relentless petit mal seizures which were refractory to medications. The plate became exposed three months later, and she underwent several debridements in the following year, till the mesh was totally removed at the age of 5 leading to the resolution of seizures. She had not received any other medical treatment until the age of 13 when she was referred to our institution.

Because no further skull growth was expected [11], the patient was a candidate to receive the definitive prosthesis. A preoperative CT scan was obtained to determine the exact size and shape of the defect (Figure 1(a)). With CAD/CAM, a 3D virtual model of the prosthesis was designed and manufactured to match the borders of defect and provide ideal contour. The titanium alloy (TiAl6V4) was used to manufacture the prosthesis by implementing 3D printing via additive manufacturing method (Figures 1(b) and 1(c)).

For placing the prosthesis, bicoronal approach with subperiosteal dissection on the surrounding bony areas was performed. Extreme caution was exercised not to penetrate the dura during dissection between the galea and dura. The defect was totally exposed, and the dura remained intact. Then, the prosthesis was placed over the dura and fixed to the surrounding bone with titanium 2.0 mm miniplates. The ideal marginal adaptability and contour are shown in Figure 2. The incision was closed in three layers, taking care to approximate the tissues in a tension-free manner. The patient received intensive care for 24 hours and was discharged in the following week. On 4.5 years of follow-up (Figure 3), the skin over the defect remained intact with no signs of inflammation or neurologic deficits.

3. Discussion

Reconstructing complex skull defects is a challenge in craniomaxillofacial surgery. Major skull defects cannot be addressed with autografts since the contour of the skull is not similar to the common osseous donor sites such as the fibula, Iliac, or ribs [2]. Therefore, these defects may be best managed with a customized prosthesis. The 3D-printed PMMA or titanium prostheses were reported to have favorable outcomes. PMMA acrylic prostheses are more susceptible to infection [12] and tissue necrosis, which not only necessitates prostheses removal [13] but also jeopardizes the soft tissue over the defect, making further reconstructions more challenging [4]. Jaberi et al. reconstructed 70 patients with PMMA custom-made implants and reported a 24% complication rate [14].

To date, titanium is the most biocompatible material available in which the rigidity, anti-inflammatory, and antibacterial nature of this metal has made it the option of choice.

Table 1: Summary of 11 included studies, reporting a total of 214 cases of skull reconstructions with custom-made CAD/CAM titanium prostheses.

Num.	Author/year	Patients	Gender	Age	Location	Titanium implant type	Follow-up	Post op complication
1	1998/E. Heissler [16]	15	12 male/3 female	21-35 years	Not mentioned	Solid	Mean 16.6 months	1 infection, 1 convulsion upon drainage removal
2	1999/J.JOFFE [17]	141	Not mentioned	6-67 years	Not mentioned	Solid	6 weeks to 1 year	1 failure
3	2009/Mario Cabraja [13]	26	Not mentioned	35.6	16 (frontotemporoparietal), 4(bifrontal), 3(frontal), 2(temporal), 1(frontoparietal)	Solid	Median 8.1 years	A transient palsy of the frontal ramus of the facial nerve postoperatively just in 1 case
4	2010/Jules Poukens [18]	1	Not mentioned	Not mentioned	Unilateral frontotemporoparietal	Solid	NM	No
5	2011/H. Sudhoff [9]	1	Male	48	Unilateral parietal, sphenoid, frontal, orbital rim, ethmoid, maxillary, zygomatic, nasal bones	Solid	1 week	No
6	2011/Juan Felipe Isaza Saldarriaga [15]	1	Male	13	Unilateral frontoparietal area	Solid	4 months	No
7	2014/S.A. Eolchiyan [19]	4	Female	24	Left fronto-orbital region	Solid	Mean 4.4 years	No
			Male	44	Right parietal-temporal region	Solid	Mean 4.4 years	No
			Female	23	Left fronto-orbital region	Solid	Mean 4.4 years	No
			Female	23	Both side frontal region	Solid	Mean 4.4 years	No
8	2015/Hyung Rok Cho [10]	3	Female	41	Left parieto-occipital area extended to right parietal area	Porous	6 months	No
			Female	32	Right frontotemporoparietal area	Porous	6 months	No
			Female	21	Left parietotemporal area	Porous	2 months	No
9	2018/Jae Yoon Kim [20]	1	Male	36	Unilateral forehead and glabella area	Solid	6 months	No
10	2019/Seong Hwan Kim [21]	2	Male	55	Right parietotemporal area	Solid	1 year	No
			Male	33	Right temporal area	Solid	NM	No
11	2019/Champeaux C [22]	19	12 male/7 female	47.4 ± 11.3	6: right side, 9: frontal side, 4: left side	Solid	Mean 1.2 year	31.6%: early postoperative complications, 1 lost to follow-up, 1 prosthesis removal, 63.1% no complication

TABLE 2: Summary of the demographic data and complication rates of the included patients.

N	214
Sex	
Female	7.47%
Male	14.02%
Not mentioned	78.50%
Age	38.93 ± 8.27
Follow-up	45.85 ± 40.01
Complication rate	5.61%

Conventional cranioplasty surgeries with prefabricated prostheses or titanium meshes usually take 4-5 hours due to the trial-and-error procedures to achieve a good fitness of the implant. By CADs, the complete procedure of the surgery is preplanned, and a customized prosthesis with excellent contour and fitness can be produced before the surgery. Therefore, not only there is no need for prosthesis adjustment during surgery but also the surgery time decreases considerably, and the outcome improves remarkably. By such a decrease in surgical time, the risk of postoperative complications such as severe pain, infection, and wound dehiscence decreases substantially. Our entire surgery lasted 1:30 hours which is approximately 70% less than conventional cranioplasty surgeries. Moreover, Saldarriaga reported the same, 85% reduction in surgery time with the similar method [15].

To get a deeper understanding, a literature review was performed. Two authors (N.N. and H.Z.) independently conducted the electronic searches using Ovid MEDLINE/-PubMed, Scopus, EMBASE, Google Scholar (first 200 results), and Cochrane Database, including articles published in March 2021. Alloplastic, titanium, and cranioplasty were used as keywords. The bibliographies of included studies were also searched for relevant articles. Preclinical studies, papers not describing cranioplasty techniques, and studies not reporting follow-up durations were excluded. Figure 4 shows the PRISMA flowchart of selection criteria for this review. Finally, 11 studies with 214 reported cases were included. Table 1 shows the extracted data, and Table 2 reports the analyses of data obtained from the included studies.

According to the results, the complication rate for titanium prosthesis reconstruction is relatively low. Among 215 cases with follow-up periods from 1 week to 8 years, 12 (5.6%) post-op complications and 2 (0.9%) prosthesis failures were reported. All studies reported excellent contour, acceptable rigidity, and high patient satisfaction rates. This rate of complications is by far more acceptable than that of PMMA prostheses.

The expenses of custom-made titanium implants are relatively high; however, the benefits definitely outweigh, such as decreased surgical time, shorter recovery and hospitalization, fewer postoperative complications, and less need to further corrective surgeries.

4. Conclusions

In conclusion, custom-made titanium implants can be considered the treatment of choice, which offers predictable aesthetic outcomes for the reconstruction of complex skull defects, with the low rate of complications and high aesthetics and patient satisfaction outcomes.

Acknowledgments

The authors wish to acknowledge Mr. Ahmad Bereimipour for his assistance in journal selection.

References

[1] D. Lindner, K. Schlothofer-Schumann, B.-C. Kern, O. Marx, A. Müns, and J. Meixensberger, "Cranioplasty using custom-made hydroxyapatite versus titanium: a randomized clinical trial," *Journal of Neurosurgery*, vol. 126, no. 1, pp. 175–183, 2017.

[2] G. F. Rogers and A. K. Greene, "Autogenous bone graft," *The Journal of Craniofacial Surgery*, vol. 23, no. 1, pp. 323–327, 2012.

[3] E.-K. Park, J.-Y. Lim, I.-S. Yun et al., "Cranioplasty enhanced by three-dimensional printing," *The Journal of Craniofacial Surgery*, vol. 27, no. 4, pp. 943–949, 2016.

[4] P. Simon, J. Mohan, S. Selvaraj, B. S. Saravanan, and P. Pari, "Craniofacial prosthetic reconstruction using polymethyl methacrylate implant: a case report," *The Journal of Indian Prosthodontic Society*, vol. 14, no. S1, pp. 303–307, 2014.

[5] J. Y. Kim, B. K. Jung, Y. S. Kim, T. S. Roh, and I. S. Yun, "Forehead reconstruction with a custom-made three-dimensional titanium implant in a Parry-Romberg syndrome patient," *Archives of Craniofacial Surgery*, vol. 19, no. 2, pp. 135–138, 2018.

[6] S. Aydin, B. Kucukyuruk, B. Abuzayed, S. Aydin, and G. Z. Sanus, "Cranioplasty: review of materials and techniques," *Journal of Neurosciences in Rural Practice*, vol. 2, no. 2, pp. 162–167, 2011.

[7] A. M. Shah, H. Jung, and S. Skirboll, "Materials used in cranioplasty: a history and analysis," *Neurosurgical Focus*, vol. 36, no. 4, article E19, 2014.

[8] Y. B. Roka, "Review of the history of materials used with experience with bone cement cranioplasty," *Nepal Journal of Neuroscience*, vol. 14, no. 1, pp. 7–13, 2017.

[9] H. Sudhoff, H. J. Hoff, and M. Lehmann, "Skull repair after major crush injury," *Case Reports in Otolaryngology*, vol. 2011, Article ID 749250, 3 pages, 2011.

[10] H. R. Cho, T. S. Roh, K. W. Shim, Y. O. Kim, D. H. Lew, and I. S. Yun, "Skull reconstruction with custom made three-dimensional titanium implant," *Archives of Craniofacial Surgery*, vol. 16, no. 1, pp. 11–16, 2015.

[11] S.-W. Jin, K.-B. Sim, and S.-D. Kim, "Development and growth of the normal cranial vault: an embryologic review," *Journal of Korean Neurosurgical Society*, vol. 59, no. 3, pp. 192–196, 2016.

[12] J. D. Oliver, J. Banuelos, A. Abu-Ghname, K. S. Vyas, and B. Sharaf, "Alloplastic cranioplasty Reconstruction," *Annals of Plastic Surgery*, vol. 82, no. 5S, pp. S289–S294, 2019.

[13] M. Cabraja, M. Klein, and T. N. Lehmann, "long-term results following titanium cranioplasty of large skull defects," *Neurosurgical Focus*, vol. 26, no. 6, article E10, 2009.

[14] J. Jaberi, K. Gambrell, P. Tiwana, C. Madden, and R. Finn, "Long-term clinical outcome analysis of poly-methyl-methacrylate cranioplasty for large skull defects," *Journal of Oral and Maxillofacial Surgery*, vol. 71, no. 2, pp. e81–e88, 2013.

[15] Saldarriaga, "Design and manufacturing of a custom skull implant," *American Journal of Engineering and Applied Sciences*, vol. 4, no. 1, pp. 169–174, 2011.

[16] E. Heissler, F. S. Fischer, S. Boiouri et al., "Custom-made cast titanium implants produced with CAD/CAM for the reconstruction of cranium defects," *International Journal of Oral and Maxillofacial Surgery*, vol. 27, no. 5, pp. 334–338, 1998.

[17] J. Joffe, M. Harris, F. Kahugu, S. Nicoll, A. Linney, and R. Richards, "A prospective study of computer-aided design and manufacture of titanium plate for cranioplasty and its clinical outcome," *British Journal of Neurosurgery*, vol. 13, no. 6, pp. 576–580, 1999.

[18] J. Poukens, P. Laeven, M. Beerens et al., "*Custom surgical implants using additive manufacturing*," *Digital Dental News*, vol. 4, no. 1, p. 72, 2010.

[19] S. A. Eolchiyan, "Complex skull defects reconstruction with CAD/CAM titanium and polyetheretherketone (PEEK) implants," *Zhurnal voprosy neirokhirurgii imeni NN Burdenko*, vol. 78, p. 3, 2014.

[20] R. S. Leão, J. R. S. Maior, C. A. A. Lemos et al., "Complications with PMMA compared with other materials used in cranioplasty: a systematic review and meta-analysis," *Brazilian Oral Research*, vol. 32, 2018.

[21] S. H. Kim, S. J. Lee, J. W. Lee, H. S. Jeong, and I. S. Suh, "Staged reconstruction of large skull defects with soft tissue infection after craniectomy using free flap and cranioplasty with a custom-made titanium mesh constructed by 3D-CT-guided 3D printing technology," *Medicine*, vol. 98, no. 6, article e13864, 2019.

[22] C. Champeaux, S. Froelich, and Y. Caudron, "Titanium three-dimensional printed cranioplasty for fronto-nasal bone defect," *The Journal of Craniofacial Surgery*, vol. 30, no. 6, pp. 1802–1805, 2019.

6

Radiographic Features of Facial Cosmetic Material: Report of Two Cases

Noura A. Alsufyani[1,2] **and Mohammed A. Alsufyani**[3]

[1]*Oral & Maxillofacial Radiology, Oral Medicine and Diagnostic Sciences Department, College of Dentistry, King Saud University, Riyadh, Saudi Arabia*
[2]*School of Dentistry, Department of Medicine and Dentistry, University of Alberta, Canada*
[3]*Cosmetic and Dermatologic Surgery, Department of Dermatology and Dermatologic Surgery, Prince Sultan Military Medical City, Riyadh, Saudi Arabia*

Correspondence should be addressed to Noura A. Alsufyani; alsufyan@ualberta.ca

Academic Editor: Alberto Delbem

Recently, the use of noninvasive facial cosmetic procedures has been widely disseminated. In the face, cosmetic fillers, threads, and implants are used to reduce or delay the effects of aging or adjust facial defects caused by trauma or disease. The dentist or dental specialist may encounter these materials in the radiographic images of their patients. There are few reports in the dental literature describing the radiographic appearance of some materials along with the diseases they mimic. As the procedures and materials advance and evolve, dentists and dental specialists must be aware of their radiographic appearance to avoid errors in diagnosis. This is a report of two cases that include panoramic radiography and CBCT scan. Among these cases, there is an unusual appearance of a cosmetic filler due to a subperiosteal injection method. Moreover, it will discuss common types of cosmetic materials used in the face and their imaginological appearance. This is the key to dentists and dental specialists due to increasing use of facial cosmetic materials and a parallel increase in the use of cone beam CT and chances to encounter such findings.

1. Introduction

With aging, changes occur in various tissues of the face resulting in cutaneous changes, volume depletion, and sagging. Fillers, autologous fat, and surgical implants are used for therapeutic or cosmetic volume correction. Suspension or lifting and threads are used to overcome the sagging and laxity. According to the American Society for Aesthetic Plastic Surgery 2018, hyaluronic acid (HA) fillers have become the second most nonsurgical procedure with a 58% increase since 2014 [1]. In 2018, the American Society for Dermatologic Surgery reports 1.6 million soft tissue filler procedures, a 78% increase since 2012, and approximately 32,000 thread lift procedures [2].

Cone beam CT has become a common diagnostic tool in dentistry; however, incidental findings pose a diagnostic challenge to dentists and dental specialists. Recently, dentists showed interest and engagement in cosmetic dermatology practices such as botulinum toxin and cosmetic filler injections. In the dental literature, several case reports presented the imaginological appearance of calcium hydroxyapatite dermal fillers, cheek and chin implants, and gold threads [3–7].

This work presents the radiographic appearance of two cases of cosmetic materials, with one unusual subperiosteal filler injection, incidentally observed in cone beam CT images. With the recent crossover from dentistry to cosmetic dermatology, this work reviews the pertinent literature of

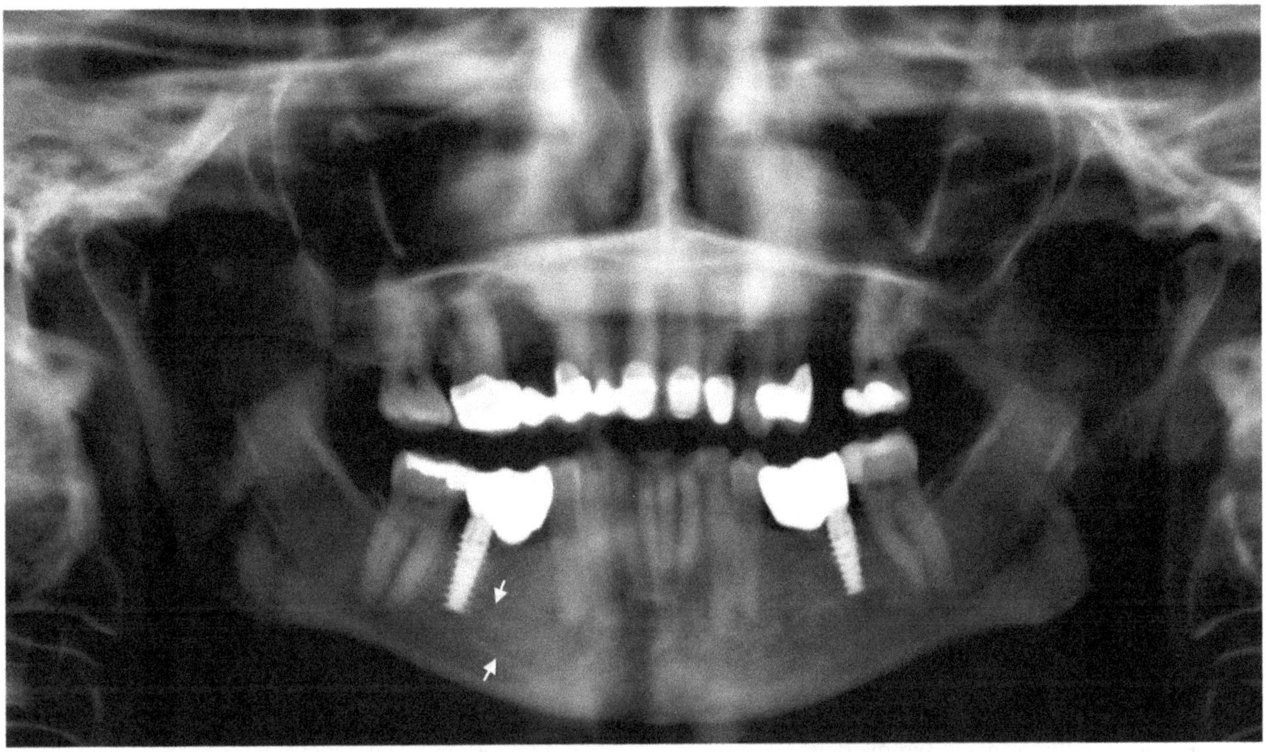

(a)

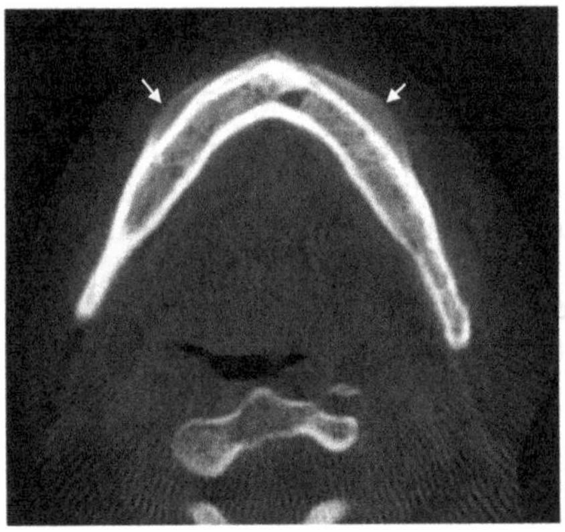

(b)

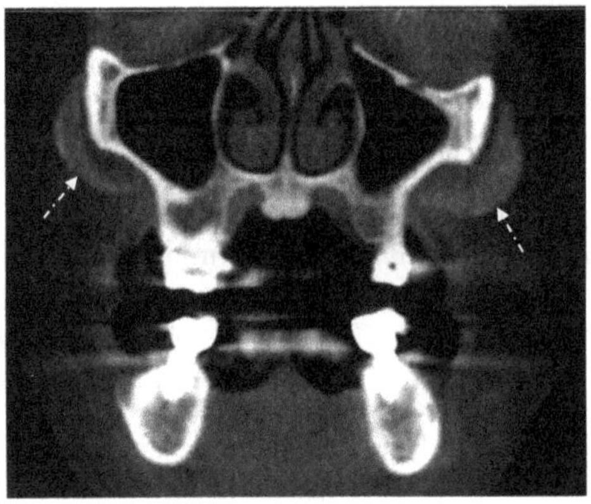

(c)

FIGURE 1: Subperiosteal cosmetic filler in the mandible (case 1): (a) panoramic radiograph showing linear radiopaque lines (arrows); (b) axial CBCT image showing a bilateral, subperiosteal cosmetic filler at the buccal cortex of the posterior mandible; (c) coronal CBCT image showing bilateral zygomatic implants (dotted arrows).

cosmetic materials that can be encountered by the dentist/-dental specialist in the facial area.

2. Case Reports

This project was approved by the Health Research Ethics Board at the University of Alberta, Canada (#00101635), and has therefore been performed in accordance with the ethical standards laid down in an appropriate version of the Declaration of Helsinki (as revised in Brazil 2013). The CBCT examination was completed at the cone beam CT services at the School of Dentistry, University of Alberta. For both cases, the i-CAT Next Generation Cone Beam (Imaging Sciences International, Hatfield, PA, USA) was used with the following protocol: 120 kVp, 20 mAs, 16 × 13 mm field of view, and 0.3 mm voxel.

2.1. Case 1. A 66-year-old female presented for maxillary and mandibular dental implant assessment. The referring clinic provided a panoramic radiography before the cone beam CT scan. On the panoramic radiograph, there were two, subtle, linear radiopaque lines extending from the apical end of implants #36 and #46 to the root apices of teeth #34 and #34, respectively, with parallel lines diverging medially and inferiorly toward the inferior border of the parasymphysis (Figure 1(a)).

The cone beam CT depicted a well-defined predominantly radiolucent entity along the buccal cortex of the mandible extending from the right mandibular molar area and crossing the midline to the left mandibular molar area (Figure 1(b)). There are few minute calcifications similar to cortical bone in density within the radiolucency. The mixed entity appears as a "subperiosteal" finding causing cortical expansion of the buccal cortex along the crestal and midalveolar levels at its distal ends and along the inferior levels at the medial ends, i.e., symphysis and parasymphysis.

In addition, there were bilateral, uniform, high-attenuation objects within the soft tissues along the outer cortex of the zygomatic process of maxilla and zygomatic bone (Figure 1(c)). The objects were fine-granular, less than cancellous bone in density. The osseous and soft tissues adjacent to these entities were unremarkable. The diagnosis was cosmetic implants of the zygoma. No differential diagnosis is offered.

The radiographic features of periphery and expansion depicted by the subperiosteal filler in the mandible based on the panoramic radiograph would suggest a benign-cystic lesion. With the presence of minute calcifications, pathological entities such as calcifying odontogenic epithelial tumor, odontogenic keratocyst with dystrophic calcifications, calcifying odontogenic cyst, and adenomatoid odontogenic tumor can be considered. The cone beam CT images revealed the uniform and symmetric shape, unusual subperiosteal location, and lack of effects on the surrounding teeth. As such, a cosmetic procedure that involves lifting the periosteum was considered rather than odontogenic pathology. The patient was contacted and has confirmed receiving cosmetic implants and fillers in the midface, mandible, and chin. A dermatology consultant confirmed that subperiosteal techniques are used in the maxillofacial and mandibular areas to deliver cosmetic fillers. Based on this information, we concluded that the entity in the mandible was a subperiosteal cosmetic filler.

2.2. Case 2. A 52-year-old female underwent a cone beam CT scan for preimplant and temporomandibular joint assessment. A cluster of multiple radiopacities was incidentally noted in the immediate soft tissues lateral to the left masseter muscle and bilaterally below the zygoma (Figures 2(a) and 2(b). The radiopacities were irregular in shape and similar to those in cortical and cancellous bone in density. Differential diagnoses considered osteoma cutis, myositis ossificans, heterotrophic/dystrophic calcifications, and foreign bodies. The patient was contacted and has confirmed receiving cosmetic fillers in the face. Nine months postbone graft for dental implant purposes, the filler material showed posterior-superior migration and reduction in size and density (Figures 2(c) and 2(d)).

3. Discussion

3.1. Soft Tissue Augmentation (Fillers). Fillers are used for a wide range of indications: correcting age-related volume loss and sagging and correction of soft tissue defects caused by trauma or disease.

Fillers used for soft tissue augmentation can be synthetic such as collagen, hyaluronic acid gel, calcium hydroxyapatite (CaHA), and poly-L-lactic acid (PLLA). These are known as temporary or semipermanent due to their biodegradability. Permanent synthetic products are polymethylmethacrylate (PMMA), polyalkylimide, and liquid silicone. The source can be as well a natural autologous one as in the case of autologous fat transfer [8–11].

The level of placement of such products depends largely on the indication intended to be addressed and facial anatomy of the target area, as well as the type of product and its approved indications. Fillers are placed intradermally, immediately subdermally, or in the subcutaneous plane [12, 13].

Injectable cosmetic fillers can have radiolucency/soft tissue density (e.g., hyaluronic acid, collagen, and fat) or varying degrees of radiopacity (e.g., calcium hydroxyapatite (CHA) and silicone).

Radiopaque fillers can be depicted on plain radiographs such as panoramic radiographs but are certainly better detailed in CT and CBCT according to several case reports in the medical and dental fields [3–7]. An example of the CaHA filler is presented in Figure 2.

Less commonly, cosmetic fillers can be injected subperiosteally, such as in case 1 (Figure 1). This method of placement showed a promising technique in the midface and chin. Less postoperative complications and desirable aesthetic outcomes partly are due to creating a skeletal support for the overlaying soft tissues thus reducing drooping or sagging [14–17].

Case 1 is the first to describe the radiographic presentation of a subperiosteal filler in the mandible. The differential diagnoses of subperiosteal fillers include intraosseous tumors or cysts rather than soft tissue lesions for dermal or subcutaneous fillers. Imaging with cone beam CT offered key features for diagnosis such as the symmetrical distribution (the extension to the left mandible was not clear in the panoramic radiograph), uniform geometry in X, Y, and Z planes, and confinement to the subperiosteal layer. The correlation with patient history to confirm cosmetic procedures was important to reach a diagnosis without surgical intervention (surgical exploration or biopsy). Patients can be reluctant to admit to cosmetic work in their initial visit to the dentist/dental specialist. The role of the oral and maxillofacial radiologist to view, analyze, investigate, and diagnose incidental findings is emphasized in case 1.

There are no direct dental implications for the cosmetic filler; however, the dental clinician must be aware of their existence and possible complications. The most common complications of fillers are transient and mild in nature such as swelling, erythema, and bruising. Other, less common, complications include infection, noninflamed nodules, biofilm, granuloma, and persistent edema (i.e., malar). And similar to case 2 (Figure 2), migration of the filler material has been reported [9, 11, 18].

3.2. Threads for Lifting. Threads are minimally invasive methods to lift saggy skin that results from increased laxity and give a more youthful appearance. Common types of threads used are polypropylene suture, poly-L-lactic acid (PLLA), polydioxanone (PDO), and polylactide/glycolide

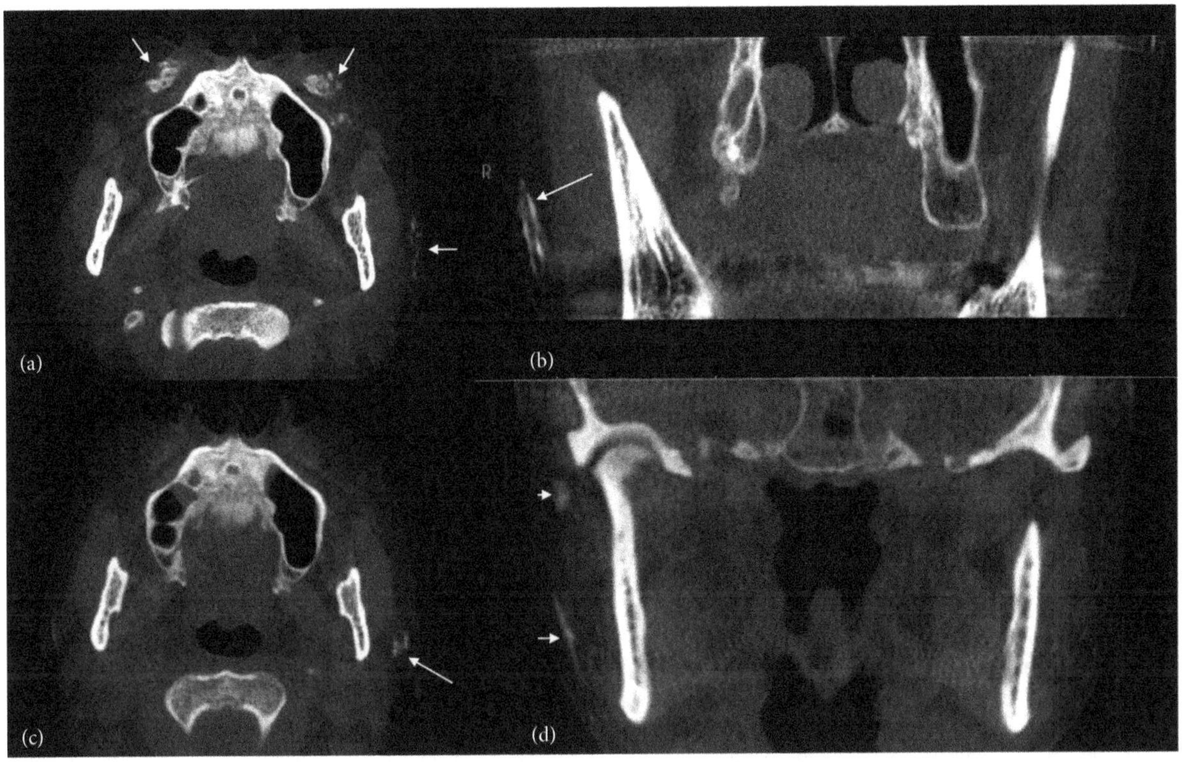

FIGURE 2: CBCT images of the subdermal CaHA filler (case 2): (a) axial and (b) coronal CBCT images showing multiple, conglomerate high-attenuation entities within the dermal layers anterior to the maxillae and lateral to the masseter muscles; (c) axial and (d) coronal CBCT images after 9 months showing resorption and posterior migration of the filler.

resorbable copolymer (PLGA) [19–21]. Gold thread therapy involves implanting pure gold threads of 0.1 mm diameter braided with polyglycolic acid or polyvinylidene difluoride into the subdermal skin. The foreign-body reaction of this therapy may trigger the production of elastin and collagen fibers and provide mechanical support to the tissues and ultimately skin rejuvenation [22, 23]. However, there is little evidence for its therapeutic efficacy [23–25].

Threads have either barbs or cons fixated on their surfaces. After marking the overlying skin with the best oriented vector to give the maximum lift effect, the threads are placed in the fibrous fatty tissue in the subcutaneous plane to lift and fix the tissue in their central part without the need to anchor either ends [20, 21, 26].

Most threads are radiolucent unless braided with gold. Tanaka Kikinzoku Kogyo KK (Tokyo, Japan) originally coated nonabsorbable cog thread with 24-carat gold [27]. Despite some commercial reports about the rejuvenation provided by gold threads, no scientific reports exist on their use except for a histological study on rats suggesting "that the gold-coated cog thread has clinical potential." [27]

Gold threads can be depicted in panoramic radiographs, in CBCT images, or in periapical radiographs if the cheek intercepts the path of the X-ray beam [23–25]. The differential diagnosis may include acupuncture needles, surgical clips, and posttrauma foreign bodies.

The cosmetic or acupuncture gold wires may cause radiographic artifacts and with time become fragmented and unevenly distributed [24, 25]. Complications that can occur with thread lifting are usually mild and temporary such as swelling, bruising, erythema, and skin dimpling. Less common complications are infection, foreign body reaction, hematoma, thread migration, and exposure [19, 21].

3.3. Surgical Implants. Implants have been used to correct deformities (congenital or acquired) and changes resulting from facial aging. Facial regions most treated are the dorsum of the nose, malar area (Figure 1), and the chin.

There are different types of implants and depending on their composition can be radiolucent (Permacol™, MERSILENE® resorbable mesh, LactoSorb®, MEDPOR®, methyl methacrylate, polyethylene, etc.) or present with a degree of radiopacity (autologous bone graft, Silastic™ silicone, titanium wire, polytetrafluoroethylene, etc.) [27, 28]. These implants need fixation by using screws or sutures or through creating pockets and contouring done at the subperiosteal plane to be immobilized [27].

Complications that may occur with placing facial implants include infection, displacement, hematoma, damage to the infraorbital or mental nerves, bone resorption, atrophy of the overlying skin, and extrusion [27, 28].

4. Conclusion

With the exponential demand of cosmetic procedures in the face, the dentists and dental specialists are bound to encounter these materials in conventional radiographs or cone beam CT images. Imaginological appearance varies widely in terms of shape and radiodensity depending on the material used. Recognizing these cosmetic materials and their imaginological appearance will improve diagnosis, avoid mismanagement or unnecessary biopsy, and anticipate any future complications of the material in the mandibular and maxillofacial area.

References

[1] American society for aesthetic plastic surgery, "2018 statistics," Accessibility verified December 2020, https://www.surgery.org/consumers/procedures.

[2] American society for dermatologic surgery, "2018 statistics," Accessibility verified December 2020, https://www.asds.net.

[3] M. A. Cabrera and F. Mulinari-Brenner, "Radiological evaluation of calcium hydroxyapatite-based cutaneous fillers," *Surgical and Cosmetic Dermatology*, vol. 3, no. 3, pp. 203–205, 2011.

[4] S. Koka, K. Shah, and S. Mallya, "Dermal filler presenting as lobular radiopacities in an edentulous patient: a clinical report," *Journal of Prosthodontics*, vol. 26, no. 8, pp. 670-671, 2017.

[5] Y. Kwon, C. An, K. S. Choi, D. Lee, and S. An, "Radiographic study of dermal fillers in the facial area: a series of 3 cases," *Imaging Science in Dentistry*, vol. 48, no. 3, pp. 227–231, 2018.

[6] P. Mundada, R. Kohler, S. Boudabbous, L. Toutous Trellu, A. Platon, and M. Becker, "Injectable facial fillers: imaging features, complications, and diagnostic pitfalls at MRI and PET CT," *Insights into imaging*, vol. 8, no. 6, pp. 557–572, 2017.

[7] J. R. Valiyaparambil, K. Rengasamy, and S. M. Mallya, "An unusual soft tissue radiopacity - radiographic appearance of a dermal filler," *British Dental Journal*, vol. 207, no. 5, pp. 211-212, 2009.

[8] J. J. Kim and G. R. D. Evans, "Applications of biomaterials in plastic surgery," *Clinics in Plastic Surgery*, vol. 39, no. 4, pp. 359–376, 2012.

[9] J. Carruthers, A. Carruthers, and S. Humphrey, "Introduction to fillers," *Plastic and Reconstructive Surgery*, vol. 136, 5 Suppl, pp. 120S–131S, 2015.

[10] J. Woodward, T. Khan, and J. Martin, "Facial filler complications," *Facial Plastic Surgery Clinics of North America.*, vol. 23, no. 4, pp. 447–458, 2015.

[11] Y. Z. Chiang, G. Pierone, and F. Al-Niaimi, "Dermal fillers: pathophysiology, prevention and treatment of complications," *JEADV*, vol. 31, no. 3, pp. 405–413, 2017.

[12] D. Mckee, K. Remington, A. Swift, V. Lambros, J. Comstock, and D. Lalonde, "Effective rejuvenation with hyaluronic acid fillers: current advanced concepts," *Plastic and Reconstructive Surgery*, vol. 143, no. 6, pp. 1277e–1289e, 2019.

[13] C. C. Surek, "Facial anatomy for filler injection: the superficial musculoaponeurotic system (SMAS) is not just for facelifting," *Clinics in Plastic Surgery*, vol. 46, no. 4, pp. 603–612, 2019.

[14] E. Martínez-Sanz, D. A. Ossipov, J. Hilborn, S. Larsson, K. B. Jonsson, and O. P. Varghese, "Bone reservoir: injectable hyaluronic acid hydrogel for minimal invasive bone augmentation," *Journal of Controlled Release*, vol. 152, no. 2, pp. 232–240, 2011.

[15] T. Pavicic, M. Yankova, T. L. Schenck et al., "Subperiosteal injections during facial soft tissue filler injections is it possible?," *Journal of Cosmetic Dermatology*, vol. 19, no. 3, pp. 590–595, 2020.

[16] R. N. Heffelfinger, K. E. Blackwell, J. Rawnsley, and G. S. Keller, "A simplified approach to midface aging," *Archives of Facial Plastic Surgery*, vol. 9, no. 1, pp. 48–55, 2007.

[17] K. Kang and C. Chai, "Subperiosteal chin augmentation with hyaluronic acid filler in patients with a small chin," *Journal of Cosmetic Medicine*, vol. 1, no. 2, pp. 120–129, 2017.

[18] T. C. Kontis, L. Bunin, and R. Fitzgerald, "Injectable fillers: panel discussion, controversies, and techniques," *Facial Plastic Surgery Clinics of North America*, vol. 26, no. 2, pp. 225–236, 2018.

[19] H. A. Gülbitti, B. Colebunders, A. Pirayesh, D. Bertossi, and B. van der Lei, "Thread-lift sutures: still in the lift? A systematic review of the literature," *Plastic and Reconstructive Surgery*, vol. 141, no. 3, pp. 341e–347e, 2018.

[20] K. A. Archer and R. E. Garcia, "Silhouette instalift: benefits to a facial plastic surgery practice," *Facial Plastic Surgery Clinics of North America*, vol. 27, no. 3, pp. 341–353, 2019.

[21] B. S. Atiyeh, S. A. Dibo, M. Costagliola, and S. N. Hayek, "Barbed sutures "lunch time" lifting: evidence-based efficacy," *Journal of Cosmetic Dermatology*, vol. 9, no. 2, pp. 132–141, 2010.

[22] K. C. Shin, T. H. Bae, W. S. Kim, and H. K. Kim, "Usefulness of gold thread implantation for crow's feet," *Archives of Plastic Surgery*, vol. 39, no. 1, pp. 42–45, 2012.

[23] G. Alsaadi, R. Jacobs, M. Quirynen, and D. van Steenberghe, "Soft tissue augmentation of the cheeks detected on intra- and extraoral radiographs: a case report," *Dentomaxillofacial Radiology*, vol. 37, no. 2, pp. 117–120, 2008.

[24] R. Negayama and T. Fujikawa, "CT appearance of gold thread facelift," *QJM*, vol. 111, no. 1, pp. 57–57, 2018.

[25] J. A. J. Keestra, R. Jacobs, and M. Quirynen, "Gold-wire artifacts on diagnostic radiographs: a case report," *Imaging Science in Dentistry*, vol. 44, no. 1, pp. 81–84, 2014.

[26] M. T. Villa, L. E. White, M. Alam, S. S. Yoo, and R. L. Walton, "Barbed sutures: a review of the literature," *Plastic and Reconstructive Surgery*, vol. 121, no. 3, pp. 102e–108e, 2008.

[27] J. D. Oliver, A. C. Eells, E. S. Saba et al., "Alloplastic facial implants: a systematic review and meta-analysis on outcomes and uses in aesthetic and reconstructive plastic surgery," *Aesthetic Plastic Surgery*, vol. 43, no. 3, pp. 625–636, 2019.

[28] D. Schwartz and F. A. Quereshy, "Combined rhytidectomy and alloplastic facial implants," *Atlas of the Oral and Maxillofacial Surgery Clinics of North America*, vol. 22, no. 1, pp. 69–73, 2014.

7

Periapical Actinomycosis: A Rare Subdivision of Cervicofacial Actinomycosis, Review of the Literature and a Case Report

Ramtin Dastgir[1] **and Maryam Sohrabi**[2]

[1]*Faculty of Dentistry, Tehran Medical Sciences, Islamic Azad University, Tehran, Iran*
[2]*Department of Oral and Maxillofacial Surgery, School of Dentistry, Tehran University of Medical Sciences, Tehran, Iran*

Correspondence should be addressed to Maryam Sohrabi; sohrabi.m.22@gmail.com

Academic Editor: Andrea Scribante

Background. Periapical actinomycosis, which is reckoned as a subgroup of cervicofacial actinomycosis, is an uncommon, more indolent, less invasive, and limited type of actinomycosis infection. However, it can be considerably underreported due to the low number of periapical surgical specimens that are submitted for histopathological analysis after excision of the lesion with the preliminary diagnosis of typical periapical infections. It is believed that during root canal treatment, the organisms are displaced from the oral cavity into the periapical regions as a result of failure to establish aseptic techniques which can further result in actinomycosis infections and, in rare instances, lead to more severe events and can even be life-threatening. *Case Presentation.* We intend to report a case of periapical actinomycosis in a 34-year-old female who presented with the chief complaint of pain and slight mobility of the mandibular right second premolar and first molar with no significant issues in the patient's medical history. Initial orthopantomography revealed a uniloculated, radiolucent lesion engulfing the apices of the aforementioned teeth. An incisional biopsy was then obtained which revealed fragments of fibroconnective tissue including few crushed bone particles severely infiltrated by acute inflammatory cells and some foamy macrophages. The suppurative exudate focally surrounds colonies of filamentous bacteria as round basophilic masses with radial configuration resembling "sulfur granules." Surgical approach consisted of curettage accompanied with peripheral ostectomy and cautious burnishing of the two involved tooth roots. *Conclusion.* This case report emphasizes the importance of aseptic techniques during endodontic and more invasive treatments, as they can cause penetration of Actinomyces into the periapical region which in some cases can lead to more serious complications and even life-threatening situations.

1. Introduction

Actinomycosis, often called the "great imitator", is a rare chronic granulomatous infection caused by Gram-positive, non-acid-fast, branched filamentous, anaerobic, or microaerophilic/capnophilic bacillus bacteria of the *Actinomyces* genus. The *Actinomyces* genus belongs to family *Actinomycetaceae* (the single member of order *Actinomycetales*) that also includes *Arcanobacterium, Actinobaculum, Mobiluncus, Trueperella*, and *Varibaculum*. They mainly colonize the oropharynx, gastrointestinal tract, and female urogenital tract [1–4]. Furthermore, *Actinomyces* spp. are normal commensals of the human oropharynx, gastrointestinal tract, and genitourinary tract [4]. Actinomycosis infection is most commonly observed in the cervicofacial region and accounts for almost 55% of all actinomycosis infection cases [5]. This infection is most commonly due to *Actinomyces israelii* or less commonly other etiologic species, such as *A. odontolyticus, A. naeslundii, A. viscosus, A. propionica, Propionibacterium propionicus*, and *A. gerencseriae* [6, 7]. The reason behind the notorious nickname of the "great imitator" can perhaps be attributed to the challenging diagnosis of this infection due to its nonspecific radiological findings and nonspecific symptoms. Despite occurring rarely, actinomycosis should be included in the differential diagnosis when encountered with a soft-tissue mass with inflammatory changes with an infiltrative nature in the cervicofacial area in radiographic images. Moreover, it should be noted that

CT scan and MRI are not sufficient for distinguishing actinomycosis from malignant tumoral masses [8]. Actinomycosis infection is characterized by suppurative and granulomatous lesions which primarily occur in soft tissues. Though rare, primary cutaneous and skeletal involvements are also probable [9–11]. Main risk factors which leave the patient vulnerable to actinomycosis infection include mucosal breach, impaired local or systemic immune defenses, poor oral hygiene, facial trauma, prior history of head and neck radiation, or oral surgeries. However, few cases of actinomycosis infection have been described where the etiology of infection could not be accurately specified [1, 5, 8]. Furthermore, this infection more commonly occurs in rural areas than urban areas [8].

We intend to report an unusual case of periapical actinomycosis which presented to our oral and maxillofacial surgery clinic with a chief complaint of pain in the posterior mandible region and further review the available literature.

2. Case Presentation

A 34-year-old female patient presented to our oral and maxillofacial surgery private practice office with the chief complaint of pain and slight mobility of the mandibular right second premolar and first molar. There were no significant issues in the patient's medical history upon presentation. The patient signed a written consent stating her approval for participation in this report and the publication of her clinical findings, photographs, radiographs, histopathologic findings, and results to be reported in this article.

Clinical examination revealed pain on percussion on the mandibular second premolar and first molar. Slight mobility of these two teeth was also evident on palpation. Overlying skin and mucosa of the region was normal and devoid of any ulcerations, erythema, suppurations, and rise in temperature. Intraoral examination did not reveal any breach in the mucosa and the integrity of it remained intact. On palpation of the oral mucosa, the consistency was bony hard on both lingual and buccal cortices.

An initial orthopantomography (OPG) was obtained which revealed a uniloculated, radiolucent lesion engulfing the apices of the mandibular right second premolar and an endodontically treated first molar, extending to the superior border of the inferior alveolar nerve canal with an irregular shape dissimilar to what is routinely observed in periapical cysts or granulomas associated with endodontically treated teeth (Figure 1). The patient claimed that the mandibular right first molar was endodontically treated almost 5 years prior to presentation. Subsequently, a cone beam computed tomography (CBCT) was ordered which further revealed the extensions of the lesion in the buccolingual aspect, almost completely obliterating the lingual cortex. The lesion measured $23.4 \times 14.2 \times 6.6$ mm at its peaks (Figure 2). Preliminary differential diagnosis based on the radiographic evaluation included odontogenic keratocyst (OKC), radicular cyst, and unicystic ameloblastoma.

Following these observations and suspicion towards something more malignant, an incisional biopsy was obtained. The incised specimen consisted of multiple fragmented and irregular pieces of soft, creamy-colored tissue. Microscopic evaluations revealed fragments of fibroconnective tissue including few crushed bone particles severely infiltrated by acute inflammatory cells and some foamy macrophages (Figure 3). The suppurative exudate focally surrounds colonies of filamentous bacteria as round basophilic masses with radial configuration resembling "sulfur granules" (Figure 4). Following the consistency between the microscopic findings of our case and of actinomycosis, the definitive diagnosis of periapical actinomycosis was made.

Upon the diagnosis, the patient was referred to an infectious diseases specialist and an endodontist for further consultations. Antibiotics were not prescribed by the infectious diseases specialist due to the limited and contained nature of the lesion. However, the endodontist endodontically retreated the tooth and the patient was referred back to us for the subsequent periapical surgery (Figure 5). After obtaining a written informed consent form from the patient, the surgery was performed under local anesthesia. Surgical procedure incorporated inferior alveolar nerve block accompanied with mental nerve block, followed by a full-thickness periosteal flap elevation with great vigilance in exposing and preserving the mental nerve and subsequent curettage accompanied with peripheral ostectomy and cautious burnishing of the two involved teeth roots. Subsequently, the flap was reapproximated and sutured in place. Furthermore, one-year follow-up of the patient did not show any evidence of recurrence.

3. Discussion and Conclusion

Actinomycosis is a rare, chronic, acute or subacute, invasive bacterial infection with an annual incidence rate of approximately 0.00003% [12, 13]. Bacteria of the genus *Actinomyces* belong to the Actinobacteria phylum and Actinomycetales order and are related to other genera such as *Corynebacterium*, *Mycobacterium*, *Nocardia*, and *Propionibacterium*. More than 30 species of *Actinomyces* have been identified. *Actinomyces israelii* is the most prevalent species isolated in human infections and is found in most clinical forms of actinomycosis infections [1, 13–18]. *A. israelii* and *A. gerencseriae* are responsible for almost 70% of actinomycotic orocervicofacial infections [17]. It should be noted that most of the *Actinomyces* spp. are present in polymicrobial flora. Hence, *Actinomyces* are often isolated with other normal commensals, such as *Aggregatibacter actinomycetemcomitans*, *Capnocytophaga*, *Eikenella corrodens*, fusobacteria, *Bacteroides*, streptococci, staphylococci, or Enterobacteriaceae, depending on the site of infection [16].

Cervicofacial actinomycosis is the most frequently observed clinical form of actinomycosis infections. Furthermore, "lumpy jaw syndrome" which is associated with odontogenic infections is its most common clinical manifestation which constitutes approximately 60% of all reported cases of actinomycosis and shows a male predominance of 1.5-3.1 times [1, 10, 15, 19]. *A. israelii* and *A. gerencseriae* are observed in almost 70% of cervicofacial actinomycosis cases; however, other species have also been described in such infections, including *A. meyeri*, *A. odontolyticus*, *A.*

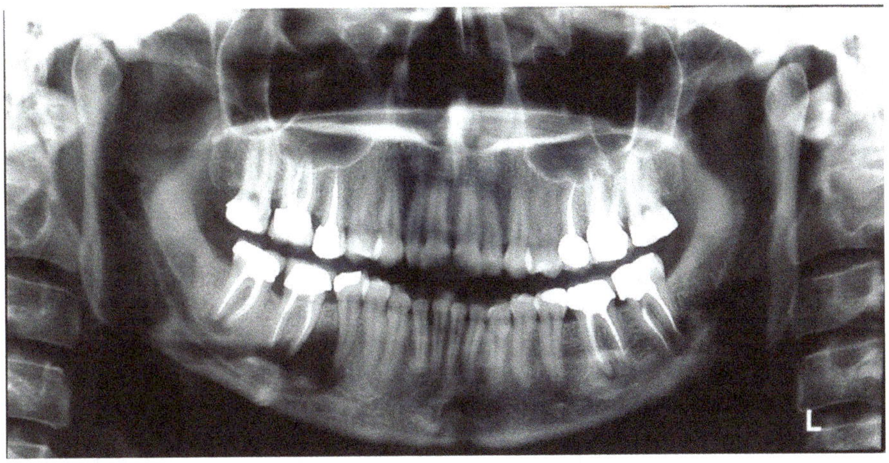

FIGURE 1: Initial OPG of the patient depicting a unilocular radiolucency encompassing the apices of the mandibular second premolar and first molar.

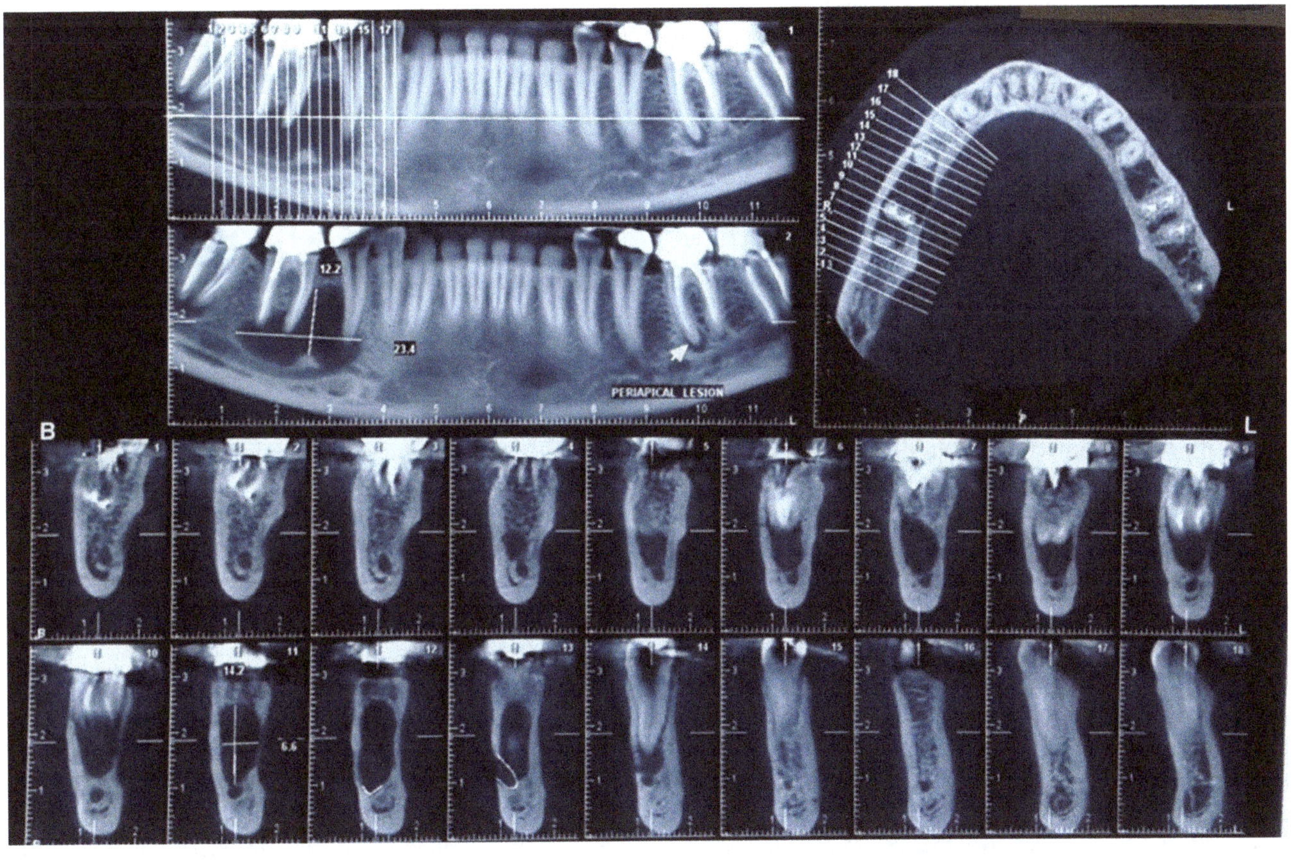

FIGURE 2: Initial CBCT obtained from the patient further revealing the extents of the lesion.

naeslundii, *Actinomyces georgiae*, *Actinomyces pyogenes*, or *A. viscosus* [17]. *Actinomyces* are also commensals of the human oropharynx, and their prevalence is particularly noted within dental plaques, gingival crevices, tonsillar crypts, and periodontal pockets and on carious teeth [1, 14, 15]. Therefore, dental procedures such as dental extractions and root canal therapy and underlying oral conditions which predispose the oral health to vulnerability such as caries, periodontal diseases, and poor oral hygiene seem to play a crucial role in its occurrence [10, 20]. Cervicofacial actinomycosis could be associated with large abscesses and/or osteomyelitis with or without sinus tract. Furthermore, cervicofacial actinomycosis can lead to invasion of the adjacent vital structures such as skull base as well as distant organ dissemination, such as the brain, lungs, and gastrointestinal tract [21, 22].

Cervicofacial actinomycosis can be further divided into central and peripheral subtypes, of which the central subtype is considerably uncommon with the incidence of just 1–2%. Periapical actinomycosis is categorized under central

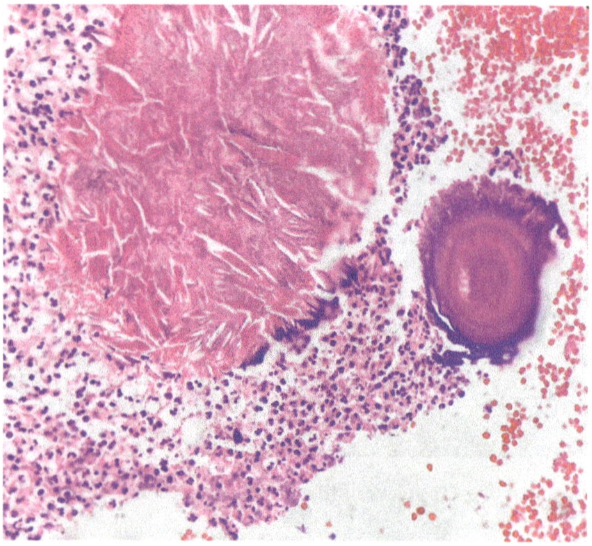

Figure 3: Microscopic findings of fibroconnective tissue containing few crushed bone particles severely infiltrated by acute inflammatory cells and some foamy macrophages (H&E staining, magnification level 10×40).

subtype which itself is very rare among central varieties [13, 23, 24]. Periapical actinomycosis, which is reckoned as a central subgroup of cervicofacial actinomycosis, is an uncommon, more indolent, less invasive, and limited type of infection that has been reported in less than just 5% of periapical lesions [25–28]. However, it can be considerably underreported due to the low number of periapical surgical specimens that are submitted for histopathological analysis after excision of the lesion with the preliminary diagnosis of typical periapical infections [20]. Most cases of periapical actinomycosis have been reported individually, and data regarding the prevalence of periapical actinomycosis among periapical lesions is limited to only a few studies [25, 27, 28]. However, there is dearth of literature supporting the mode of entry of actinomycosis into the periapical region. Nevertheless, it is believed that during root canal treatment, the organisms are displaced from the oral cavity into the periapical regions as a result of failure to establish aseptic techniques. Since the majority of actinomycosis cases described in the literature have been reported in endodontically treated teeth, it can further cement the aforementioned hypothesis [24, 25, 29]. Penetration of the bacteria through the impaired periodontium has also been hypothesized to play an important role in periapical actinomycosis [30].

Radiologically, periapical actinomycosis usually presents as well-defined radiolucent lesion located in the apical region of an endodontically treated maxillary or mandibular teeth which does not entail a pivotal diagnostic value as it can be misinterpreted with a variety of odontogenic lesions, most specifically a periapical granuloma or abscess [25]. As seen in our case, it presented as a uniloculated, radiolucent lesion encompassing apices of the right mandibular first molar and second premolar.

Histopathologically, microscopic findings for actinomycosis indicate two zones: an outer zone of granulation and a central zone with multiple granules representing colonies of Actinomyces. Histopathological analysis discloses one to three sulfur granules in about 75% of cases, described as basophilic masses with eosinophilic terminal clubs on staining with hematoxylin and eosin. Classic microscopic findings include necrosis with yellowish sulfur granules and filamentous Gram-positive fungal-like pathogens. Yellow sulfur granules are established by aggregation of bacteria trapped in biofilm [31–33]. However, sulfur granules are not pathognomonic, as they are only present in 35–55% of actinomycosis cases and are also seen with *Nocardia*, *Streptomyces*, and *Peptostreptococcus* [3, 9, 23]. Tissue culture is the most precise method of diagnosis of actinomycosis. However, it is limited in practice since *Actinomyces* species have difficulty growing due to their anaerobic nature [9]. More recently, molecular and genetic techniques involving immunofluorescence, fluorescent in situ hybridization, and 16S rRNA analysis with polymerase chain reaction (PCR) have been utilized to aid diagnosis of actinomycosis [15, 34–37].

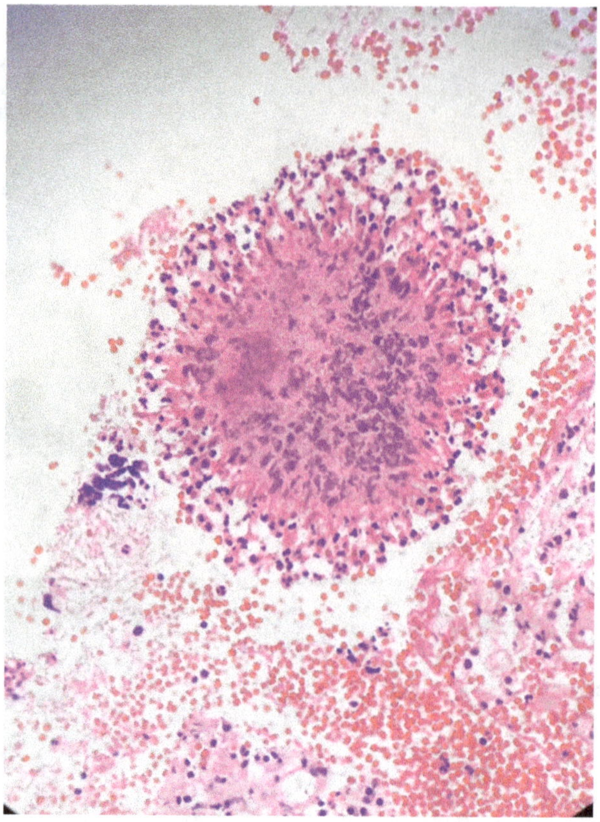

Figure 4: The suppurative exudate focally surrounding colonies of filamentous bacteria as round basophilic masses with radial configuration resembling "sulfur granules" (H&E staining, magnification level 10×40).

Treatment of cervicofacial actinomycosis primarily consists of surgery of incision and drainage in conjunction with long-term antibiotic therapy. *Actinomyces* spp. are usually extremely susceptible to beta-lactams, especially penicillin G or amoxicillin. As a result, penicillin G or amoxicillin is considered a drug of choice for the treatment of

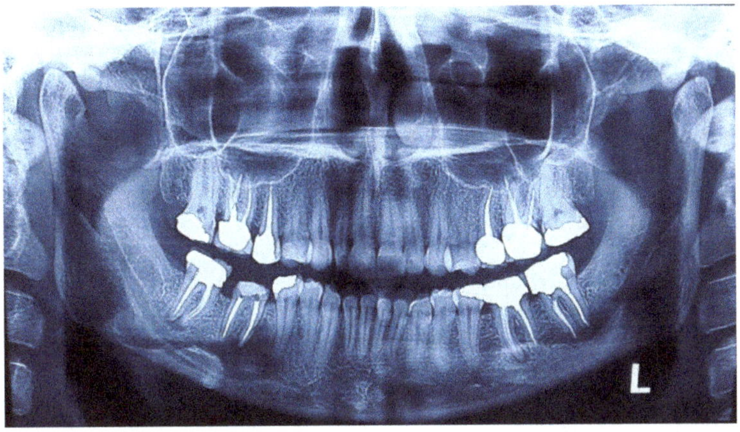

FIGURE 5: Mandibular second molar was endodontically retreated and referred back to us for further evaluation.

actinomycosis. It should be noted that inadequate short-term antibiotic therapy can result in the relapse of infection. Furthermore, drug resistance is not an issue in treatment of actinomycosis [2, 14, 15, 38]. Treatment of periapical actinomycosis however differs from the treatment of other cervicofacial actinomycosis infections. Endodontic treatment or retreatment is usually recommended for elimination of the intrapulpal source of infection, with or without periradicular surgery when an extraradicular infection is believed to have established a periapical lesion. Furthermore, dental extraction can also be of value in elimination of the local infection. Therefore, antibiotic therapy may be of limited value, with regard to evidences that it cannot sufficiently reach the infected necrotic periapical regions at adequate concentrations [13, 39]. For this same reason, the infectious diseases specialist we consulted did not prescribe any antibiotic regimen for our patient and insisted on avoiding overusing antibiotics. In a recent study, Butera et al. evaluated the efficacy of probiotics/paraprobiotics in periodontal diseases. In their study, it was demonstrated that hyaluronic acid and lactoferrin appear as reliable approaches for the management of periodontal disease. Furthermore, paraprobiotics are likely to demonstrate the most important benefit due to their immunomodulating mechanism of action [40]. The results of this study can be considered for future evaluation on the role of probiotics/paraprobiotics for actinomycosis infections as well as different oral infections mainly due to their immunomodulation effects.

Periapical actinomycosis is a very rare subtype of cervicofacial actinomycosis that presents with nonspecific clinical and radiological manifestations. Though not totally accurate, conventional biopsies and hematoxylin and eosin (H&E) staining in addition to histochemical stains and in conjunction with clinical signs and symptoms can be beneficial in reaching a definitive diagnosis. The current evidence is not adequate to determine a definitive treatment for periapical actinomycosis; however, surgical resection of the lesion seems to be the treatment of choice as antibiotic treatment seems to be unnecessary in such cases.

Our case report further emphasizes the importance of aseptic techniques during endodontic and more invasive treatments, as they can cause penetration of Actinomyces into the periapical region which in some cases can lead to more serious complications and even life-threatening situations.

Abbreviations

A. odontolyticus:	Actinomyces odontolyticus
A. naeslundii:	Actinomyces naeslundii
A. viscosus:	Actinomyces viscosus
A. propionica:	Actinomyces propionica
A. gerencseriae:	Actinomyces gerencseriae
A. meyeri:	Actinomyces meyeri
OPG:	Orthopantomography
CBCT:	Cone beam computed tomography
OKC:	Odontogenic keratocyst
spp.:	Species
rRNA:	Ribosomal RNA
PCR:	Polymerase chain reaction
H&E:	Hematoxylin and eosin.

Consent

A written consent form was obtained from the patient. The patient consents to her clinical findings, photographs, radiographs, histopathologic findings, and results to be reported in this article. The patient understands that her name or initials will not be mentioned anywhere in this report and due efforts will be made to completely conceal her identity. The patient signed a written consent stating her approval for participation in this report.

Authors' Contributions

MS conducted the surgery. RD was responsible for data collection and writing of the manuscript. RD and MS were responsible for editing and revising the manuscript. All authors discussed the results and contributed to the final manuscript.

References

[1] T. A. Russo, "Agents of actinomycosis," in *Mandell, Douglas, and Bennett's Principles and Practiceof Infectious Diseases*, J. E. Bennett and R. Dolin, Eds., pp. 2864–2873, Saunders, Philadelphia, 8th edition, 2015.

[2] J. R. Hupp, M. R. Tucker, and E. Ellis III, *Contemporary Oral and Maxillofacial Surgery*, Mosby, St. Louis, MO, 7th edition, 2018.

[3] I. Brook, "Actinomycosis," in *Goldman's Cecil Medicine*, L. Goldman and A. I. Schafer, Eds., Saunders Elsevier, PA, USA, 24th edition, 2011.

[4] L. Goldman and A. I. Schafer, *Goldman's Cecil Medicine*, Grune & Stratton, London, England, 24th edition, 2011.

[5] K. Zhao, W. Li, C. Kang et al., "Phylogenomics and evolutionary dynamics of the family Actinomycetaceae," *Genome Biology and Evolution*, vol. 6, no. 10, pp. 2625–2633, 2014.

[6] E. Könönen and W. G. Wade, "Actinomyces and related organisms in human infections," *Clinical Microbiology Reviews*, vol. 28, no. 2, pp. 419–442, 2015.

[7] R. Nagler, M. Peled, and D. Laufer, "Cervicofacial actinomycosis: a diagnostic challenge," *Oral Surgery, Oral Medicine, Oral Pathology, Oral Radiology, and Endodontics*, vol. 83, no. 6, pp. 652–656, 1997.

[8] B. Vidaković, D. Macan, B. Perić, and M. Spomenka, "Actinomycosis of the cheek," *Srpski Arhiv za Celokupno Lekarstvo*, vol. 142, no. 7-8, pp. 472–475, 2014.

[9] M. Volante, A. M. Contucci, M. Fantoni, R. Ricci, and J. Galli, "Cervicofacial actinomycosis: still a difficult differential diagnosis," *Acta Otorhinolaryngologica Italica*, vol. 25, no. 2, pp. 116–119, 2005.

[10] A. A. Sharkawy, "Cervicofacial actinomycosis and mandibular osteomyelitis," *Infectious Disease Clinics of North America*, vol. 21, no. 2, pp. 543–556, 2007.

[11] Y. J. Jeong, H. W. Suh, and H.-S. Shim, "Cervicofacial primary cutaneous actinomycosis: surgical treatment for complete remission of the disease," *The Journal of Craniofacial Surgery*, vol. 28, no. 3, pp. e269–e271, 2017.

[12] M. Gajdács, E. Urbán, and G. Terhes, "Microbiological and clinical aspects of cervicofacial Actinomyces infections: an overview," *Dental Journal*, vol. 7, no. 3, p. 85, 2019.

[13] D. Ricucci and J. F. Siqueira Jr., "Apical actinomycosis as a continuum of intraradicular and extraradicular infection: case report and critical review on its involvement with treatment failure," *Journal of Endodontia*, vol. 34, no. 9, pp. 1124–1129, 2008.

[14] R. A. Smego Jr. and G. Foglia, "Actinomycosis," *Clinical Infectious Diseases*, vol. 26, no. 6, pp. 1255–1261, 1998.

[15] V. K. Wong, T. D. Turmezei, and V. C. Weston, "Actinomycosis," *BMJ*, vol. 343, no. oct11 3, p. d6099, 2011.

[16] K. P. Schaal and H. J. Lee, "Actinomycete infections in humans - a review," *Gene*, vol. 115, no. 1-2, pp. 201–211, 1992.

[17] G. Pulverer, H. Schütt-Gerowitt, and K. P. Schaal, "Human cervicofacial actinomycoses: microbiological data for 1997 cases," *Clinical Infectious Diseases*, vol. 37, no. 4, pp. 490–497, 2003.

[18] R. H. Eng, M. L. Corrado, D. Cleri, C. Cherubin, and E. J. Goldstein, "Infections caused by Actinomyces viscosus," *American Journal of Clinical Pathology*, vol. 75, no. 1, pp. 113–116, 1981.

[19] O. Oostman and R. A. Smego, "Cervicofacial actinomycosis: diagnosis and management," *Current Infectious Disease Reports*, vol. 7, no. 3, pp. 170–174, 2005.

[20] I. Kaplan, K. Anavi, Y. Anavi et al., "The clinical spectrum of _Actinomyces_ -associated lesions of the oral mucosa and jawbones: correlations with histomorphometric analysis," *Oral Surgery, Oral Medicine, Oral Pathology, Oral Radiology, and Endodontics*, vol. 108, no. 5, pp. 738–746, 2009.

[21] A. McCann, S. A. Alvi, J. Newman et al., "Atypical form of cervicofacial actinomycosis involving the skull base and temporal bone," *The Annals of Otology, Rhinology, and Laryngology*, vol. 128, no. 2, pp. 152–156, 2019.

[22] F. Valour, A. Sénéchal, C. Dupieux et al., "Actinomycosis: etiology, clinical features, diagnosis, treatment, and management," *Infection and Drug Resistance*, vol. 7, pp. 183–197, 2014.

[23] A. Lancella, G. Abbate, A. M. Foscolo, and R. Dosdegani, "Two unusual presentations of cervicofacial actinomycosis and review of the literature," *Acta Otorhinolaryngologica Italica*, vol. 28, no. 2, pp. 89–93, 2008.

[24] B. G. Jeansonne, "Periapical actinomycosis: a review," *Quintessence International*, vol. 36, no. 2, pp. 149–153, 2005.

[25] A. Hirshberg, I. Tsesis, Z. Metzger, and I. Kaplan, "Periapical actinomycosis: a clinicopathologic study," *Oral Surgery, Oral Medicine, Oral Pathology, Oral Radiology, and Endodontics*, vol. 95, no. 5, pp. 614–620, 2003.

[26] P. L. Sakellariou, "Periapical actinomycosis: report of a case and review of the literature," *Dental Traumatology*, vol. 12, no. 3, pp. 151–154, 1996.

[27] P. N. Ramachandran Nair and H. E. Schroeder, "Actinomicosis periapical," *Journal of Endodontia*, vol. 10, no. 12, pp. 567–570, 1984.

[28] A. Bystrom, R.-P. Happonen, U. Sjogren, and G. Sundqvist, "Healing of periapical lesions of pulpless teeth after endodontic treatment with controlled asepsis," *Dental Traumatology*, vol. 3, no. 2, pp. 58–63, 1987.

[29] S. Oppenheimer, G. S. Miller, K. Knopf, and H. Blechman, "Periapical actinomycosis: an unusual case report," *Oral Surgery, Oral Medicine, and Oral Pathology*, vol. 46, no. 1, pp. 101–106, 1978.

[30] S. P. Pasupathy, D. Chakravarthy, S. Chanmougananda, and P. P. Nair, "Periapical actinomycosis," *BML Case Reports*, vol. 2012, no. jul31 1, pp. bcr2012006218–bcr 2012006218, 2012.

[31] D. F. Bennhoff, "Actinomycosis: diagnostic and therapeutic considerations and a review of 32 cases," *The Laryngoscope*, vol. 94, no. 9, pp. 1198–1217, 1984.

[32] J. E. Heffner, "Pleuropulmonary manifestations of actinomycosis and nocardiosis," *Seminars in Respiratory Infections*, vol. 3, no. 4, pp. 352–361, 1988.

[33] J. R. Brown, "Human actinomycosis: a study of 181 subjects," *Human Pathology*, vol. 4, no. 3, pp. 319–330, 1973.

[34] W. C. Weese and I. M. Smith, "A study of 57 cases of actinomycosis over a 36-year period. A diagnostic "failure" with good prognosis after treatment," *Archives of Internal Medicine*, vol. 135, no. 12, pp. 1562–1568, 1975.

[35] M. Hotchi and J. Schwarz, "Characterization of actinomycotic granules by architecture and staining methods," *Archives of Pathology*, vol. 93, no. 5, pp. 392–400, 1972.

[36] K. Kuyama, K. Fukui, E. Ochiai et al., "Identification of the actinomycete 16S ribosomal RNA gene by polymerase chain reaction in oral inflammatory lesions," *Oral Surgery, Oral Medicine, Oral Pathology, Oral Radiology*, vol. 116, no. 4, pp. 485-491, 2013.

[37] L. Pine, G. B. Malcolm, E. M. Curtis, and J. M. Brown, "Demonstration of Actinomyces and Arachnia species in cervicovaginal smears by direct staining with species-specific fluorescent-antibody conjugate," *Journal of Clinical Microbiology*, vol. 13, no. 1, pp. 15–21, 1981.

[38] A. J. Smith, V. Hall, B. Thakker, and C. G. Gemmell, "Antimicrobial susceptibility testing of Actinomyces species with 12 antimicrobial agents," *The Journal of Antimicrobial Chemotherapy*, vol. 56, no. 2, pp. 407–409, 2005.

[39] W. Gomes-Silva, D.-L. Pereira, E.-R. Fregnani, O.-P. Almeida, L. Armada, and F.-R. Pires, "Clinicopathological and ultrastructural characterization of periapical actinomycosis," *Medicina Oral, Patología Oral y Cirugía Bucal*, vol. 25, no. 1, pp. e131–e136, 2020.

[40] A. Butera, S. Gallo, C. Maiorani et al., "Management of gingival bleeding in periodontal patients with domiciliary use of toothpastes containing hyaluronic acid, lactoferrin, or paraprobiotics: a randomized controlled clinical trial," *Applied Sciences*, vol. 11, no. 18, p. 8586, 2021.

8

Mammary Analogue Secretory Carcinoma of the Palate: Case Report and Review of the Literature

Christian Boliere ,[1] James Murphy,[1,2] Mohammed Qaisi,[1,3] Frances Manosca,[4] and Henry Fung[1]

[1]*Division of Oral & Maxillofacial Surgery, John H. Stroger Hospital of Cook County, Chicago, IL, USA*
[2]*Division of Plastic and Reconstructive Surgery, Rush University Medical Center, Chicago, IL, USA*
[3]*Division of Otolaryngology, John H. Stroger Hospital of Cook County, Chicago, IL, USA*
[4]*Department of Pathology, John H. Stroger Hospital of Cook County, Chicago, IL, USA*

Correspondence should be addressed to Christian Boliere; cboliere26@gmail.com

Academic Editor: Andresa Borges Soares

Mammary analogue secretory carcinoma (MASC) is a recently described salivary gland tumor, with a limited number of published reports. Less than three hundred cases have been reported in the literature and only 18 of these cases have been reported in minor palatal salivary glands, though publication bias is likely a factor. We present a case of a 57-year-old male who was diagnosed with MASC tumor presenting in a minor salivary gland and briefly review the current literature. MASC has a variety of histological features and different range of clinical behaviors. The histopathological diagnosis of MASC can be difficult, and the immunohistochemical profile of MASC is still being updated. The gold standard for MASC diagnosis is cytogenetics, with the majority having a translocation t(12;15)(p133;q25). Presently, there is no conclusive evidence that MASC should be treated differently than any other low-grade malignant salivary gland tumors, though high-grade transformation has been described.

1. Introduction

Mammary analogue secretory carcinoma (MASC) is a rare salivary gland neoplasm that was first reported in 2010 by Skalova et al. [1]. In the original report, 16 cases of salivary gland tumors were reexamined and were found to have similar histological and molecular features as breast secretory carcinoma. Breast secretory carcinoma is a slow-growing, low-grade ductal carcinoma which is a subtype of infiltrating ductal carcinoma of the breast. It occurs primarily in adolescent women [2]. Both MASC and breast secretory carcinoma are associated with translocation t(12;15)(p13;q25), which is a fusion of the ETV6 gene on chromosome 12 and the NTRK3 gene on chromosome 15. The fusion gene encodes a chimeric tyrosine kinase, which has potential transformation activity and plays a role in carcinogenesis [3]. This fusion has also been shown in other tumors including infantile fibrosarcoma, acute myeloid leukemia, and congenital mesoblastic nephroma [4]. Fluorescence in situ hybridization for the ETV6 rearrangement, with close to 99% of MASC tumors showing this mutation, is the gold standard to arrive at a definitive diagnosis of MASC [5]. The financial burden of this cytogenetic test can be prohibitive for some institutions, and there have been reports of cases not demonstrating *ETV6-NTRK3* fusion gene but were diagnosed as MASC based on the results of immunohistochemistry [6].

According to Khurram et al., immunohistochemistry can accurately diagnose MASC tumors [7]. Refinement of the immunohistochemical panel for the diagnosis of MASC could potentially completely reduce the cytogenic need in diagnosing MASC tumor [8]. To complicate matters, Mariano et al. recently reported that some cases of MASC, whose profile was NTRK3 split-negative and ETV6 split-positive, unknown (non-NTRK) genes appeared to fuse with ETV6 (ETV6-X fusion) [9].

A significant proportion of MASC tumors reported in the literature was cases that were reclassified when they were secondarily reviewed. MASC tumors have a wider morphological and immunohistochemical spectrum than previously recognized. Diagnosis and differentiation of MASC from other salivary gland tumor are aided by histological features and immunohistochemistry. MASC rarely shows perineural invasion or lymphovascular invasion, and necrosis is not typical [8]. MASC shows immunoreactivity for S100 and mammaglobin (70% of the time [9]) which are rarely positive in acinic cell carcinoma. DOG-1 is predominantly negative in MASC but usually positive in acinic cell carcinoma. Mammary analogue secretory carcinoma of the salivary glands is a lipid-rich tumor, and adipophilin can be valuable in its identification [10]. There is a multitude of markers which is beyond the scope of this paper.

Seventy percent of MASC tumors are found in the major salivary glands, predominantly the parotid. Less than a quarter of the cases arise from minor salivary glands within the oral cavity [3]. We present a case of a MASC tumor presenting in the hard palate. To our knowledge, this is one of the few case reports of palatal MASC, which was diagnosed by immunohistochemistry from an incisional biopsy from the hard palate, and prospectively definitively treated as a MASC tumor. Twelve cases of MASC on the hard palate and six on the soft palate have been reported in the literature worldwide to date [11]. The clinical course, presentation, and immunohistological findings are discussed.

2. Case Presentation

A 57-year-old male presented to the oral and maxillofacial surgery clinic at our institution with more than a 20-year history of a painless mass in the hard palate region. He elected to have the lesion evaluated due to its increase in size, although indolent. He reported no other symptoms.

His past medical history was significant for hypertension and hyperlipidemia. He denies any past surgical history, he was not taking any medications, and he has no known drug allergies. He presently denies any social history but admits to tobacco use for 15 years and stopped almost 20 years ago.

On examination, it was noted that the patient had a firm, erythematous, raised lesion with a central area of ulceration located at the junction of the hard and soft palate on the right side. The lesion was roughly 2.0 cm × 1.0 cm in size (Figure 1). There was no palpable lymphadenopathy on head and neck examination.

Computed tomography (CT) and magnetic resonance imaging (MRI) showed a mass involving the right palate measuring 39 mm in the greatest dimension. The CT showed a focal area of bone thinning and focal dehiscence at the floor of the right maxillary sinus without evidence for frank tumor extension into the sinus (Figures 2(a) and 2(b)).

An incisional biopsy was performed and sent for pathology. On hematoxylin and eosin stain, the tumor comprised of cells forming microcystic and glandular spaces containing eosinophilic homogenous material. The secretory material from the glandular spaces was noted to be periodic acid Schiff- (PAS-) positive and diastase-resistant (Figure 3).

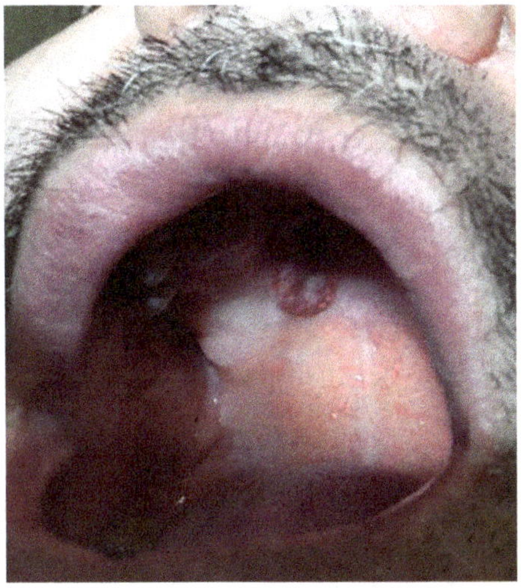

Figure 1: Preoperative image of MASC tumor right palate.

The tumor cells had eosinophilic granular cytoplasm with low-grade vesicular nuclei and visible nucleoli (Figures 4 and 5). There were rare mitotic figures, and scattered inflammatory cells were present. A broad front pattern of invasion was noted. Immunohistochemical stains showed positivity for cytokeratin 7, SMA, p53, and CK5/6. The tumor was also diffusely positive for both mammaglobin and S100, supportive for the diagnosis of MASC [7] (Figures 6 and 7). DOG-1 staining was negative. Cytogenic testing was not performed in this case.

Treatment consisted of wide local excision of the lesion with 1 cm margins and a right selective neck dissection levels 1-3. Hemostasis of the greater palatine neurovascular bundle was achieved with bipolar electrocautery and bone wax. The surgical site was allowed to heal by secondary intention with granulation tissue (Figure 8).

A total of 42 lymph nodes were harvested and all lymph nodes were negative. No lymphovascular and no perineural invasion was noted. All margins were negative with the closest margins at 0.5 mm. The final pathologic diagnosis was MASC with the tumor size measuring $1 \times 0.7 \times 0.6$ cm. Given the negative margins and the lack of consensus regarding the utility of adjuvant therapy in this disease entity, no further treatment was administered.

Patient's postoperative course was uneventful, although a biopsy was done 6 months later which showed no evidence of disease. At his most recent follow-up, 36 months after surgery, the patient was free of tumor (Figure 9). The patient had no neurologic deficit. He had no range of motion issues with his shoulder, however complained of slight numbness over his right shoulder. He denied any change in speech or swallowing issues. The nasal mucosa was preserved; levator muscles and palatal muscles were preserved. The hard palate site healed well by secondary intention.

3. Discussion

MASC involves the parotid gland in approximately 70% of cases. Less than 25% of MASC tumors have been reported

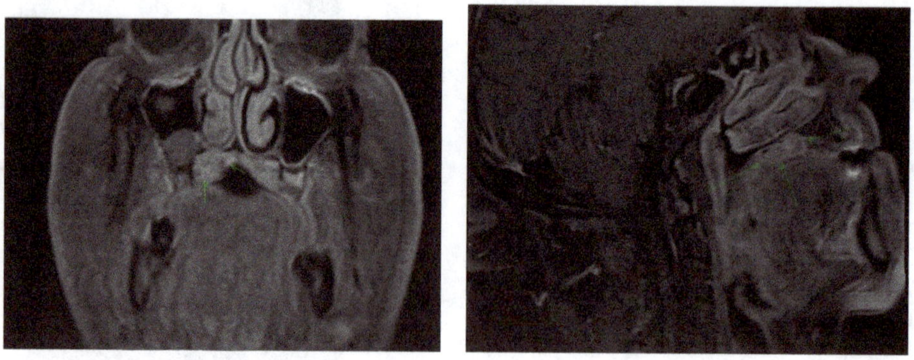

(a) (b)

FIGURE 2: (a) MRI coronal T1image with MASC tumor. (b) MRI sagittal T1 image with MASC tumor.

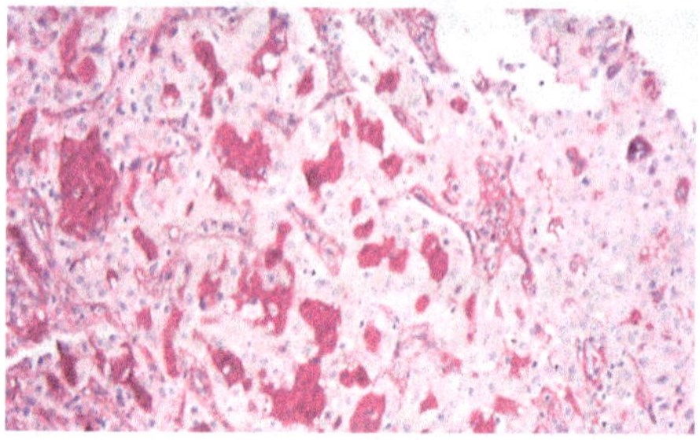

FIGURE 3: MASC tumor with PAS stain and diastase (magnification ×200).

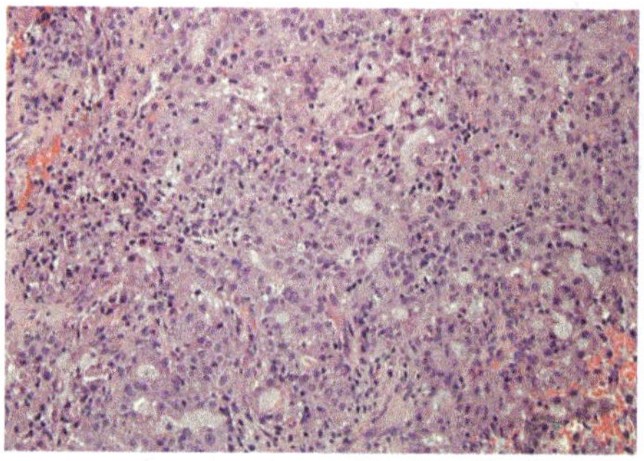

FIGURE 4: MASC tumor comprised of cells forming microcystic and glandular spaces containing eosinophilic homogenous material (H&E, magnification ×200).

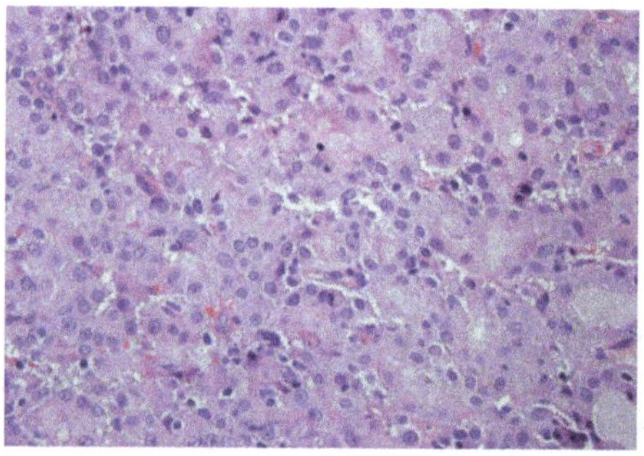

FIGURE 5: MASC tumor cells with eosinophilic granular cytoplasm and low-grade vesicular nuclei (H&E, magnification ×400).

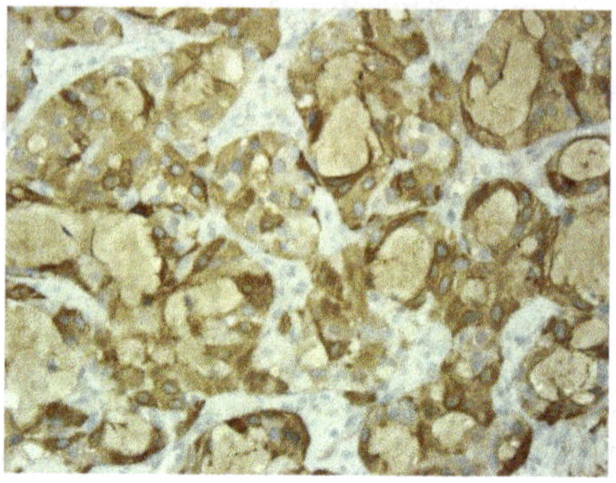

FIGURE 6: Mammaglobin highlights the neoplastic cells and secretions (magnification ×400).

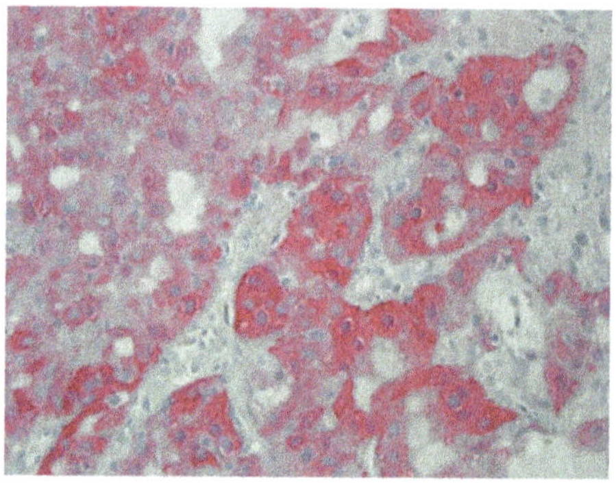

FIGURE 7: S100 protein staining is present in the tumor cells (magnification ×400).

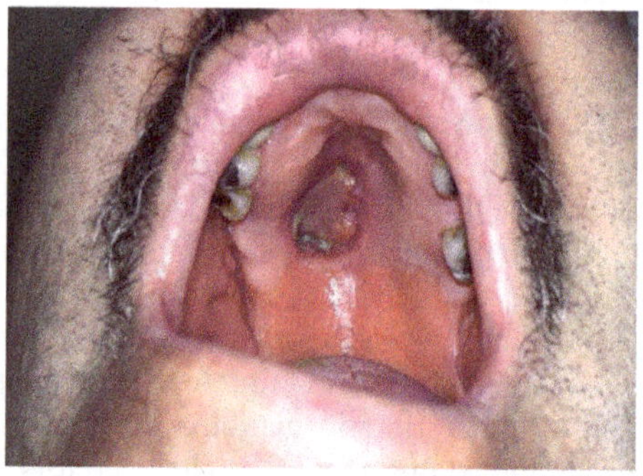

FIGURE 8: Postoperative image of surgical site healing by secondary intention.

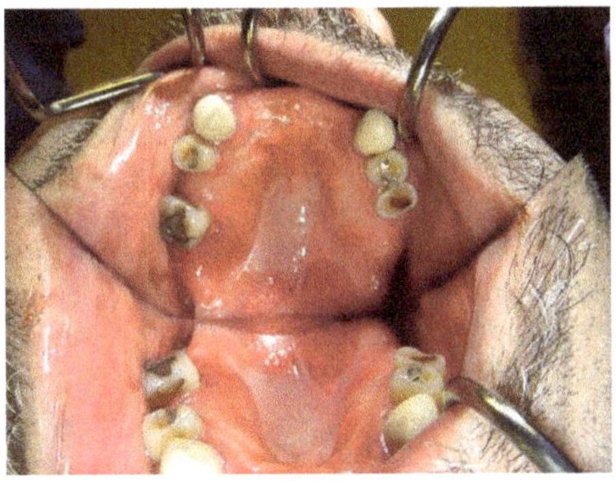

FIGURE 9: Surgical site at 36 months. No evidence of recurrence.

in minor salivary glands, at sites including the palate, buccal mucosa, base of the tongue, and lips [12]. There has also been a case report on a lymph node with MASC of unknown primary origin [10].

The average age of patients presenting with MASC is in the fourth or fifth decade. The tumor is very rare in children and adolescents, but few cases have been reported [13]. MASC has been reported to have a slight male predilection [9], but no racial predisposition has been documented. The disease typically follows an indolent course. The most common presentation is a slowly enlarging and painless nodule, often detected incidentally on physical examination [12]. Our case presented with a similar description. There has been a report of one patient with facial paralysis from a bulky parotid gland MASC tumor.

The exact incidence of MASC is unknown. It is reported that MASC accounts for <0.3% of all salivary gland tumors [14]. Luk et al. and Majewska et al. reported that MASC makes up 4 and 4.5%, respectively, of malignant salivary gland disease processes [15]. The percentage of MASC tumors involving the minor salivary glands is unknown. In the most recent update, there has been a total of 279 MASC cases reported in the literature, and 68 (24%) cases of MASC reported in minor salivary glands [11].

In the current case, polymorphous low-grade adenocarcinoma (PLGA) was ruled out based on histopathological features including a well-defined broad front invasive pattern seen in this case as opposed to an infiltrative cord-like one typical in PLGA [16]. The presence of microcystic areas with abundant vacuolated colloid-like PAS-positive secretory material within the microcystic spaces, low-grade vesicular nuclei with a distinctive centrally located small nucleolus, the lack of perineural invasion, and the diffuse pattern of staining seen with S100 protein and mammaglobin were further features which support the diagnosis of MASC. Further histopathological evidence supporting the diagnosis of MASC was the fact that the luminal secretions were PAS-positive and diastase-resistant, and cytoplasmic granules were not present. Bishop et al. reported [17] that approximately 80% of extra parotid acinic cell carcinoma needed to be reclassified as MASC on the basis of an ETV6 translocation together with strong staining for S100 and mammaglobin. Pinto et al. reported in their study that 3 out of 6 MASC tumors were initially classified as acinic cell carcinoma [18]. In addition to acinic cell carcinoma, other cases of cystadenocarcinoma, mucoepidermoid carcinoma, or signet ring adenocarcinoma were reclassified as MASC [19]. Griffith et al. prospectively diagnosed a case of MASC based on cytogenetic study of a parotid mass fine needle aspiration (FNA), which was subsequently confirmed on final pathology [20]. The use of FNA in the diagnosis of MASC is still of questionable value [21]. Takeda et al. state that MASC cannot be diagnosed only from cytology alone [22]. Histopathological findings of MASC overlap with other salivary gland tumors, most commonly acinic cell carcinoma and adenocarcinoma not otherwise specified [12]. The histologic findings of MASC can include solid, microcystic, tubular, and papillary-cystic patterns in varying proportions. The case described in this report presented predominantly with microcystic features. MASC usually shows evidence of mucin production, a feature not seen in acinic cell carcinoma [23]. In MASC, the cells show vacuolated or foamy cytoplasm devoid of basophilic coarse zymogen granules, which may histologically resemble zymogen-poor acinic cell carcinoma. Many histologic findings seen in MASC and other salivary gland tumors overlap; therefore, the use of ancillary studies to aid in the distinction among the entities is important. New cytomorphology features were recently added to those of the original description though their clinical usefulness has not been studied extensively yet [9].

There is no data in the literature showing a difference in clinical behavior or rates of regional metastasis between minor and major salivary gland MASC. It is not uncommon for MASC to metastasize to regional lymph nodes. In one study, the rates of lymph node metastasis for MASC and acinic cell carcinoma were 17.6% (6/34) and 7.9% (3/38), respectively, with a mean disease-free survival, including death and recurrence, for MASC and acinic cell carcinoma being 92 and 121 months, respectively [24]. Although limited in numbers, other studies have explored treatment outcomes and prognosis of MASC and acinic cell carcinoma and concluded they can be treated similarly [25]. With regard to treatment, neck dissection is presently a surgeon preference based on clinical, radiological, and histological parameters. Sethi et al. reviewed 86 patients with MASC and reported 21 patients underwent neck dissections, 17 patients received postoperative radiotherapy (PORT), and 2 patients received PORT and chemotherapy (agents unspecified). No reported patients have received RT without prior surgical resection [12]. The rate of occult nodal metastasis for MASC is not well documented and we possibly need more reported cases, but one study reported that 4 out of 18 patients treated with neck dissections at the University of Pittsburg had nodal involvement [25].

MASC usually has an overall favorable prognosis; however, high-grade transformation has been described which results in a more aggressive tumor [14]. Stevens et al. noted high-grade transformation in 3/100 MASC cases reviewed [26]. Currently, MASC tumors with necrosis [24] tend to demonstrate a more aggressive nature and ultimately a poorer prognosis. Sethi et al. reported that of 91 cases of MASC documented at the time of writing, only 4 cases of death from the disease were reported, although survival data were variably reported, and follow-up was minimal.

4. Conclusion

We encountered a MASC tumor presenting in the region of the hard palate. The patient underwent complete excision of the lesion and a selective neck dissection without adjuvant therapy. No local recurrence or metastatic disease has been detected during a follow-up period of 36 months. This patient, with a prospectively diagnosed and treated MASC in the hard palate, is presented to add to the existing limited body of literature regarding this entity. The diagnosis in this case was based on the morphology with supporting S100 protein/mammaglobin immunoreactivity. Due to the histopathological findings, absence of unusual morphology, and the immunohistochemical profile, the financial burden associated with cytogenetic analysis to diagnose MASC was determined to be unnecessary. To the best of our knowledge, this is one of the few cases to report this method to prospectively diagnose a hard palate MASC tumor. This is an important finding for modern fiscally conservative medical systems to minimize escalating costs.

References

[1] A. Skálová, T. Vanecek, R. Sima et al., "Mammary analogue secretory carcinoma of salivary glands, containing the ETV6-NTRK3 fusion gene: a hitherto undescribed salivary gland tumor entity," *The American Journal of Surgical Pathology*, vol. 34, no. 5, pp. 1–608, 2010.

[2] F. Aktepe, D. Sarsenov, and V. Özmen, "Secretory carcinoma of the breast," *Journal of Breast Health*, vol. 12, no. 4, pp. 174–176, 2016.

[3] J. A. Bishop, "Unmasking MASC: bringing to light the unique morphologic, immunohistochemical and genetic features of the newly recognized mammary analogue secretory carcinoma of salivary glands," *Head and Neck Pathology*, vol. 7, no. 1, pp. 35–39, 2013.

[4] J. A. Bishop, R. Yonescu, D. A. S. Batista, W. H. Westra, and S. Z. Ali, "Cytopathologic features of mammary analogue secretory carcinoma," *Cancer Cytopathology*, vol. 121, no. 5, pp. 228–233, 2013.

[5] A. Skalova, "Mammary analogue secretory carcinoma of salivary gland origin: an update and expanded morphologic and immunohistochemical spectrum of recently described entity," *Head and Neck Pathology*, vol. 7, no. S1, pp. 30–36, 2013.

[6] M. L. Serrano-Arevalo, A. Mosqueda-Taylor, H. Dominguez-Malagon, and M. Michal, "Mammary analogue secretory carcinoma (MASC) of salivary gland in four Mexican patients," *Medicina Oral Patología Oral y Cirugia Bucal*, vol. 20, pp. e23–e29, 2015.

[7] S. A. Khurram, J. Sultan-Khan, N. Atkey, and P. M. Speight, "Cytogenetic and immunohistochemical characterization of mammary analogue secretory carcinoma of salivary glands," *Oral Surgery, Oral Medicine, Oral Pathology, Oral Radiology*, vol. 122, no. 6, pp. 731–742, 2016.

[8] A. Skalova, M. Michal, and R. H. W. Simpson, "Newly described salivary gland tumors," *Modern Pathology*, vol. 30, no. s1, pp. S27–S43, 2017.

[9] F. V. Mariano, H. dos Santos, W. D. Azañero et al., "Mammary analogue secretory carcinoma of salivary glands is a lipid-rich tumour, and adipophilin can be valuable in Its identification," *Histopathology*, vol. 63, no. 4, pp. 558–567, 2013.

[10] K. Suzuki, M. Yagi, A. Kanda et al., "Mammary analogue secretory carcinoma presenting as a cervical lymph node metastasis of unknown primary site: a case report," *Case Reports in Oncology*, vol. 10, no. 1, pp. 192–198, 2017.

[11] B. A. Khalele, "Systematic review of mammary analog secretory carcinoma of salivary glands at 7 years after description," *Head & Neck*, vol. 39, no. 6, pp. 1243–1248, 2017.

[12] R. Sethi, E. Kozin, A. Remenschneider et al., "Mammary analogue secretory carcinoma: update on a new diagnosis of salivary gland malignancy," *Laryngoscope*, vol. 124, no. 1, pp. 188–195, 2014.

[13] A. L. Ngouajio, S. M. Drejet, D. R. Phillips, D. J. Summerlin, and J. P. Dahl, "A systematic review including an additional pediatric case report: pediatric cases of mammary analogue secretory carcinoma," *International Journal of Pediatric Otorhinolaryngology*, vol. 100, pp. 187–193, 2017.

[14] I. M. Zardawi and P. Hook, "Mammary analogue secretory carcinoma of minor salivary glands," *Pathology*, vol. 46, no. 7, pp. 667–669, 2014.

[15] I. Damjanov, F. Skenderi, and S. Vranic, "Mammary analogue secretory carcinoma (MASC) of the salivary gland: a new tumor entity," *Bosnian Journal of Basic Medical Sciences*, vol. 16, no. 3, pp. 237-238, 2017.

[16] J. C. Prera, "Historical evolution of the polymorphous adenocarcinoma," *Head and Neck Pathology*, 2018.

[17] J. A. Bishop, R. Yonescu, D. Batista, D. W. Eisele, and W. H. Westra, "Most Nonparotid "Acinic Cell Carcinomas" Represent Mammary Analog Secretory Carcinomas," *The American Journal of Surgical Pathology*, vol. 37, no. 7, pp. 1053–1057, 2013.

[18] A. Pinto, V. Nosé, C. Rojas, Y.-S. Fan, and C. Gomez-Fernandez, "Searching for mammary analog secretory carcinoma of salivary gland among Its mimics," *Modern Pathology*, vol. 27, no. 1, pp. 30–37, 2014.

[19] M. J. Hwang, P. R. Wu, C.-M. Chen, C.-Y. Chen, and C.-J. Chen, "A rare malignancy of the parotid gland in a 13-year-old Taiwanese boy: case report of a mammary analogue secretory carcinoma of the salivary gland with molecular study," *Medical Molecular Morphology*, vol. 47, no. 1, pp. 57–61, 2014.

[20] C. C. Griffith, E. B. Stelow, A. Saqi et al., "The cytological features of mammary analogue secretory carcinoma: a series of 6 molecularly confirmed cases," *Cancer Cytopathology*, vol. 121, no. 5, pp. 234–241, 2013.

[21] H. Salat, R. Mumtaz, M. Ikram, and N. U. Din, "Mammary analogue secretory carcinoma of the parotid gland: a third world country perspective – a case series," *Case Reports in Otolaryngology*, vol. 2015, Article ID 697254, 4 pages, 2015.

[22] M. Takeda, T. Kasai, K. Morita et al., "Cytopathological features of mammary analogue secretory carcinoma–review of literature," *Diagnostic Cytopathology*, vol. 43, no. 2, pp. 131–137, 2015.

[23] T. D. Samulski, V. A. LiVolsi, and Z. Baloch, "The cytopathologic features of mammary analog secretory carcinoma and Its mimics," *CytoJournal*, vol. 11, no. 1, p. 24, 2014.

[24] S. I. Chiosea, C. Griffith, A. Assaad, and R. R. Seethala, "Clinicopathological characterization of mammary analogue secretory carcinoma of salivary glands," *Histopathology*, vol. 61, no. 3, pp. 387–394, 2012.

[25] T. M. Stevens and V. Parekh, "Mammary analogue secretory carcinoma," *Archives of Pathology & Laboratory Medicine*, vol. 140, no. 9, pp. 997–1001, 2016.

[26] T. M. Stevens, A. O. Kovalovsky, C. Velosa et al., "Mammary analog secretory carcinoma, low-grade salivary duct carcinoma, and mimickers: a comparative study," *Modern Pathology*, vol. 28, no. 8, pp. 1084–1100, 2015.

9

A Hybrid Oral Rehabilitation of Hypohidrotic Ectodermal Dysplasia: A Conservative Approach with Three-Year Follow-Up

Aryen Kaushik ,[1] HarshVardhan Sinha ,[2] M. N. Hombesh ,[3] Pooja Rani ,[4] and Taranjeet Kaur [3]

[1]*Department of Prosthodontics, ITS Dental College, Greater Noida, India*
[2]*Department of Prosthodontics, Saraswati Dental College, Lucknow, India*
[3]*Department of Prosthodontics, College of Dental Sciences, Davangere, India*
[4]*Department of Prosthodontics, Buddha Institute of Dental Sciences and Hospital, Patna, India*

Correspondence should be addressed to Aryen Kaushik; aryaenkaushik@gmail.com

Academic Editor: Konstantinos Michalakis

This case report presents a 19-year-old male patient with hypohidrotic ectodermal dysplasia, having a chief complaint of multiple missing teeth. Atraumatic extraction of the teeth with hopeless prognosis was done, and teeth with grade 2 mobility were submerged using cast dowel and coping. Following this, incremental increase in the vertical dimension was made using removable flexible splint of two-millimeter thickness. After facebow transfer and making appropriate eccentric bite records to program the semiadjustable articulator, wax-up was done at the desired vertical dimension (VD). The upper arch was finally restored using a long-span fixed partial denture and lower arch using bilateral attachment (Rhein 83) retained cast removable partial denture as a definitive prosthesis. Therefore, in conditions like hypodontia or oligodontia caused due to ectodermal dysplasia, attachment retained removable partial denture may prove beneficial by effectively distributing the occlusal forces. In clinical scenarios where implant is not feasible or not opted by the patient, this combination treatment may be a viable option.

1. Introduction

Ectodermal dysplasias (EDs) are a heterogeneous group of rare congenital disorders (incidence at birth-1 in 100,000 males), which involve primary developmental defects of two or more tissues derived from the ectoderm like skin, nails, teeth, and eccrine glands. The disorder can be classified as hidrotic type (Clouston syndrome) inherited as autosomal dominant condition and hypohidrotic or anhidrotic type (Christ-Siemens-Touraine syndrome) which is inherited as X linked recessive attribute [1]. Although the National Foundation for Ectodermal Dysplasia has listed twenty different types of such disorders, severity may differ within the same type of ED [1]. In these cases, the prosthodontic interventions mainly focus to enhance the esthetics, phonetics, and function, by various fixed or removable treatment approaches [1–4].

This specific case was unique from the previous case studies reported as the patient had hyposalivation and severe gag reflex and presented with mixed dentition, posing a problem in treatment planning. Moreover, there was a marked loss in occlusal vertical dimension. Although every treatment option has its own advantages and disadvantages, we have tried to manage this case using a hybrid approach by rehabilitating the upper arch with a long-span fixed partial denture and lower arch with bilateral attachment retained removable partial denture, a treatment approach which has not been documented in previous case report literature.

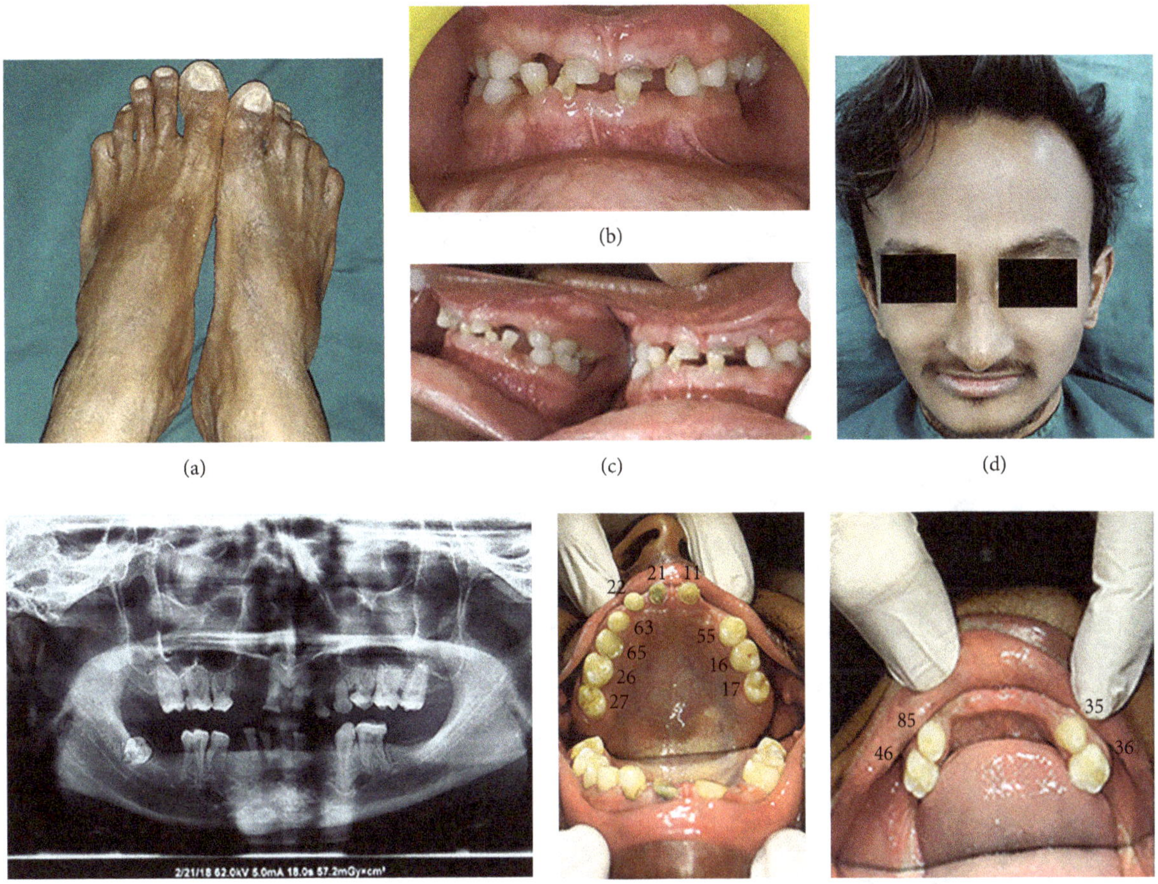

(a) (b) (c) (d) (e) (f) (g)

FIGURE 1: (a) Dystrophy of toe nails, (b–d) pretreatment occlusal vertical dimension loss, (e) pretreatment orthopantomogram, (f) pretreatment maxillary, and (g) mandibular arch.

2. Case Presentation

A 19-year-old male with a chief complaint of multiple missing teeth and difficulty in chewing food was referred to the Department of Prosthodontics by his physician. On extraoral clinical examination, he had frontal bossing, depressed nasal bridge, thick everted lower lips, sparse facial hair, sunken cheeks, and dystrophy of toe nails. The patient was concerned regarding his esthetics and seemed to have a low self-esteem. Previous health reports had mentioned the diagnosis as hypohidrotic type of ectodermal dysplasia. Extraoral examination revealed sunken cheeks, deep nasolabial fold, mild frontal bossing, thin sparse facial hair, and normal nails (Figure 1(a)). Various treatment modalities like direct composite restorations, fixed partial dentures, and removable prosthetic options like overdentures, endosseous implants, mini-implants, and zygomatic implants have been advocated by various authors [1–4].

Intraoral examination revealed dry oral mucosa (later confirmed by sialometry test) and residual ridge with adequate width and height. The teeth present were 17, 16, 55, 11, 21, 22, 63, 65, 26, 27, 71, 81, 82, 36, 35, 85, and 46 (Figures 1(b)–1(g)). A thorough oral prophylaxis was done, and the patient was recalled after 2 weeks to assess the periodontal prognosis of each tooth. Bearing in mind the existing crown root ratio and number of teeth which would remain after extraction of grade three mobile teeth, a single unit long-span porcelain fused to metal fixed partial denture was planned for the maxillary arch. After assessing the periodontal health of the lower teeth and crown height space of 6.5 millimeters (mm), a bilateral attachment retained cast removable partial denture was planned for lower arch.

Vertical dimension (VD) of face was assessed using phonetics along with the Niswonger's physiologic method. This step was done by placing an adhesive tape in the shape of a small equilateral triangle at the tip of nose and chin and then asking the patient to repeat words ending with sound "m." At least six to seven readings were recorded between the two points, and an average of all was considered as vertical dimension at rest. The patient was then asked to occlude all teeth, and the distance between two points revealed the vertical dimension at occlusion. Subtracting the latter from former resulted in a freeway space of seven to eight millimeters (with normal range of three to four millimeters), which was evident clinically in premolar region, indicating a loss in occlusal vertical dimension.

An incremental increase in VD up to 4 mm over a period of 3 months was planned to assess the physiologic comfort and ensure an adequate adaptation time for temporomandibular joint [5]. Therefore, conforming to the "two splint

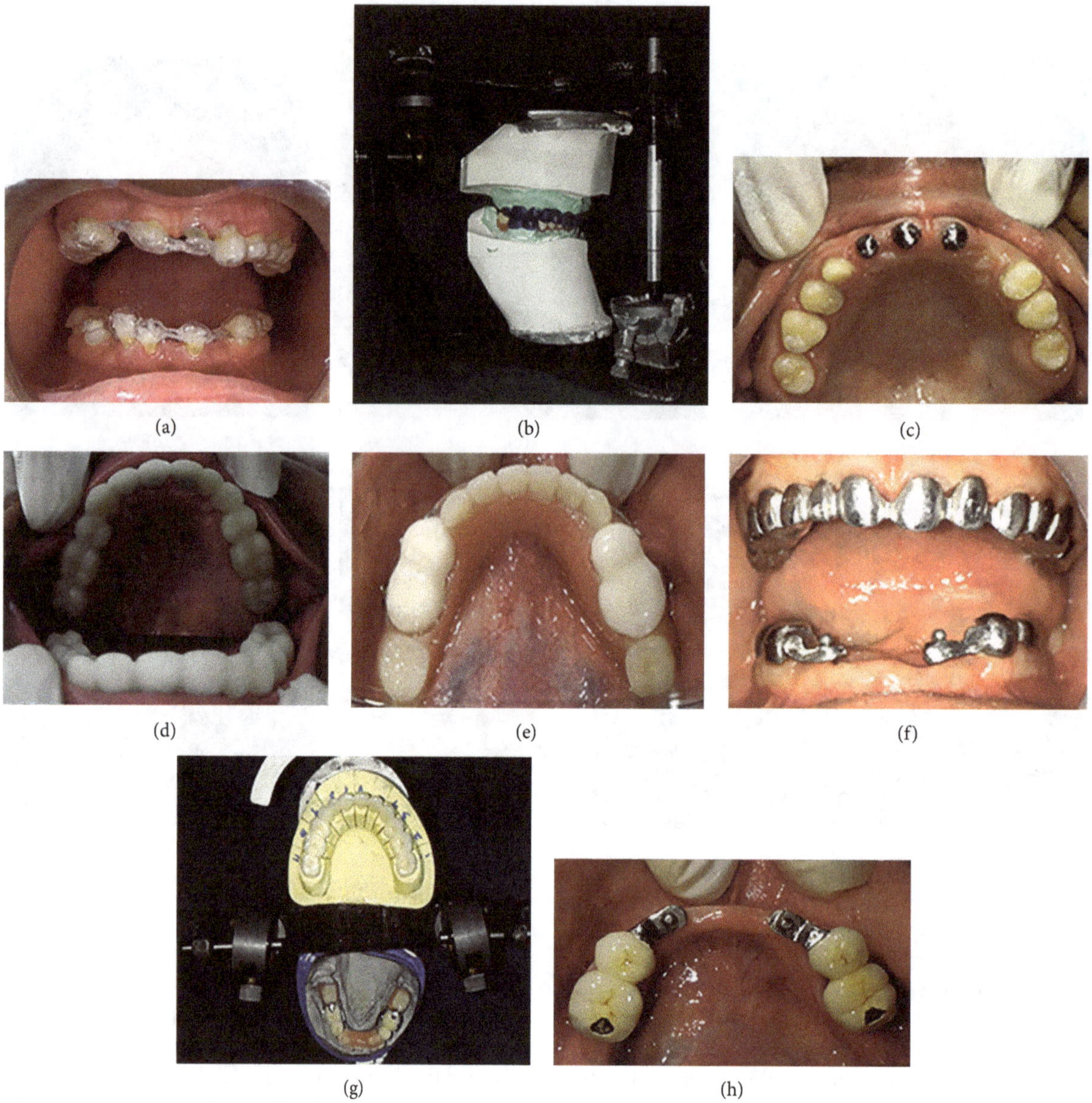

FIGURE 2: (a) Flexible occlusal splint, (b) final wax-up at desired vertical dimension, (c) minimal tooth preparation with polished metal copings, (d) maxillary and (e) mandibular provisional restorations, (f) metal coping try-in, (g) ceramic layering of prosthesis, and Rhein 83 attachment.

concept," a removable flexible splint of 2 mm thickness was worn by the patient in mandibular arch for initial 6 weeks and in the maxilla for next 6 weeks (Figure 2(a)) [5, 6]. Alternatively, a second mandibular splint of 4 mm thickness could have been given to the patient as a substitute for maxillary 2 mm thickness splint. Either ways, the desired VD increase of 4 mm would have been achieved. Initially, a hard splint was tried for the same procedure but later, a soft splint was used as the patient was more comfortable and compliant to it. Moreover, recent studies show that both hard and soft splints are equally effective in achieving the desired results of treatment [7, 8]. The soft splint in this case was not intimately adapted on the teeth with grade 2 mobility, to prevent any further detrimental effect due to occlusal forces.

Teeth with grade 3 mobility and poor crown root ratio, i.e., 71, 81, and 82, were extracted. Following 2 weeks of socket healing, diagnostic impressions were made using irreversible hydrocolloid and casts were poured. Upper diagnostic cast was mounted on Hanau wide-vue articulator using Hanau springbow transfer. Centric jaw relation record was obtained by guiding patient's jaw as per bimanual manipulation method and using 4.5 mm thickness of warm Aluwax for recording the cusp indentations (Aluwax Dental Products Co), followed by mounting of the mandibular casts. A complete tentative wax-up was performed on diagnostic mounting and putty index (Dentsply Aquasil) were made (Figure 2(b)). Teeth with inadequate crown surface area, i.e., 11, 21, and 22, were endodontically treated followed by cast post and metal coping (root submergence technique). Meanwhile, an intraoral mockup was performed using these putty indices and a provisional restorative material (Protemp4). Protrusive record (up to six millimeters) was now

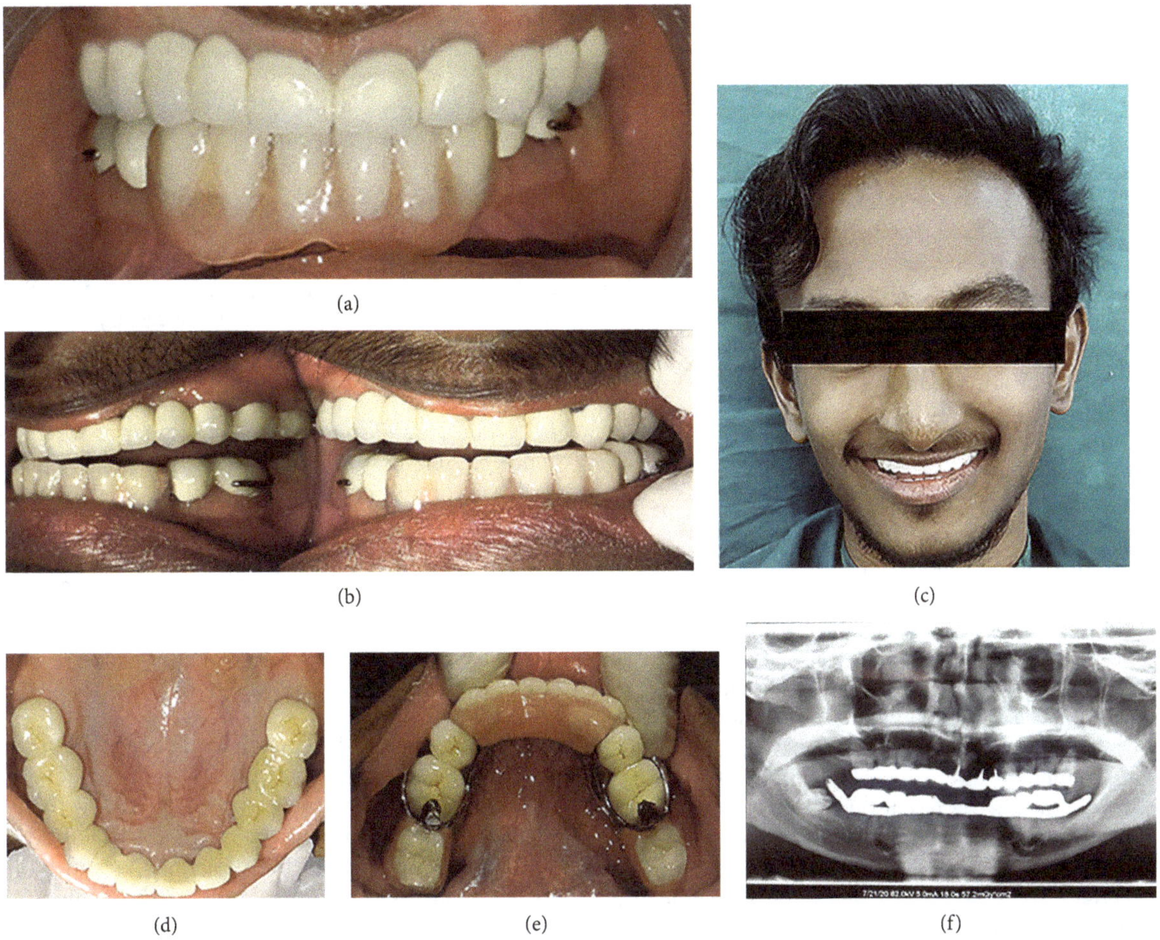

FIGURE 3: (a) Final prosthesis in maximum intercuspation, (b) group function occlusion on lateral excursion movement. (c) Posttreatment esthetics, (d, e) 3-year periodic review intraoral photographs, and (f) follow-up orthopantomogram.

obtained intraorally, to program the horizontal condylar guidance on the articulator.

Conservative tooth preparation was done on maxillary teeth, using the intraoral mockup as a tooth preparation guide. As teeth were hypoplastic in nature and had a tendency to chip, only minor refinement was done using extra-fine diamond bur. No occlusal reduction was attempted as increase in vertical dimension was planned (Figure 2(c)). As tapered cone shaped and malformed teeth were present, achieving the parallelism by excessive tooth reduction was not clinically challenging.

Final impressions were made using two-stage putty wash impression technique, and provisional restorations were fabricated directly using the final putty indices and luted with noneugenol temporary luting cement (3M ESPE RelyX Temp NE) (Figures 2(d) and 2(e)). Mounting of the master casts was done in centric relation at desired VD as mentioned above. Metal trial made using direct metal laser sintering technique was tried in patient's mouth to ensure marginal adaptation (Figure 2(f)). The ceramic layering with feldspathic porcelain established the occlusion plane using the final wax-up as a reference (Figure 2(g)). In this, case ceramic baked over direct metal laser sintered coping was used instead of single unit zirconia bride due to various reasons. First, the patient had an average smile line (exposing slightly more than 75% of central incisors), hence minimizing the probability of slight metal discolored margin visibility in future. Second, the retrievability of resin cement luted single unit zirconia bridge would have been challenging. Third, due to the milling process used for fabricating the metal coping substructure, the 2 mm thickness of porcelain layering could be easily standardized, hence resulting in more predictive metal porcelain bond. Fourth, it was more cost-effective for the patient when discussed.

A mandibular cast removable partial denture framework (Co-Cr alloy) was then designed over Rhein 83 attachment using yellow extrasoft nylon retentive cap, and passive circumferential clasps were given (Figures 2(g) and 2(h)). Occlusal contacts in maximum intercuspation position were checked before luting the fixed restoration (Figure 2(a)). Finally, the luting of the fixed partial denture using glass ionomer cement (GC Gold Label 1 Luting & Lining Cement) and final denture insertion was done after ensuring Christensen's phenomenon as well as bilateral group function occlusion intraorally (Figure 2(b)). The esthetics and phonetics of the patient were verified (Figure 3(c)).

As a part of maintenance therapy for hyposalivation, a lemon-flavored synthetic saliva spray (Glandosane Synthetic saliva spray by Fresenius Kabi Oncology Pvt. Ltd) was used by the patient four to five times a day. This would ensure timely lubrication of the mouth, hence minimizing complications like dry and rough tongue, mouth sores, caries, and halitosis. As susceptibility to enamel caries is more in these conditions due to reduced saliva, a 1.1% sodium fluoride toothpaste (Colgate PreviDent 5000 ppm Booster Plus) was prescribed once a day. Additionally, a water flosser in pulsed mode was recommended twice a day, to enhance effective cleansability in the pontic and connector region of the fixed prosthesis.

The patient was advised for a regular follow-up every 6 months. Figures 3(d) and 3(e) depict a healthy periodontal condition and good oral hygiene maintenance at a periodic recall visit after 3 years. An orthopantomogram taken after 2.5 years showed healthy abutments with minimal alveolar changes (Figure 3(f)).

3. Discussion

Although occlusal stops in posterior teeth are present in this case, the teeth are peg shaped, malformed, and widely spaced. Due to the lack of tooth bud formation, the alveolar bone is minimally formed and is hypoplastic in ED cases [1]. All these factors contribute to dentoalveolar tissue deficiency and severely reduced vertical dimension of occlusion.

All possible implant treatment options were initially discussed to the patient but were denied by him due to financial restrains. Dry oral mucosa has always been associated with soreness in denture bearing tissues and patient dissatisfaction with removable oral prosthesis [9]. Therefore, considering the hyposalivation, severe gag reflex, and psychological discomfort expressed by the patient, removable prosthodontic options were precluded from treatment plan for the maxillary arch. Many authors do not advocate fixed partial dentures (FPDs) with rigid connectors, especially if the prosthesis crosses the midline as only few abutments are present in most of the cases reported and the patients were in their growth phase during the treatment [10]. However, a single unit long-span FPD was planned for the maxillary arch as sufficient healthy abutment teeth were present to support the prosthesis and the patient was in late adolescence. The growth of maxilla in males has been reported to be consistent after the age of 18 [11].

Due to the abutment conditions with respect to 11, 21, and 22, root submergence technique was applied in the maxillary anterior region, as it is a promising method of maintaining the alveolar ridge dimensions at the pontic site of an FPD especially in esthetic zones [12]. For effective cleansability, a uniform clearance of 1 mm was ensured between the modified ridge lap pontic and the metal copings.

Considering the resilient nature of the extrasoft nylon retentive cap used over Rhein 83 attachment, the occlusal forces are better distributed between the lower fixed partial denture and alveolar ridge mucosa. Hence, attributing to this "stress breaker effect," masticatory overload on the lower fixed prosthesis is circumvented, contributing to the periodontal health of the lower abutments.

As the canine teeth were missing in both the arches, a group function occlusion was provided bilaterally, ensuring the absence of premature contacts on nonworking side. The patient has been followed up for 3 years, and so far, there have been no complications.

4. Conclusion

In conditions like hypodontia or oligodontia caused due to ectodermal dysplasia, attachment retained cast removable partial denture may prove beneficial by effectively distributing the occlusal forces. As evident in the follow-up orthopantomogram, although the prognosis of the rehabilitation is good, a regular follow-up is necessary to assess the intraoral force factors and ensure the comfort and longevity of the prosthesis.

4.1. Clinical Significance. In clinical scenarios where implant is not feasible or not opted by the patient, a combination treatment of long-span fixed partial denture and an attachment retained cast removable partial denture can prove beneficial. This case gives an excellent treatment outcome in terms of esthetics as well as function, hence improving the quality of life.

Consent

The authors certify that they have obtained all appropriate patient consent forms. In the form, the patient(s) has/have given his/her/their consent for his/her/their images and other clinical information to be reported in the journal. The patients understand that their names and initials will not be published, and due efforts will be made to conceal their identity, but anonymity cannot be guaranteed.

Acknowledgments

The authors thank Dr. Shashidhara HS, who served as a scientific advisor.

References

[1] A. J. Hickey and T. J. Vergo Jr., "Prosthetic treatments for patients with ectodermal dysplasia," *The Journal of Prosthetic Dentistry*, vol. 86, no. 4, pp. 364–368, 2001.

[2] D. Schnabl, I. Grunert, M. Schmuth, and I. Kapferer-Seebacher, "Prosthetic rehabilitation of patients with hypohidrotic ectodermal dysplasia: a systematic review," *Journal of Oral Rehabilitation*, vol. 45, no. 7, pp. 555–570, 2018.

[3] B. Z. Mello, T. C. Silva, D. Rios, M. A. Machado, F. P. Valarelli, and T. M. Oliveira, "Mini-implants: alternative for oral rehabilitation of a child with ectodermal dysplasia," *Brazilian Dental Journal*, vol. 26, no. 1, pp. 75–78, 2015.

[4] F. Goker, E. Grecchi, E. G. Mancini, M. Del Fabbro, and F. Grecchi, "Zygomatic implant survival in 9 ectodermal dysplasia patients with 3.5- to 7-year follow-up," *Oral Diseases*, vol. 26, no. 8, pp. 1803–1809, 2020.

[5] D. Edelhoff, J. Schweiger, O. Prandtner, J. Trimpl, M. Stimmelmayr, and J. F. Güth, "CAD/CAM splints for the functional and esthetic evaluation of newly defined occlusal dimensions," *Quintessence International*, vol. 48, no. 3, pp. 181–191, 2017.

[6] K. A. Turner and D. M. Missirlian, "Restoration of the extremely worn dentition," *The Journal of Prosthetic Dentistry*, vol. 52, no. 4, pp. 467–474, 1984.

[7] S. A. Seifeldin and K. A. Elhayes, "Soft versus hard occlusal splint therapy in the management of temporomandibular disorders (TMDs)," *The Saudi dental journal*, vol. 27, no. 4, pp. 208–214, 2015.

[8] A. Amin, R. Meshramkar, and K. Lekha, "Comparative evaluation of clinical performance of different kind of occlusal splint in management of myofascial pain," *The Journal of the Indian Prosthodontic Society*, vol. 16, no. 2, pp. 176–181, 2016.

[9] K. Ikebe, K. Morii, J. Kashiwagi, T. Nokubi, and R. L. Ettinger, "Impact of dry mouth on oral symptoms and function in removable denture wearers in Japan," *Oral Surgery, Oral Medicine, Oral Pathology, Oral Radiology, and Endodontics*, vol. 99, no. 6, pp. 704–710, 2005.

[10] R. Ladda, S. Gangadhar, V. Kasat, and A. Bhandari, "Prosthodontic management of hypohidrotic ectodermal dysplasia with anodontia: a case report in pediatric patient and review of literature," *Annals of Medical and Health Sciences Research*, vol. 3, no. 2, pp. 277–281, 2013.

[11] R. J. Love, J. M. Murray, and A. H. Mamandras, "Facial growth in males 16 to 20 years of age," *American Journal of Orthodontics and Dentofacial Orthopedics*, vol. 97, no. 3, pp. 200–206, 1990.

[12] S. Choi, I. S. Yeo, S. H. Kim, J. W. Lee, C. W. Cheong, and J. S. Han, "A root submergence technique for pontic site development in fixed dental prostheses in the maxillary anterior esthetic zone," *Journal of periodontal & implant science*, vol. 45, no. 4, pp. 152–155, 2015.

Management of Oroantral Fistulae and Communications: Our Recommendations for Routine Practice

Mahamadou Konate, Dounia Sarfi, Mounia El Bouhairi, and Ihsane Benyahya

Department of Oral Surgery, Université Hassan II, Casablanca, Morocco BP: 9157

Correspondence should be addressed to Mahamadou Konate; mahamadoukonate370@gmail.com

Academic Editor: Darko Macan

Oroantral communication (OAC) is one of the main complications of extracting antral or sinus teeth. OAC is a gap between the maxillary sinus and the oral cavity. When left untreated, it causes maxillary sinusitis and dramatically impairs the patient's quality of life. Numerous surgical treatment techniques have been described, from mucosal techniques to using bone substitutes or very conservative alternative means. Many cases of recurrence after treatment have been reported, and the choice of the method adapted to the clinical situation remains challenging. Therefore, it is necessary to establish a correct diagnosis and choose the surgical technique best adapted to the case. This work is aimed at reviewing several techniques for the treatment of OAC and at describing our recommendations for use in daily practice for each of them through four clinical cases.

1. Introduction

Oroantral communication (OAC) is a gap between the maxillary sinus and the oral cavity. When left untreated, it can lead to an oroantral fistula and maxillary sinusitis [1]. Oroantral communications are often iatrogenic following the extraction of antral or sinus teeth. Indeed, the inferior wall of the maxillary sinus has an anatomical relationship with the maxillary premolar area (antral teeth) (Figure 1). The distance between the apex and the sinus is 1 to 7 mm for a sinus floor thickness of 2 to 3 mm. Thus, sinus effraction can be observed in 3.8% to 1.3% of cases after maxillary molar extraction [2]. OACs can also be induced by tumor surgery, implant surgery, trauma, or orthognathic surgery involving the maxilla.

Surgical treatment of OACs should be performed as early as possible. Indeed, in the face of extensive untreated oroantral communication, 50% of patients develop sinusitis after 48 hours and 90% after two weeks with a filling of the sinus on radiological examination [3] (Figure 2). In the healthy sinus, OACs less than 5 mm close spontaneously [4]. Nevertheless, it is difficult, if not impossible, to evaluate the diameter of an OAC in the clinical setting, which is why it is necessary to intervene surgically in the majority of clinical situations. Different surgical techniques have been described, such as surrounding soft tissues (vestibular flap, palatal flap, buccal fat pad).

The high recurrence rate for significant bone defects and the increasing need to obtain closure for implant rehabilitation has led practitioners to develop new bone closure techniques using new materials that allow for new therapeutic perspectives.

The choice of the appropriate treatment depends on several factors, including the time of consultation, the presence of associated sinusitis, or the size of the communication.

This work is aimed at describing the different therapeutic options of OACs through some clinical cases and at presenting the decision factors of these treatments.

2. Observations

2.1. Observation 1. A 41-year-old female patient with no particular medical history was referred to the Surgical Odontology Department of the Casablanca Dental Consultation and

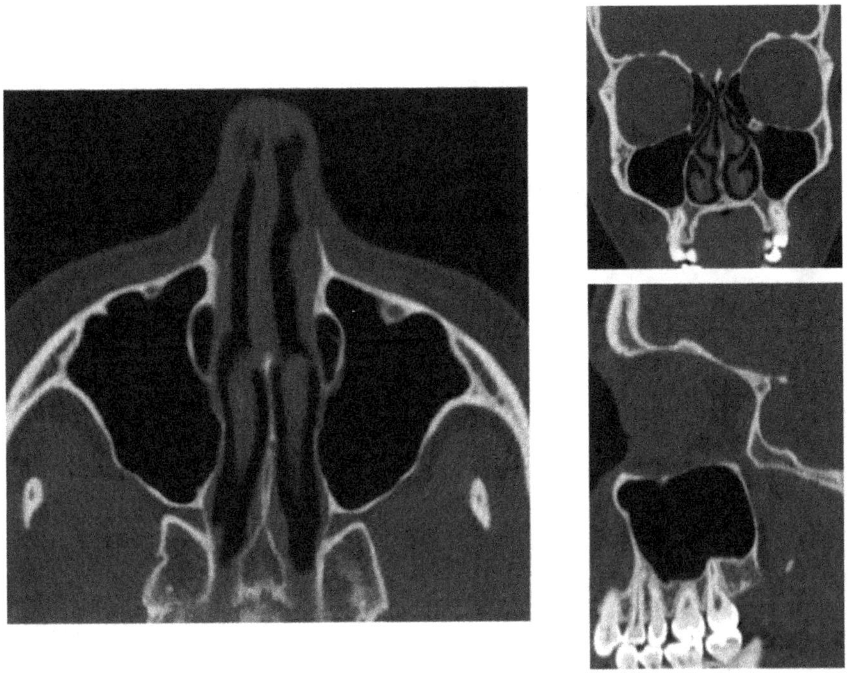

FIGURE 1: CT scan of the maxillary sinuses showing the anatomy of the sinuses and their relationship to the teeth.

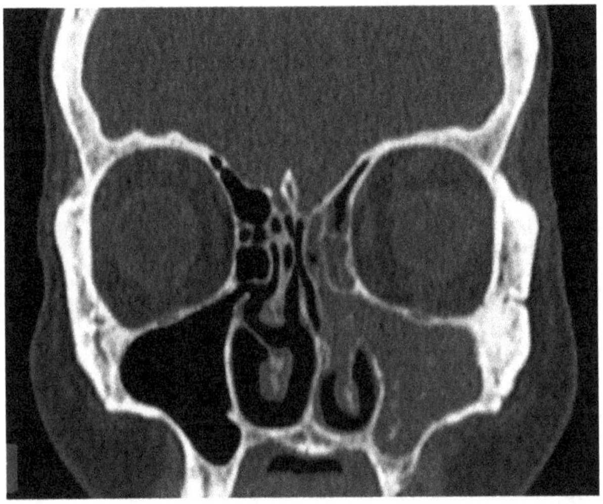

FIGURE 2: Frontal CT section showing the filling of the left maxillary sinus.

Treatment Center by her private dentist following the persistence of a right maxillary oroantral fistula (OAF) for one month. The patient reported pain in the right upper maxillary area accentuated by gravity and associated with oronasal fluid reflux. The extraoral examination was unremarkable. The intraoral examination showed a fistula about 3 mm in diameter on the right posterior maxillary ridge with normal mucosa (Figure 3). The panoramic radiograph showed a bony discontinuity in the fistula area with a relationship to the right maxillary sinus. We confirmed the diagnosis of oroantral fistula associated with maxillary sinusitis. The management consisted initially in the sanitation of the maxillary sinus, which an otolaryngologist performed. The surgical treatment for closure of the OAC consisted of traction of a vestibular flap following the Rehrmann technique associated with a resorbable collagen membrane (Figure 4).

Follow-up at 15 days and then at one month showed good mucosal healing and disappearance of clinical signs (Figure 5). At six-month follow-up, the patient did not present any clinical symptoms.

2.2. Observation 2. A 35-year-old patient presented to the Oral Surgery, Clinical Department of the Consultation Center and Dental Treatment in Casablanca, following complications of extraction of the upper left second molar, performed in a liberal dental office. The patient reports air passage via the extraction site to the nasal cavity associated with slight pain in the upper left infraorbital region accentuated by gravity. The extraoral examination was without particularity. The intraoral examination showed a persistent fistula of about one centimeter opposite the vestibular site's extraction site. The panoramic X-ray showed a bone discontinuity in the left posterior maxillary zone, which is intimately related to the left maxillary sinus. The medical care consisted initially in the sanitation of the maxillary sinus by medical treatment based on amoxicillin/clavulanic acid at a rate of 3 g per day for ten days. We managed this case using a Rehrmann flap associated with the buccal fat pad graft. Follow-up of the patient at six months and one year reported clinical silence.

2.3. Observation 3. A 53-year-old patient presented to the Oral Surgery, Clinical Department of the Consultation Center and Dental Treatment in Casablanca, following complications from the extraction of a maxillary wisdom tooth from a week ago, performed in a liberal dental office.

The patient reports a passage of air and food between the oral and nasal cavity, associated with pain in the left

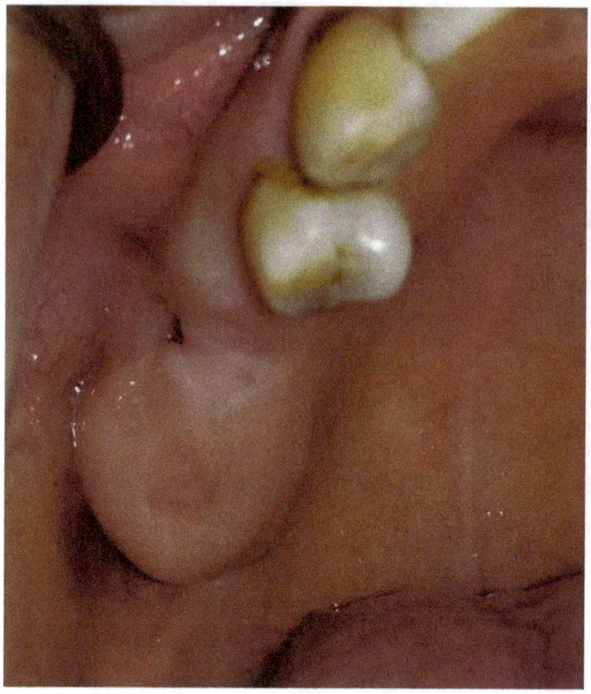

FIGURE 3: Intraoral view showing a 3 mm diameter oroantral fistula on the right maxillary ridge.

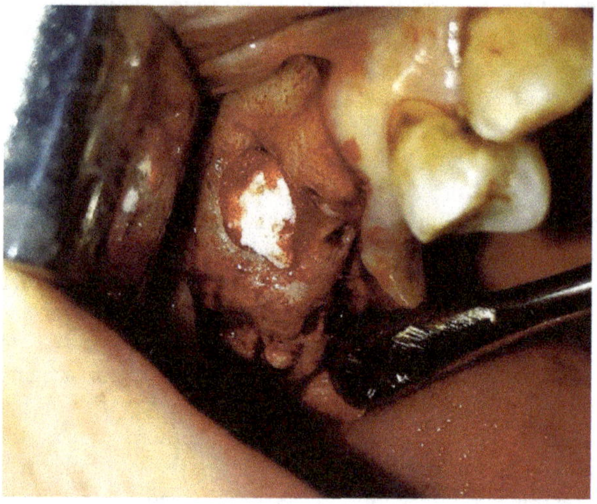

FIGURE 4: Intraoral view showing the closure of the OAC by a collagen membrane.

infraorbital area accentuated by gravity. In addition, the patient was treated with antibiotics at the rate of 2 g of amoxicillin a day for four days. The extraoral examination was in an unremarkable condition.

The intraoral examination demonstrated that the socket of the left maxillary wisdom tooth was persistent and with serosity all around (Figure 6). The panoramic X-ray has shown a residual root-like radioopacity of the left maxillary quadrant and a discontinuity of the bone cortex at this level, responsible for a close relationship between the oral cavity and the left maxillary sinus. The treatment consisted initially of medical treatment associated with daily nasal wash and rinse of

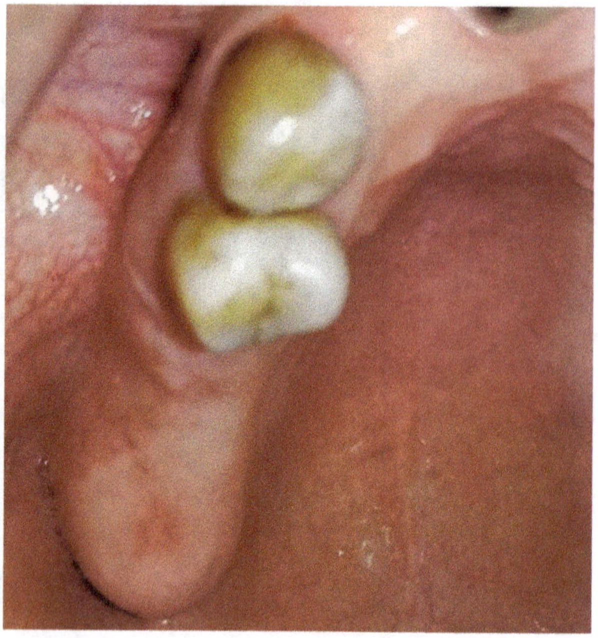

FIGURE 5: Intraoral view showing healing at one month.

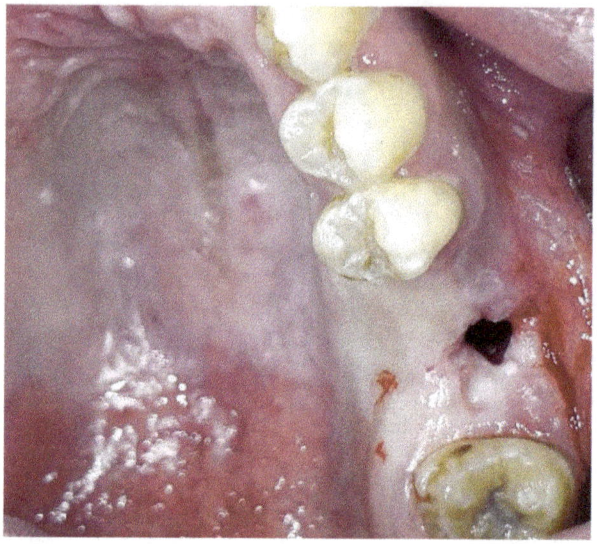

FIGURE 6: Intraoral view showing a left maxillary OAC of 7 mm diameter.

OAC. After the signs of infection had disappeared, the surgical closure of the OAC, as in the previous case, consisted of performing a Rehrmann flap associated with a buccal fat pad graft (Figure 7). After one month and then six months, there was a complete cure and no clinical symptoms.

2.4. Observation 4. A 34-year-old patient presented in consultation to the Oral Surgery, Clinical Department of the Consultation Center and Dental Treatment in Casablanca, three days after the extraction by her dentist practicing in the liberal sector. The patient reports having had a first attempt to extract her first left maxillary molar a week earlier, with persistent roots. During the interrogation, we

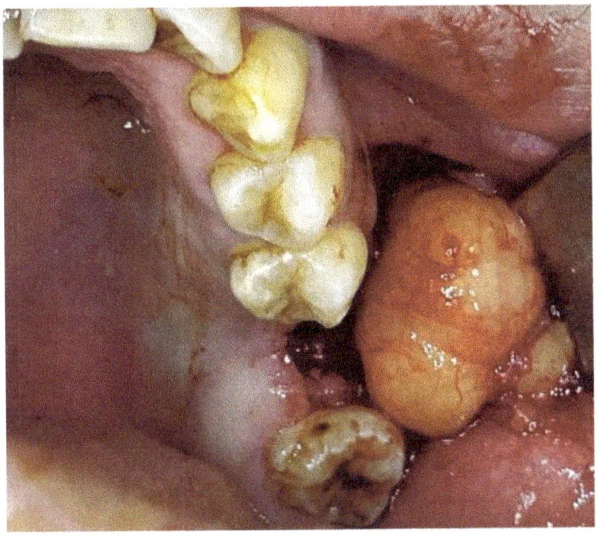

FIGURE 7: Intraoral view showing access to the buccal fat pad in treating a left maxillary OAC.

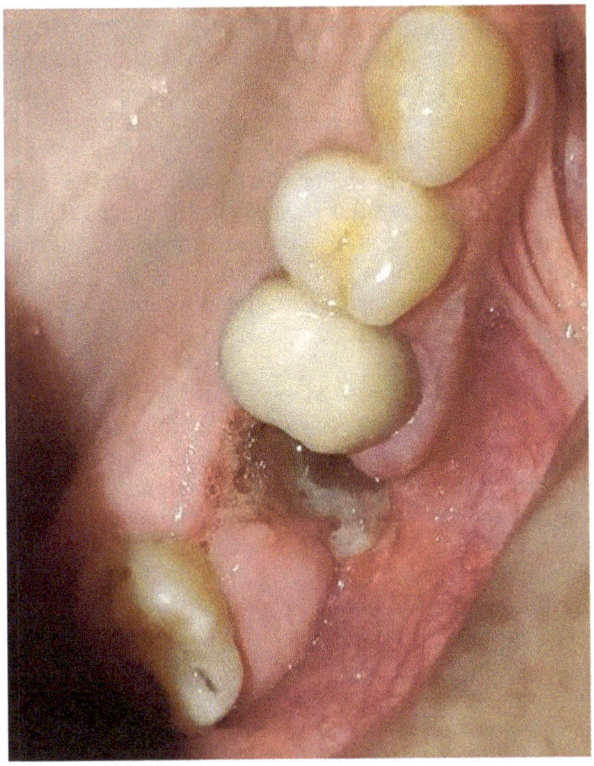

FIGURE 8: Intraoral view of a recent purulent left maxillary OAC.

noted that the oroantral communication (OAC) appeared during a second intervention by her doctor for extraction of the residual roots four days later. The patient reported the passage of air through the dental socket during respiratory exhalation and a slight feeling of heaviness concerning the left sinus. The extraoral examination has not shown anything unusual. The intraoral view showed a fistula of 10 mm with exposed bone (Figure 8). The Valsalva maneuver highlights the presence of bubbles in the bottom of the tooth

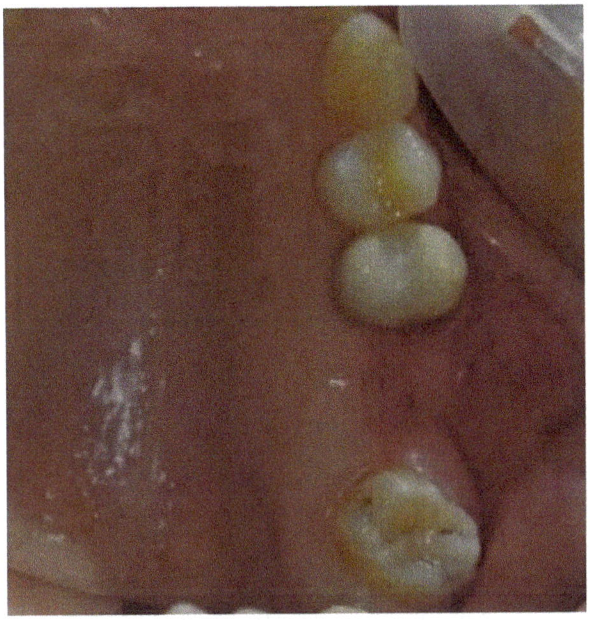

FIGURE 9: Intraoral view showing healing at 40 days.

socket. The radiological examination shows continuity between the dental socket and the left maxillary sinus.

The patient had received medical treatment based on amoxicillin at a rate of 3 g per day and 1.5 g of metronidazole per day.

On the other hand, the patient's fear of undergoing surgery, given her history, and the delay in consultation, led us to opt for a nonsurgical, conservative technic. After a thorough site cleaning, the fistula was closed by a eugenol-free periodontal dressing type COE-PAK*. The patient came back regularly to change the dressing until the area healed entirely and there were no clinical symptoms after 40 days (Figure 9). After one year of follow-up, the patient did not present any clinical signs.

3. Discussion

Several techniques can treat OAC. the choice of method must take different factors into account: the size of the communication, the presence or absence of an infection, and, especially, the time of exposure.

Indeed, in the presence of a healthy sinus, when the treatment is early (within 48 hours), the management will only be surgical to close the OAC. In the case of deferred care, treatment has two stages:

First of all, medical treatment to cleanse the sinus [5]. Some authors recommend the following protocol: antibiotic therapy: association of amoxicillin/clavulanic acid twice a day; clindamycin 300 mg 4 times a day or moxifloxacin 400 mg once a day for at least ten days combined with a decongestant and rinse of the sinus with physiological serum through OAC [3]. Other treatment methods are possible and must be discussed in collaboration with an otolaryngologist. We will not develop this aspect of care in this work.

On the other hand, with the cleaned sinus, the treatment is surgical, closing the OAC. There is no consensus

Table 1: Recommendations for the choice of surgical techniques according to the clinical situation.

Clinical situation			Surgical technique
Suspicion of OAC postextraction			Collagen sponges + sutures
Confirmed OAC	Unplanned implant*	<10 mm of diameter	Rehrmann's flap or conservative nonsurgical technique
		10-15 mm of diameter or failure of anterior treatment	Buccal fat pad
		>15 mm of diameter or failure of anterior treatment	Combination of techniques: double or triple thickness closure technique: (i) Buccal fat pad + Rehrmann's flap (ii) Buccal fat pad + allogenic membrane + Rehrmann's flap
	Planned implant*	Autogenic or xenogenic bone graft	

*The implant placements described in the table are for the exact areas of the OACs without considering the probably healthy adjacent areas.

regarding a specific technique. Each of these techniques has its pros and cons. It is therefore essential to choose the method according to the clinical situation.

Before describing the different surgical options, it is essential to remember that in the presence of a healthy sinus, OACs smaller than 5 mm tend to close spontaneously [4]. Therefore, after tooth extraction, when an OAC is suspected, it would be wise to suture the surgical site with or without collagen sponges. The patient is advised to avoid all iatrogenic movements, such as the violent blowing of the nose, which could increase the size of the OAC.

3.1. Rehrmann's Flap. The coronally advanced flap is the most common and oldest technique known in the treatment of OAC [3, 6]. It was described by Rehrmann in 1936 and remains today the most accepted technique by the authors [7]. This technique consists of making a vestibular flap of trapezoidal shape advanced coronally to close the bone defect. Its broad base would provide the necessary vascular supply for the success of this technique. This technique has a success rate of 93% [7]. The disadvantages of this technique are postoperative pain and edema associated with a reduction in the depth of the vestibule concerned. Indeed, a second vestibule deepening surgery is often necessary after six months unless you opt for an implant solution.

3.2. Buccal Fat Pad Graft. This technique is suitable for small and medium volume OAC. The Buccal fat pad graft is located between the masticatory muscles with three arterial trunks to ensure vascularization: the superficial temporal, maxillary, and facial arteries. One of its extensions, called the buccal extension, is close to the maxillary premolar-molar zone. The size of this ball is constant regardless of the body mass [7]. This technique was described for the first time by Egyedi in 1977 [8]. After making a full-thickness vestibular flap around the OAC, it consists of incising in the periosteum in the posterior zone opposite the maxillary tuberosity to discover the buccal extension of the Bichat ball. This ball of fat is pulled and sutured to cover the OAC [3]. The produced flap is sutured and repositioned in its starting position. This ball of pedunculated fat left bare in the oral cavity has been shown to epithelialize after two weeks [9]. This technique has the advantage of keeping the vestibule intact. However, the buccal fat pad may necrose. Egyedi had recommended for this purpose to cover the buccal fat with a free skin graft [3, 8]. Other variants of this technique are informed, in particular the double thickness closure technique. It consists of covering the buccal fat of the cheek with the buccal mucoperiosteal flap [10].

We have presented this technique in two of the patients presented in this work, and it reports promising results. Nevertheless, it is essential to note that the amount of fat tissue obtained can be variable. According to Visscher et al. [7], this quantity is constant regardless of the patient's body weight, so that this variability may depend on the operator's clinical experience. For this reason, we recommend reinforcing the buccal fat pad graft with a Rehrmann flap whenever possible. This method also has the advantage of limiting the possible necrosis associated with the exposure of the buccal fat pad to the oral cavity.

3.3. Autogenic Bone Graft. In 1969, Proctor. was the first to suggest the use of autogenous iliac bone grafts in the closure of large OACs [7]. Given the additional costs and comorbidity linked to this technique, it was abandoned. Haas et al. recommend using monoblock bone grafts for the closure of OAC [11]. These blocks are prepared to adapt to the bone defect and remain stable. Otherwise, they will have to be stabilized using miniscrews.

A Rehrmann-type vestibular flap covers both the bone defect and the graft.

3.4. Allogenic and Xenogenic Materials. Some authors use these materials for closing oral communications. Marković reported a case of OAC treated with a collagen membrane. After completing a mucoperiosteal vestibular flap and elimination of the mucosal pathway of the fistula, the technique consists of placing the membrane on the bone defect. The flap is thus returned to its original position without covering the collagen membrane [12]. This technique differs slightly from the first case reported in this work, where the mucoperiosteal flap covers the membrane. We placed an allogenic membrane that we covered with the vestibular flap drawn coronally. Clinical experience has shown us an increased risk of secondary infection when the membrane is exposed to the oral cavity, hence the decision to cover it entirely with the mucoperiosteal flap. This method is known as a double-layer closure technique. It is close to the triple-layer closure technique reported by George [13], which closes an oroantral communication by three levels of structure: the mucoperiosteal flap associated with a buccal fat pad and a fibrin membrane rich in platelets. The cost of this therapy remains a critical limit.

On the other hand, OAC may be effectively closed using lyophilized fibrin glue of human origin. After preparing fibrin for 15 to 20 minutes, it is placed at the level of the OAC associated with a collagen membrane [7]. The advantage of this technique is the absence of a flap and, therefore, of postoperational effects. In the same way, the anatomy of the oral cavity also remains intact. On the other hand, the risk of disease transmission and the preparation time are significant drawbacks.

3.5. Laser Therapy. The use of laser by the LLLT (low-level laser therapy) technique has also been reported in the treatment of OAC. Grzesiak-Janas and Janas reported using a laser with a wavelength of 830 nm with power at 30 mW in continuous mode at the rate of 3 cycles of intraoral and extraoral. The same cycle is repeated for four consecutive days [14].

The cost and lack of clinical hindsight of this technique come as a significant limit.

3.6. Conservative Nonsurgical Treatment. In certain circumstances, surgical treatment turns out to be difficult or even impossible for the closure of OAC. In patients with general conditions or pathologies leading to immunosuppression, postoperative infection is more significant, and scarring may be altered. Logan and Coates reported a case of conservative treatment in a patient presenting with an HIV infection [15]. The authors used a surgical splint such as a palatal plate made of acrylic resin covering the defect. After continuously wearing the plate for two weeks, satisfactory results were visible. After eight weeks, the authors emphasize the complete healing of the bone defect. This technique is similar to the one used in the last case reported in this work. Indeed, the difference is using an alloplastic material (COE-PACK) to isolate the defect instead of a palatal plate locally. This conservative technique has significant advantages but requires good patient cooperation, given the healing time and the discomfort.

Faced with this plethora of techniques, it can be challenging to choose a good strategy. For this reason, we propose some recommendations based on the clinical situation (Table 1).

4. Conclusion

Today, there is no best treatment or consensus regarding oroantral communication. Each technique has its advantages and disadvantages. The choice of a method must be made on a case-by-case basis, considering all factors regarding the act and the patient. According to Visscher et al. [7], the ideal treatment for OAC is fast, secure, simple, and well-tolerated by patients, at low cost, resulting in good bone and mucosal healing.

References

[1] U. Demetoglu, H. Ocak, and S. Bilge, "Closure of oroantral communication with plasma-rich fibrin membrane," *Journal of Craniofacial Surgery*, vol. 29, no. 4, pp. e367–e370, 2018.

[2] J. Lerat, K. Aubry, J. Brie, A.-F. Perez, S. Orsel, and J.-P. Bessede, *Communications bucco-naso-sinusiennes. /data/traites/or/20-56402/ [internet]*, Elsevier Masson, 2010, 2020, https://www.em-consulte.com/en/article/276381.

[3] H. Dym and J. C. Wolf, "Oroantral communication," *Oral and Maxillofacial Surgery Clinics of North America*, vol. 24, no. 2, pp. 239–247, 2012.

[4] N. von Wowern, "Closure of oroantral fistula with buccal flap: *Rehrmann* versus *M oczar*," *International Journal of Oral Surgery*, vol. 11, no. 3, pp. 156–165, 1982.

[5] P. Parvini, K. Obreja, R. Sader, J. Becker, F. Schwarz, and L. Salti, "Surgical options in oroantral fistula management: a narrative review," *International Journal of Implant Dentistry*, vol. 4, no. 1, p. 40, 2018.

[6] D. L. Wells and J. O. Capes, "Complications of dentoalveolar surgery," in *Oral and maxillofacial surgery, vol 1*, WB Saunders Co, Philadelphia (PA), 2000.

[7] S. H. Visscher, B. van Minnen, and R. R. M. Bos, "Closure of oroantral communications: a review of the literature," *Journal of Oral and Maxillofacial Surgery*, vol. 68, no. 6, pp. 1384–1391, 2010.

[8] P. Egyedi, "Utilization of the buccal fat pad for closure of oro-antral and/or oro-nasal communications," *Journal of Maxillofacial Surgery*, vol. 5, pp. 241–244, 1977.

[9] H. Tideman, A. Bosanquet, and J. Scott, "Use of the buccal fat pad as a pedicled graft," *Journal of Oral and Maxillofacial Surgery*, vol. 44, no. 6, pp. 435–440, 1986.

[10] M. Konate, M. Haitami, and I. Benyahya, "Approche combinée lambeau de Rehrmann et boule graisseuse de la joue dans le traitement de la communication bucco-sinusienne. A propos d'un cas clinique," *JACCR Africa*, vol. 4, p. 6, 2020.

[11] R. Haas, G. Watzak, M. Baron, G. Tepper, G. Mailath, and G. Watzek, "A preliminary study of monocortical bone grafts for oroantral fistula closure," *Oral Surgery, Oral Medicine, Oral Pathology, Oral Radiology, and Endodontics*, vol. 96, no. 3, pp. 263–266, 2003.

[12] A. Markovic, S. Colic, R. Drazic, L. Stojcev, and B. Gacic, "Closure of large oroantral fistula with resorbable collagen membrane-case report," *Serbian Dental Journal*, vol. 56, no. 4, pp. 201–206, 2009.

[13] E. George, "Triple-layered closure of an oroantral fistula: a case report," *The International Journal of Oral & Maxillofacial Implants*, vol. 33, no. 2, pp. e33–e36, 2018.

[14] G. Grzesiak-Janas and A. Janas, "Conservative closure of antro-oral communication stimulated with laser light," *Journal of Clinical Laser Medicine & Surgery*, vol. 19, no. 4, pp. 181–184, 2001.

[15] R. M. Logan and E. A. Coates, "Nonsurgical management of an oro-antral fistula in a patient with HIV infection," *Australian Dental Journal*, vol. 48, no. 4, pp. 255–258, 2003.

11

Osteoblastoma and Osteoid Osteoma of the Mandible: Review of the Literature and Report of Two Cases

Taylor Ellingsen,[1] Andrew Nalley,[2] Dolphine Oda,[3] Thomas B. Dodson,[3] and Peggy P. Lee[4]

[1]*School of Dentistry, University of Washington, Box 356370, 1959 NE Pacific St, Seattle, WA 98195, USA*
[2]*Clinical Instructor, Division of Radiology, Department of Oral Medicine, School of Dentistry, University of Washington, Box 356370, 1959 NE Pacific St, Seattle, WA 98195, USA*
[3]*Department of Oral and Maxillofacial Surgery, School of Dentistry, University of Washington, Box 357131, 1959 NE Pacific St, Seattle, WA 98195, USA*
[4]*Department of Oral Medicine, School of Dentistry, University of Washington, Box 356370, 1959 NE Pacific St, Seattle, WA 98195, USA*

Correspondence should be addressed to Peggy P. Lee; plee@uw.edu

Academic Editor: Pia L. Jornet

Osteoblastoma and osteoid osteoma are rare benign neoplasms of the jaws. We reviewed current literature surrounding the ongoing debate over similarities and differences of osteoblastoma and osteoid osteoma and present two cases. Both cases are well-demarcated mixed radiodensity mandibular lesions with histological features of osteoblastoma. They exhibit, however, distinctly unique and contrasting clinical and imaging characteristics suggesting that the first case is osteoblastoma and the second is osteoid osteoma. The first case of a 37-year-old male presents with a large, expansile lesion at posterior mandible, surrounded by a thick sclerotic band. Unusual features include significant buccal/lingual expansion, extensive new bone apposition, and soft tissue edema in the masseter muscle. This is in contrast to the second case of a much smaller lesion in a 17-year-old male with history of recent third molar extraction in the left posterior mandible. In this case, CT imaging revealed a circular, nonexpansile lesion with a sclerotic border surrounded by a radiolucent rim. Both patients underwent surgical excision of the lesion with extraction of the adjacent tooth. We discuss herein the distinct clinical and imaging features.

1. Introduction

Osteoblastoma and osteoid osteoma are benign and slow-growing neoplasms of the bone with similar, if not identical, histopathological features. Some have proposed that any benign neoplasm of the maxilla or mandible that is composed of osteoblasts forming osteoid and bone trabeculae set in a well-vascularized connective tissue stroma be classified as a single entity, osteoblastoma [1, 2]. However, the World Health Organization (WHO) continues to classify them as two separate entities [3, 4]. Osteoid osteoma was initially described by Heine in 1927 with Jaffe the first to recognize it as a unique entity in 1935 [5]. Osteoblastoma was first described in1932 by Jaffe and Mayer as "an osteoblastic-osteoid tissue forming tumor" [6].

Osteoblastoma is a rare tumor of the bone, accounting for approximately 3% of all benign bone tumors and 1% of primary bone tumors [7]. Osteoblastoma is most commonly found in the spine or areas of cancellous bone [8]. It is rare in the maxillofacial region with only 10% of osteoblastomas occurring in the skull [9]. When they do occur in the maxillofacial region, there is a marked predilection for the mandible, specifically the posterior mandible [7]. Osteoblastoma has a reported 2 : 1 male to female ratio; however, there is no gender predilection in the summary report of 77 cases in maxilla or mandible [2]. They are more common in

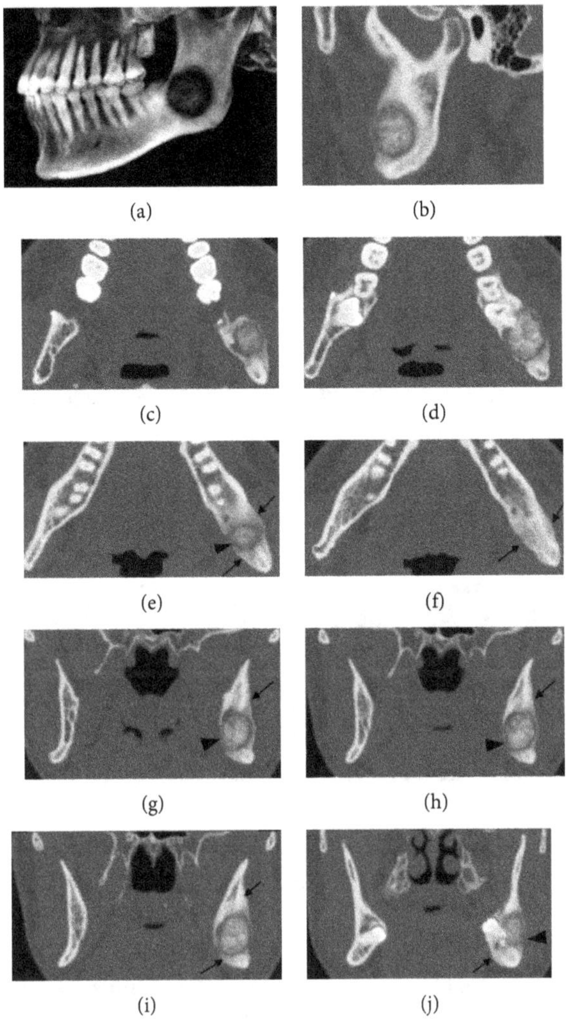

FIGURE 1: Case #1 3D CT reconstruction (a) and bone window CT sagittal view (b) showing the mixed density lesion associated with impacted #17 measuring 1.6 × 2.1 × 2 cm. The border of the lesion is well circumscribed with a broad sclerotic rim surrounding a lucent halo. Axial views ((c-f) from superior to inferior) and coronal views ((g-j) from posterior to anterior) showing buccal and lingual expansion, thinning, and areas of perforation at buccal and lingual cortices (arrowheads). Extensive sclerotic reactive bone is seen surrounding the lesion. New bone formation can be seen at buccal, lingual cortical, and inferior to the lesion (arrows). The lucent rim of the lesion extends into the left mandibular canal, with potential involvement of the inferior alveolar nerve (g–j).

younger patients, generally presenting in the second through fourth decades of life with a mean age of 24 [2, 10, 11].

Osteoid osteomas are more common than osteoblastomas accounting for approximately 10-12% of all benign bone tumors and 3% of primary bone tumors [7]. These lesions are more common in the lower extremity long bones, where more than 50% of lesions are reported to occur [7]. Osteoid osteoma, by contrast, is commonly located within cortical bone [8]. Like osteoblastoma, these lesions are exceptionally rare in the maxillofacial region with a tendency for the mandible when they do occur [10, 12, 13]. Osteoid osteoma has a characteristic nocturnal pain pattern and limited growth potential usually presenting small in size. Gender predilection and average age range in the maxillofacial region are similar to that of osteoblastoma [2, 10, 12].

Radiographically, both lesions usually appear as well-circumscribed, mixed density lesions surrounded by a sclerotic rim. Osteoid osteoma usually displays a larger area of sclerotic bone formation than osteoblastoma [7, 10]. Osteoblastoma is known to expand and erode the surrounding bone. In osteoid osteoma, a discrete central area of lucency known as the nidus with patchy mineralization and an ovoid shape can be appreciated [7, 10, 12]. This radiographic presentation of the central nidus is most easily appreciated in cortical lesions and may be more difficult to distinguish if the lesion arises from medullary bone [7].

Histologically, osteoblastoma and osteoid osteoma appear similarly and are characterized by the abnormal proliferation of osteoblasts forming osteoid and woven bone superimposed on a well-vascularized fibrous connective tissue stroma [1, 7, 10]. Additionally, immunohistochemical staining was similar in both osteoid osteoma and osteoblastoma [1]. Others believe that there are subtle histological and immunological differences between the two bony neoplasms such as the presence of epithelioid osteoblasts in more aggressive types of osteoblastoma, the presence of S-100

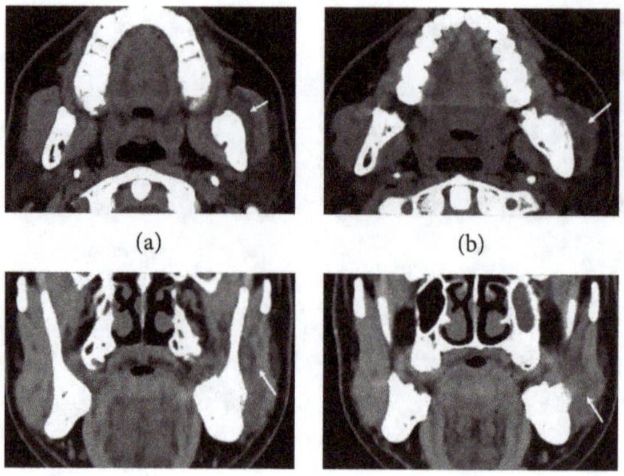

FIGURE 2: Case #1, soft tissue window CT images. Axial views (a–b) and coronal views (c–d) showing edema within the adjacent left masseter muscle (arrows).

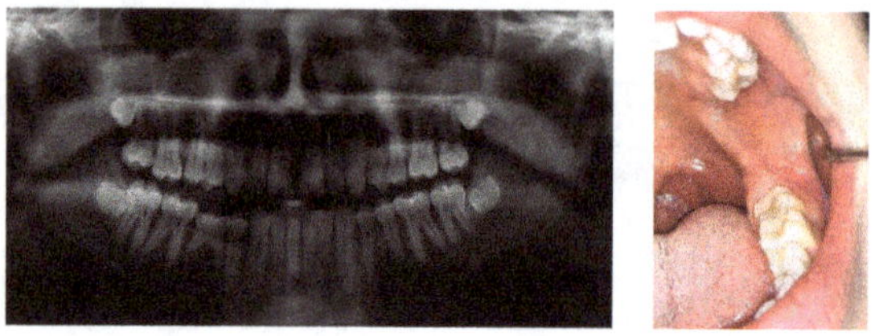

FIGURE 3: (a) Panoramic radiograph of case #2 prior to third molar extraction showing partially developed and bony impacted #1, 16, 17, and 32. No signs of pathology noted around the impacted #17. (b) Clinical photo post extraction with noted scar tissue at #17 extraction site but otherwise no abnormalities or swelling.

protein in osteoid osteoma, and the increased COX-2 expression in osteoid osteoma [10, 14].

We report herein the details of two cases with histological features of osteoblastoma with distinct clinical and imaging characteristics. We will review case reports of osteoblastoma and osteoid osteoma in the maxilla and mandible. The literature search was conducted using PubMed and Google Scholar search. The search term for osteoblastoma literature was "osteoblastoma AND mandible OR jaw". The search term for osteoid osteoma literature was "osteoid osteoma AND mandible OR jaw". We will further discuss the ongoing debate over the similarities and differences between osteoblastoma and osteoid osteoma.

2. Case Presentation

2.1. Case #1

2.1.1. Clinical Presentation. A 37-year-old male presented to the clinic with pain in the left posterior mandible and preauricular area that had been progressively worsening over the past four months. Pain was managed with nonsteroidal anti-inflammatory drugs (NSAID) and acetaminophen at the time of initial exam.

Clinically, there were no changes to occlusion or paresthesias. The range of motion was within normal limits. Both intraoral and extraoral exam demonstrated swelling in the ascending ramus area of the left mandible with pain on palpation. All four wisdom teeth are impacted and not visible clinically. Probing depths were less than 4 mm in the lower left quadrant.

Past medical history is significant for treatment of a mandibular fracture 11 years prior to presentation with no complications but is otherwise noncontributory.

2.1.2. Imaging Features. Medical grade CT revealed a well-defined, mixed radiodensity lesion within the body of left mandible, measuring 1.6 × 2.1 × 2.0 cm. The lesion is located in the left posterior mandibular angle, involving the root of full bony impacted #17 and extending to the inferior third of the mandibular ramus. The internal structure was mixed but predominantly densely mineralized with a surrounding lucent halo. Buccal and lingual expansion, thinning, and areas of perforation at buccal and lingual cortices can be appreciated. There was a broad zone of reactive sclerotic bone surrounding this lesion (Figure 1). Large periosteal bone formation can be seen at buccal, lingual cortical, and inferior aspects of the lesion. The lucent rim of the lesion extends into the left mandibular canal, with potential involvement of the inferior alveolar nerve (Figure 1). Edema was noted within the adjacent masseter muscle (Figure 2).

2.1.3. Differential Diagnosis. Due to size and radiographic presentation, the differential diagnosis for this lesion in the

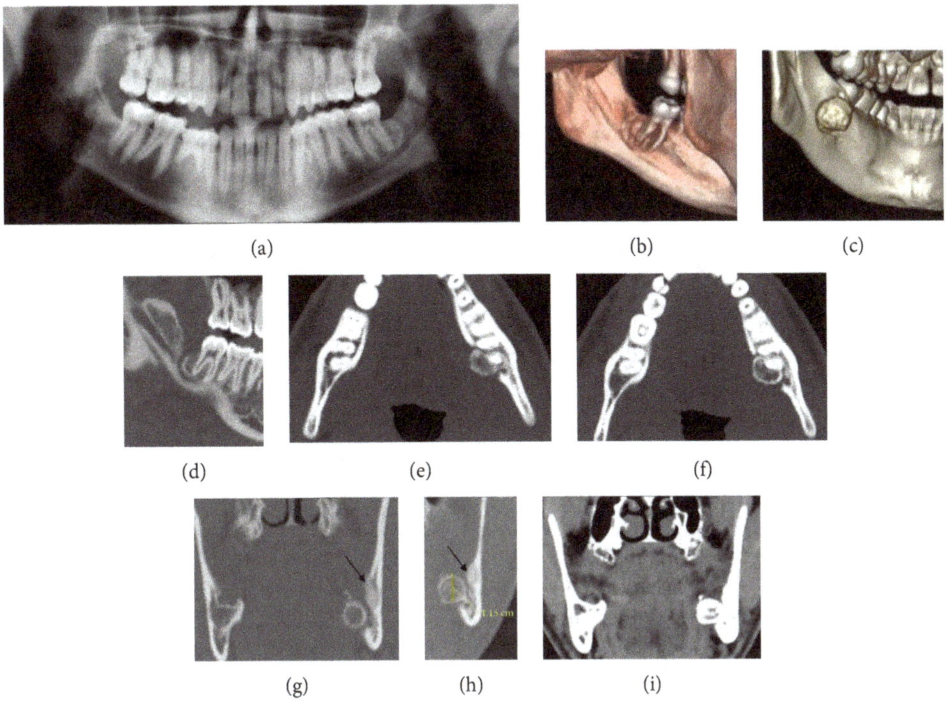

FIGURE 4: (a) Case #2 panoramic radiograph. (b and c) 3D CT reconstruction, viewed from the lingual aspect. (d) CBCT sagittal view. (e–f) Bone window CT axial views. (g–h) Bone window CT coronal views. (i) Soft tissue window CT coronal view. Panoramic radiograph was taken 8 months postsurgical extraction of the impacted tooth #17. An exophytic mixed density lesion, measuring $1.2 \times 1.0 \times 1.1$ cm, emanated from the distal root of tooth #18. The border of the lesion is well-demarcated with a sclerotic rim surrounded by a lucent rim. Small area of bony sclerosis is noted at buccal and superior of the lesion (arrows) (g and h). There was no evidence of root resorption at associated root of #18. Unlike case 1, there is no evidence of expansion, new bone formation, or adjacent soft tissue edema (i).

left posterior mandible includes osteoblastoma, osteosarcoma, osteoid osteoma, ossifying fibroma, focal cemento-osseous dysplasia or calcifying odontogenic cyst with odontoma. Radiographically, osteosarcoma usually presents with poorly delineated borders, making an osteosarcoma diagnosis less likely for the lesion in question. Given the large size of the lesion, a diagnosis of osteoid osteoma would be unlikely. Ossifying fibroma does not typically present with a wide zone of sclerotic bone formation as seen in this lesion. Due to the expansile nature of the lesion, focal cemento-osseous dysplasia is unlikely in this case.

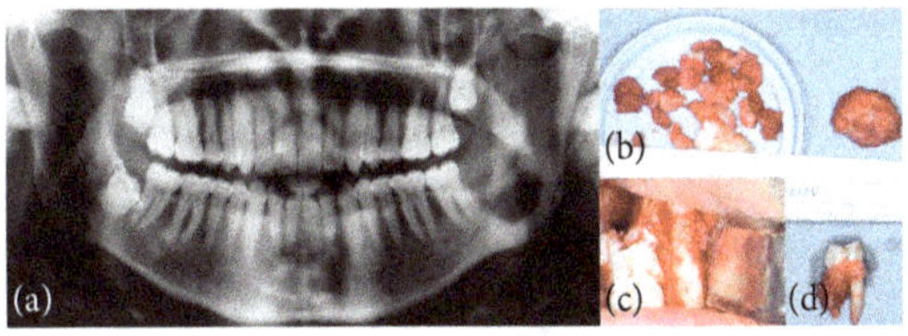

FIGURE 5: (a) Case #1 panoramic radiograph one month post excisional biopsy showing the lesion and #17 completely removed with bony sclerosis still visible. (b) Case #1 surgical specimen. (c) Case #1 intraoperative clinical photo. (d) Case #2 surgical specimen showing the lesion in association with the distal root of #18.

2.2. Case #2

2.2.1. Clinical Presentation. A 17-year-old male was referred to an oral surgeon for surgical extraction of complete bony impacted third molars (Figure 3(a)). For his third molar extractions, a full thickness mucoperiosteal flap was opened with crestal bone removal and buccal trough for delivery. The sockets were irrigated, and the surgeon reported no direct visualization of any adjacent structures. 4-0 chromic sutures were placed, and gauze packs were applied over sockets to obtain hemostasis. Eight days later, the patient returned for a post-op appointment where healing was within normal limits and pain levels were minimal. Three months after the initial follow-up appointment, the patient started feeling pain in the area of #17 that progressively worsened over the next 5 months.

Panoramic and CBCT imaging revealed a small well-circumscribed lesion distal and lingual of tooth #18 (Figures 4(a) and 4(d)). The oral surgeon did a surgical exploration of the area to obtain a biopsy of the tissue. The initial biopsy returned as fibrous tissue with retained foreign materials, stating that there was a "golden-brown pigmented material with lipid vacuoles likely represents an intrasocket medication."

The patient initially said he was feeling better after the surgical exploration, but by the next month, the pain had returned and was continually worsening. The patient was then referred to the Oral and Maxillofacial Surgery Department at the University of Washington for further evaluation and treatment. Upon exam at the University of Washington, the patient was found to have radiating pain to his ear. The

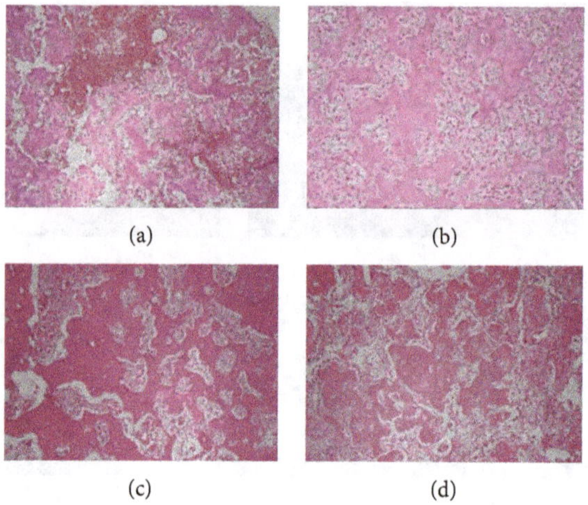

FIGURE 6: Histological features of case #1 (a and b). (a) Decalcified bone with evident reversal lines with prominent osteoblastic activity. Note the vascular connective tissue stroma with dilated blood vessels and hemorrhage (H&E stain, ×40). (b) A higher magnification of panel (a) showing the bone with prominent and large osteoblasts with abundant cytoplasm and epithelioid morphology (H&E stain, ×100). (c and d) Histological features of case #2. (c) Decalcified bone with reversal lines with prominent osteoblastic activity. Note the vascular connective tissue stroma with dilated blood vessels and small foci of hemorrhage (H&E stain, ×40). (d) A higher magnification of panel (c) showing the bone with prominent and large osteoblasts with abundant cytoplasm and vascular connective tissue stroma with dilated blood vessels and scattered erythrocytes (H&E stain, ×100).

TABLE 1: Characteristics of osteoblastoma and osteoid osteoma as previously summarized [7, 8, 10] comparing to current cases.

	Sex	Chief complaint	Imaging features	Size (cm)
Osteoblastoma [7, 8, 10]	M ≥ F	Mild to moderate pain. Less relief from aspirin (unlike osteoid osteoma).	Mixed to radiopaque, variable. Surrounded by sclerotic bone. Expansile, erosive. Arises in medullary bone.	≥1.5-2
Case #1	M	Progressively worsening pain and swelling. Pain managed by NSAID.	Mostly radiopaque mass. Surrounded by sclerotic bone. Expansile, erosive. Arises in medullary bone.	2.1
Osteoid osteoma [7, 8, 10]	M ≥ F	Moderate to severe pain. Progressive pain worsening at night and responds well to NSAIDs.	Lucent or mixed nidus. Surrounded by sclerotic bone. Arises in cortical bone.	<1.5-2
Case #2	M	Progressively worsening pain beginning 8 months post surgical extraction. Shooting pain worse at night and controlled with ibuprofen.	Lucent nidus with patchy mineralization. Arises in lingual cortex.	1

patient described it as "shooting nerve pain that gets worse at night." Patient reported intermittent vague swelling, but no bad taste. At this time, he was controlling the pain with ibuprofen. Intraoral examination revealed scar tissue at extraction site but no swelling, erythema, drainage, or abnormally appearing tissue (Figure 3(b)).

2.2.2. Imaging Features. Panoramic imaging 8 months post extraction when the patient began feeling pain in the area revealed a small mixed density lesion associated with the distal root of #18 which was not present in the panoramic image prior to #17 extraction (Figures 3(a) and 4(a)).

Cone beam CT image obtained by the oral surgeon prior to initial biopsy revealed a well-defined, mixed density lesion with a soft tissue capsule surrounding a cortical border on the distal and lingual aspects of #18. The lesion has eroded and expanded beyond the lingual cortical plate (Figure 4). No root resorption associated with #18 distal root was appreciated.

A medical CT scan was obtained several months after the CBCT to evaluate the changes from the CBCT as well as potential soft tissue involvement. Imaging revealed a 1.2 × 1.0 × 1.1 cm lesion emanated from the distal root of #18 that had eroded and expanded beyond the lingual cortical plate. A small area of bony sclerosis is noted at the buccal and superior aspects of the lesion. The lesion appeared similarly on bone window CT as the previous CBCT. There was no soft tissue involvement (Figure 4).

2.2.3. Differential Diagnosis. Given the radiographic findings and characteristic pain presentation, osteoid osteoma was considered to be high on the differential diagnosis followed by osteoblastoma. Close relation the distal root of #18 added cementoblastoma to the differential. However, the distal root

Table 2: Characteristics of previously reported osteoblastoma of the maxilla and mandible ($n = 29$).

Case	Author (year)	Age	Sex	Chief complaint	Site	Imaging features	Size (cm)
1	Yamada (2009) [23]	29	M	Pain, swelling	Maxilla, hard palate	Mixed density mass with narrow radiolucent zone	2
2*	Lin (2012) [24]	10	M	Pain, swelling	Mandible, anterior	Radiopaque mass with an irregular border and an ill-defined margin	4 × 3
3	Lin (2012) [24]	26	F	Pain	Mandible, anterior	Expansile, mixed radiolucent, and radiopaque lesion with a radiolucent rim	.5 × .5
4	Bokhari (2012) [25]	18	M	Swelling, slight pain	Maxilla	Well-circumscribed, radiopaque mixed with areas of radiolucency. Surrounded by a well-defined radiolucent rim. There was no reactive bone forming rim	3 × 2
5	Pérez (2012) [26]	7	F	Painless facial asymmetry	Mandible, body to condyle	Well-defined multilocular mass with honeycomb areas	NS
6	Rawal (2006) [27]	30	F	Pain	Mandible, body to parasymphysis	Well-defined radiolucency	2 × 2
7	Rawal (2006) [27]	31	F	Pain	Mandible, body	Well-defined radiolucency	2 × 2
8	Rawal (2006) [27]	16	M	Pain	Maxilla, canine to premolar	Well-defined radiolucency	5 × 4
9	Rawal (2006) [27]	29	F	Pain	Mandible, body	Poorly defined, mixed radiodensity	3 × 2
10†	Rawal (2006) [27]	18	F	Pain	Mandible, body	NS	5 × 5
11†	Rawal (2006) [27]	15	F	Pain	Mandible, body	Well-defined radiopaque	2 × 1 × 1
12†	Rawal (2006) [27]	78	M	Pain	Mandible, body	Soft tissue opacity overlying residual alveolus	2.5 × 1.75 × 1
13	Mahajan (2013) [28]	45	F	Swelling, lymphadenopathy	Mandible, posterior body	NS	5 × 3.5
14	More (2012) [16]	40	F	Swelling, hx of extraction	Mandible, posterior body	Well-defined compact trabecular pattern, with dense bone in certain areas of the lesion	4.5
15	Sheikh (2014) [29]	45	F	Pain and swelling	Mandible, posterior body	Mixed radiolucent-radiopaque lesion with sclerotic borders. Loss of trabeculation with normal surrounding bone	2 × 3.5
16	Shah (2013) [30]	7	M	Pain and swelling	Mandible, posterior body	Homogeneous radiopaque expansile. The adjacent tooth germs were displaced Recurrent: large well-defined mass composed of two locules with multiple internal calcifications	Original: 3.5 Recurrent: 2.5 × 2 × 1.5 and 3 × 3 × 1.5
17*	Kaur (2012) [31]	26	F	Pain and swelling	Mandible, posterior body	Well-delineated expansile radiolucency contained calcified mass and few radiopaque flecks scattered within the radiolucency. Expansion and thinning of the lower border of the mandible	3 × 3
18*	Castro (2016) [32]	7	F	Pain and swelling	Mandible, posterior body	Poorly defined mixed radiolucent-radiopaque	8
19*	Vinuth (2013) [33]	25	M	Pain and swelling	Mandible, posterior body	Ill-defined radiolucency with internal radiodensities	5 × 4
20*	Harrington (2011) [34]	25	M	Mild pain and swelling	Maxilla	Ill-defined radiolucency with internal radiodensities	4

Table 2: Continued.

Case	Author (year)	Age	Sex	Chief complaint	Site	Imaging features	Size (cm)
21	Woźniak (2010) [35]	30	M	Swelling	Mandible, body	Poorly marginated from adjacent tissue. Small, irregular radiolucent foci of bone destruction with a few patchy calcifications are visible centrally	4 × 5
22	Angiero (2006) [36]	24	M	Swelling	Mandible, posterior body	Poorly defined, "ground-glass" radiopaque lesion	1
23	Angiero (2006) [36]	8	M	Swelling, missing teeth	Maxilla	Mixed pattern of radiolucency and radiopacity	1.5
24**	Mardaleishvili (2014) [20]	12	F	Pain, swelling	Mandible, body	Well-defined, radiolucent with minimal calcification	3.5
25	Capodiferro (2005) [9]	16	F	Pain and swelling	Mandible, posterior body	Deformity of the bone architecture and containing large amounts of calcified material. The lesion is not associated with sclerotic borders or periosteal alteration	3
26	Capodiferro (2005) [9]	10	M	Pain and swelling	Mandible, body	NS	2.5
27	Capodiferro (2005) [9]	21	F	Pain and swelling	Mandible, body	NS	2
28	Capodiferro (2005) [9]	20	M	Pain and swelling	Mandible, posterior body	Radiolucent lesion of the left mandibular molar area, in close association with an unerupted tooth, with regular contours and containing fine calcifications	3
29	Capelozza (2005) [37]	8	M	Failure of eruption	Mandible, anterior	Ill-defined borders, displaying varied degrees of radiopacity, surrounded by a radiolucent halo	1 × 1

This summary does not include 67 osteoblastoma cases summarized by Jones et al. in 2006. *Aggressive osteoblastoma. †Periosteal osteoblastoma. **Lesions described as predominantly RL with some calcifications were classified as RL. NS: not stated; hx: history.

of #18 showed no evidence of root resorption making this diagnosis unlikely.

3. Treatment and Histopathology

Case #1 was treated with enucleation and full bony extraction of #17. The lesion was removed in pieces (Figures 5(b) and 5(c)). Cauterization was used to obtain hemostasis and the defect was closed using running 3-0 chromic sutures.

Panoramic radiograph obtained one month post excisional biopsy demonstrated complete removal of the lesion and #17 with evidence of bony sclerosis still visible (Figure 5(a)).

Case #2 was treated with enucleation, curettage, and extraction of #18. The site was irrigated and closed using multiple interrupted 3-0 chromic sutures. Adequate hemostasis was obtained with primary closure. Figure 5(d) depicts the surgical specimen, showing the lesion in association with the distal root of #18.

Histopathological interpretation of both biopsy samples obtained from excisional biopsy was consistent with osteoblastoma. Biopsy specimens were represented by multiple fragments of decalcified hard and soft tissue made up of bone at different stages of development (Figures 6(a), 6(c), and 6(d)), some mineralized with other areas made up of new bone formation. The mineralized bone showed reversal lines. All bone fragments showed prominent osteoblastic activity with abundant cytoplasm in some areas (Figures 6(a), 6(b), and 6(d)). Scattered osteoclastic activity was noted. The connective tissue stroma in both specimens was loose and vascular. It contained many dilated blood vessels and foci of hemorrhage (Figures 6(a), 6(b), and 6(d)).

4. Discussion and Literature Review

Though both cases presented were diagnosed as osteoblastoma histopathologically, they differ significantly in both clinical presentation and imaging characteristics. Taken together, case #1 is considered osteoblastoma and case #2 is considered osteoid osteoma (Table 1). It has been reported that clinical presentation, size, location, and imaging features are the most important factors in determining the definitive diagnosis of these two similar lesions [7]. The clinical and radiographic features of reported osteoblastoma and osteoid osteoma cases not included in the previous reviews by Jones et al. and An et al. are presented in Tables 2 and 3 [2, 12]. Table 4 summarizes the characteristics of all cases reviewed here (see Table 2 and Table 3), those reviewed by Jones et al., An et al., and our two new cases.

Clinically, both osteoblastoma and osteoid osteoma commonly present with pain; however, the pain pattern is specific for each neoplasm. Pain reported in osteoblastoma is described as dull, aching, and progressively worsening over time. It is thought to be caused by local expansion of

Table 3: Characteristics of previously reported osteoid osteoma of the maxilla and mandible (n = 12).

Case	Author (year)	Age	Sex	Chief complaint	Site	Imaging features	Size (cm)
1	Singh (2011) [13]	20	M	Radiating pain and swelling, hx of extraction	Mandible, posterior body	Well-defined radiopacity with a radiolucent rim showing a central radiopaque nidus surrounded by a radiolucent border	3.5
2	Mohammed (2013) [38]	20	NS	Pain and swelling, NSAIDs effective	Mandible, posterior body	Mixed radiopaque radiolucent lesion. The roots of the second premolar and the first molar appeared to be involved	3 × 2
3	Thopte (2018) [39]	21	M	Swelling, reduced mouth opening	Mandible, condyle	Solitary ill-defined homogeneous mixed radiopaque-radiolucency with a thin sclerotic border on the left mandibular condyle.	4.5 × 3
4	Matthies (2019) [40]	18	M	Pain, worse at night, response to NSAIDs	Mandible, posterior	Unclear tumor mass, radiopaque with lucent rim	.9x.8 × .5
5	Betz (2017) [15]	18	M	Swelling, slight pain	Mandible, posterior body	Well-defined, noncorticated borders and a surrounding radiolucency, internally radiodense material showed a laminated pattern, focal destruction of the cortical plate	1 × .6 × .6
6	Porto (2007) [41]	23	F	Severe pain nonresponsive to NSAIDs, limited opening	Mandible, condyle	Well-circumscribed and predominantly radiopaque	1.1 × .8
7	Infante-Cossio (2017) [42]	44	F	Mild pain worse at night, response to NSAIDs	Mandible, posterior body	Sclerotic lesion with a well delineated central calcified nidus surrounded by a radiolucent band and reactive sclerosis	1
8	Devathambi (2017) [43]	13	F	Dull progressive pain with response to NSAIDs	Mandible, posterior body and ramus	Well-defined radiopaque mass	1.4 × 1.5
9	Díaz-Rengifo (2019) [44]	69	F	Incidental finding	Maxilla	Well-delimited radiopaque mass	.5 × .8
10	Roscher (2018) [45]	21	M	Severe pain, swelling	Maxilla	Radiopaque lesion with a radiolucent core and peripheral reactive sclerosis	.5
11	Khaitan (2016) [46]	40	M	Pain, swelling, loose tooth, bleeding	Maxilla	Ill-defined homogenous periarticular radiolucency	2 × 1
12	Bajpai (2018) [47]	54	M	Pain, swelling	Mandible, posterior	Well-defined radiopaque w central radiolucency	NS

This summary does not include 21 osteoid osteoma cases summarized by An et al. in 2013. NS: not stated; hx: history.

the tumor and does not typically respond to treatment with NSAIDs [15]. A typical pain presentation of osteoid osteoma, seen in around 80% of patients, involves localized pain which worsens at night and is usually greatly relieved by the use of NSAIDs [2, 14]. The unique pain pattern of osteoid osteoma can be explained by an abundance of nerve fibers in the nidus matrix, elevated levels of prostaglandins, and increased expression of COX-2. These features are not found in osteoblastoma or other benign osseous lesions [7, 14]. The pain presentation of case #2 was consistent with a classic osteoid osteoma presentation endorsing worsening pain at night that was well controlled with NSAIDs. In our review, nocturnal pain was only reported in two of the 11 osteoid osteoma cases and one of the 31 osteoblastoma cases. The reason for the low incidence of nocturnal pain in case reports maybe due to underreporting by the clinicians or patients, which underscores the limitation of reviews of published case reports.

Another important difference between the two lesions is size. Osteoblastoma typically presents as >1.5-2 cm in diameter and is known for its tendency to cause bony expansion [7, 8]. The average size of osteoblastoma in our review was 2.97 cm (Table 4). Case #1 fits these criteria measuring 2.1 cm at its greatest dimension. Osteoid osteoma has a more limited growth potential, usually presenting smaller than 1.5-2 cm with the nidus generally <1 cm [7]. The average size of osteoid osteomas in our review was 1.16 cm (Table 4). Case #2 fits these criteria measuring at 1 cm in diameter.

The average age of patients in our review diagnosed with osteoid osteoma was similar but slightly older than those diagnosed with osteoblastoma with averages of 26.63 years and 22.76 years, respectively. This is consistent with previous reports of these lesions predominantly arising in the first and second decades of life [2, 10, 11]; however, rare case reports included older patients as well (Table 3). Male to female ratios were close to 1 : 1 for both lesion types,

Table 4: Summary of all reported cases of osteoblastoma and osteoid osteoma of the maxilla and mandible, including current cases.

		Osteoblastoma ($n = 97$)	Osteoid osteoma ($n = 33$)
Age, mean (range)		22.76 (3-78)	26.63 (4-77)
Male, female, NS		42, 55	16, 15, 2
Maxilla		22	7
Mandible	Posterior	56	19
	Anterior	12	1
	Condyle	7	6
Symptoms	Asymptomatic	7	3
	Pain	67	25
	Swelling	63	17
Size (cm), mean (range)		2.93 (0.5-5)	1.16 (0.4-4.5)
History of trauma	Yes	4	1
	NS	93	32
Radiographic description	Radiolucent	25	2
	Radiopaque	20	11
	Mixed	42	18
	Surrounding sclerosis	3	15
	NS	10	2

This summary excludes one case from An et al. in 2013 due to location on the temporal bone. NS: not stated.

differing from WHO classification which state a 2 : 1 male to female ratio [3, 4]. It is possible that the gender predilection for these lesions is different for the maxillofacial region than it is for the rest of the body.

Radiographically, most osteoblastoma and osteoid osteoma cases reviewed in Table 4 were described as mixed density. Lesions diagnosed as osteoblastoma were more likely to present as predominantly radiolucent than lesions diagnosed as osteoid osteoma. 25 osteoblastoma cases were reported as predominantly radiolucent compared to only two lesions diagnosed as osteoid osteoma. Lesions diagnosed as osteoid osteoma were more likely to have a surrounding area of sclerosis. As summarized in Table 4, sclerosis was seen in 15/33 (45%), of osteoid osteoma cases compared to only 3/97 (3%) of osteoblastoma cases. These findings are similar to previous reports [7, 10]. Of the lesions reviewed in Tables 2 and 3, 6 osteoblastoma and 4 osteoid osteoma cases were found to have an area of surrounding radiolucency. Cases reviewed by An et al. and Jones et al. did not include this information and therefore cannot be compared.

Case #1 demonstrated a unique degree of soft tissue edema in the adjacent masseter muscle as well as the extensive formation of new, reactive bone (Figures 1(c)–1(f) and 2). To the best of our knowledge, this is the first report of muscle edema and extensive new bone formation associated with osteoblastoma. These unusual features cannot be related to the aggressiveness of the tumor as histologic analysis did not indicate aggressive osteoblastoma. It is possible that soft tissue edema has been underreported in the past due to the choice of image modality.

The lesion in case #2 developed shortly after routine third molar extractions. While history of extraction has been reported in other cases of osteoblastoma and osteoid osteoma, the timing of this presentation is closer to time of extraction, occurring only 8 months after the procedure [13, 16]. It is possible that this lesion may have formed in response to third molar extraction or the associated healing process; however, there is a lack of evidence to justify this hypothesis. Other osteoblastoma cases, including case #1, have a history of nonspecific facial trauma which again may or may not be associated with the formation their lesions [11]. Many cases reviewed in this paper did not state whether or not there was a history of trauma. Given the anecdotal association, further investigation is required to determine if trauma is a contributing factor to the formation of these lesions.

With so few reports of these benign bony neoplasms available in the literature, misdiagnoses can be common and preoperative diagnoses are often variable. In 24 cases of osteoblastoma, Jones et al. found 37.5% of preoperative diagnoses to be a fibro-osseous process such as fibrous dysplasia, ossifying fibroma, or focal osseous dysplasia, 25% to be a bone tumor or bone disease, 20.8% to be an odontogenic cyst, 12.5% to have no preoperative diagnosis, and 4.2% to be a salivary gland neoplasm [2]. This initial misdiagnosis can be seen in case #2 where foreign body reaction was suspected from initial biopsy results.

The recommended treatment for osteoblastoma and osteoid osteoma can be very different, thus highlighting the importance of distinguishing between the two lesions despite similar histopathological features. Our reviews here as well as previous case reports support that osteoid osteoma and osteoblastoma can and should be distinguished from one another based on reported features [3, 4, 17]. For osteoid osteoma, nonsurgical management with NSAIDs is an option as it can effectively relieve pain in some cases [7]. There are few studies on the long-term effectiveness of nonsurgical management. Some studies have indicated that conservative treatments can be as effective as surgical management [18]. Some reports have even claimed that lesions can spontaneously regress while being treated nonsurgically with NSAIDs [19]. Osteoblastoma on the other hand is always treated surgically due to a lack of responsiveness to nonsurgical pain management and potential for aggressive behavior [20]. Though the relationship is not well understood, many have noted similarities between aggressive type osteoblastoma and osteosarcoma [1, 5, 21]. This relationship contributes to the urgency seen in treatment methods of osteoblastoma as compared to those of osteoid osteoma.

Recurrences of both lesions have been described in the literature. It has been found that osteoid osteomas recur slightly less often than osteoblastomas, with a recurrence rate of 4.5% compared to 9.8%, respectively [8]. Additionally, osteoblastoma may have other closely related lesions such as atypical sclerosing osteoblastic neoplasm that have an even higher recurrence rate of about 10-21% [14, 20]. To further complicate the relationship, there have been several reports of osteoid osteoma transforming into or recurring as osteoblastoma [1, 7, 22]. Some believe that osteoid osteoma is simply an immature osteoblastoma that happened to be discovered earlier in its developmental course. To the best of our knowledge, both cases #1 and #2 remain disease free today.

While the WHO still classifies osteoblastoma and osteoid osteoma as separate tumors, it has been recommended by some to reclassify these two neoplasms as single and separate disease processes [1–4]. Others suggest that the nomenclature should be changed to reflect distinct clinical presentations of the same pathological process [8]. Still more, some believe that the current classification should remain, keeping the neoplasms as separate entities. Further investigation of the benign bony lesions including clinical and radiographic presentation, location, size, demographics, history of trauma, and behavior is needed in order to better understand the relationship between osteoblastoma and osteoid osteoma. A better understanding of this relationship will aid in the diagnosis and management of these lesions in the maxillofacial region. In this paper, we shared two cases of osteoblastoma. They each had unique imaging and clinical characteristics as well as some previously unreported attributes. Along with the existing literature, these cases can contribute to the ongoing research, treatment, and debate behind these lesions.

Consent

Informed consent was obtained from all patients for which identifying information is included in this article.

References

[1] E. Barlow, A. M. Davies, W. P. Cool, D. Barlow, and D. C. Mangham, "Osteoid osteoma and osteoblastoma : novel histological and immunohistochemical observations as evidence for a single entity," *Journal of Clinical Pathology*, vol. 66, no. 9, pp. 768–774, 2013.

[2] A. C. Jones, T. J. Prihoda, J. E. Kacher, N. A. Odingo, P. D. Freedman, and S. Antonio, "Osteoblastoma of the maxilla and mandible : a report of 24 cases , review of the literature , and discussion of its relationship to osteoid osteoma of the jaws," *Oral Surgery, Oral Medicine, Oral Pathology, Oral Radiology, and Endodontology*, vol. 102, no. 5, pp. 639–650, 2006.

[3] C. Fletcher and V. Y. Jo, "WHO classification of soft tissue tumours: an update based on the 2013 (4th) edition," *Royal College of Pathologists of Australasia*, vol. 46, pp. 95–104, 2014.

[4] C. Fletcher, J. Bridge, P. Hogendoorn, and E. Al, *World Health Organisation classification of tumours. Pathology and genetics. Tumours of soft tissue and Bone*, World Health Organization, 4th edition, 2013.

[5] H. L. Jaffe, "Osteoid osteoma: a benign osteoblastic tumor composed of osteoid and atypical bone," *Archives of Surgery*, vol. 31, no. 5, pp. 709–728, 1935.

[6] H. Jaffe and L. Mayer, "An osteoblastic osteoid tissue-forming tumor of metacarpal bone," *Archives of Surgery*, vol. 24, no. 4, pp. 550–564, 1932.

[7] K. Atesok, B. Alman, E. Schemitsch, A. Peyser, and H. Mankin, "Osteoid Osteoma and Osteoblastoma," *Journal of the American Academy of Orthopaedic Surgeons*, vol. 19, no. 11, pp. 678–689, 2011.

[8] R. Jackson, F. Reckling, and F. Mantz, "Osteoid osteoma and Osteoblastoma," *Clinical Orthopaedics and Related Research*, vol. 128, pp. 303–313, 1977.

[9] S. Capodiferro, E. Maiorano, C. Giardina, M. G. Lacaita, M. L. Lo, and G. Favia, "Osteoblastoma of the mandible: clinicopathological study of four cases and literature review," *Head & Neck: Journal for the Sciences and Specialties of the Head and Neck*, vol. 27, no. 7, pp. 616–621, 2005.

[10] G. P. Nielsen and A. E. Rosenberg, "Update on bone forming tumors of the head and neck," *Head and Neck Pathology*, vol. 1, no. 1, pp. 87–93, 2007.

[11] M. S. Ahmed and A. L. Nwoku, "Benign osteoblastoma of the mandibular ramus : review of the literature and report of a case," *Journal of Oral and Maxillofacial Surgery*, vol. 58, no. 11, pp. 1310–1317, 2000.

[12] S. An, H. Shin, K. Choi et al., "Unusual osteoid osteoma of the mandible : report of case and review of the literature," *Oral Surgery, Oral Medicine, Oral Pathology and Oral Radiology*, vol. 116, no. 2, pp. e134–e140, 2013.

[13] A. Singh and M. C. Solomon, "Osteoid osteoma of the mandible: a case report with review of the literature," *Journal of Dental Sciences*, vol. 12, no. 2, pp. 185–189, 2017.

[14] D. V. Mungo, X. Zhang, R. J. O. Keefe, R. N. Rosier, J. E. Puzas, and E. M. Schwarz, "COX-1 and COX-2 expression in osteoid osteomas," *Journal of Orthopaedic Research*, vol. 20, no. 1, pp. 159–162, 2002.

[15] S. J. Betz, Z. Lim, A. D. Flores-hidalgo, R. J. Riggs, and A. E. Curran, "Tender swelling of the posterior mandible," *Oral surgery, oral medicine, oral pathology and oral radiology*, vol. 124, no. 4, pp. 327–332, 2017.

[16] C. B. More, S. K. Das, K. S. Bhavsar, and M. N. Tailor, "Benign osteoblastoma- an unusual rare clinical presentation," *Journal of Advanced Oral Research*, vol. 3, no. 1, pp. 21–24, 2012.

[17] F. Schajowicz, H. A. Sissons, and L. H. Sobin, "The World Health Organization's histologic classification of bone tumors A commentary on the second edition," *Cancer Journal*, vol. 75, pp. 1208–1214, 1995.

[18] J. Kinsel and M. Simon, "Medical management compared with operative treatment for osteoid-osteoma," *Journal of Bone and Joint Surgery*, vol. 74, no. 2, pp. 179–185, 1992.

[19] T. Goto, Y. Shinoda, T. Okuma et al., "Administration of non-steroidal anti-inflammatory drugs accelerates spontaneous healing of osteoid osteoma," *Archives of Orthopaedic and Trauma Surgery*, vol. 131, no. 5, pp. 619-625, 2011.

[20] K. Mardaleishvili, Z. Kakabadze, A. Machavariani et al., "Benign osteoblastoma of the mandible in a 12-year-old female: a case report," *Oncology Letters*, vol. 8, no. 6, pp. 2691–2694, 2014.

[21] K. E. Mchugh, J. D. Reith, D. R. Lucas, C. L. Emory, N. W. Mesko, and S. E. Kilpatrick, "Atypical "sclerosing" osteoblastic neoplasm: a tumor of intermediate biological potential between usual osteoblastoma and conventional osteosarcoma," *The American Journal of Surgical Pathology*, vol. 43, no. 5, pp. 610–617, 2019.

[22] M. B. Bruneau, M. Polivka, J. F. Cornelius, and B. George, "Progression of an osteoid osteoma to an osteoblastoma," *Journal of Neurosurgery. Spine*, vol. 3, no. 3, pp. 238–241, 2005.

[23] S. Yamada, G. Kawasaki, N. Shiraishi et al., "Osteoblastoma in the maxilla : report of a case," *Oral Medicine & Pathology*, vol. 14, no. 1, pp. 37–40, 2009.

[24] B. Lin, Z. G. Cai, G. Y. Yu, and L. F. Jia, "A report of 2 cases and literature review," *Chinese Journal of Dental Research*, vol. 15, no. 2, pp. 153–158, 2012.

[25] K. Bokhari, M. S. Hameed, M. Ajmal, and R. A. Togoo, "Benign osteoblastoma involving maxilla: a case report and review of the literature," *Case Reports in Dentistry*, vol. 2012, Article ID 351241, 4 pages, 2012.

[26] P. C. Pérez and J. J. Segura, "Osteoblastoma of mandible," *International Journal of Surgical Pathology*, vol. 20, no. 4, pp. 375-376, 2012.

[27] Y. B. Rawal, F. Angiero, C. M. Allen, J. R. Kalmar, P. P. Sedghizadeh, and A. M. Steinhilber, "Gnathic osteoblastoma: Clinicopathologic review of seven cases with long-term follow-up," *Oral Oncology*, vol. 42, no. 2, pp. 123–130, 2006.

[28] A. Mahajan, P. Kumar, K. Desai, and R. P. Kaul, "Osteoblastoma in the retromolar region - report of an unusual case and review of literature," *Journal of Oral and Maxillofacial Surgery*, vol. 12, no. 3, pp. 338–340, 2013.

[29] S. Sheikh, S. Pallagatti, I. Singla, S. Kaur, and A. Aggarwal, "Osteoblastoma of mandible : a case report," *Journal of Pioneering Medical Sciences*, vol. 4, no. 2, pp. 60–63, 2014.

[30] S. Shah, J. Kim, K. Huh, W. Yi, M. Heo, and S. Lee, "Recurrent osteoblastoma of the maxilla," *Dentomaxillofacial Radiology*, vol. 42, no. 5, pp. 20100263–20100266, 2013.

[31] H. Kaur, S. Verma, M. K. Jawanda, and A. Sharma, "Aggressive osteoblastoma of the mandible : a diagnostic dilemma," *Dental Research Journal*, vol. 9, no. 3, pp. 334–337, 2012.

[32] P. H. S. Castro, D. L. Molinari, H. Q. Stateri, A. H. Borges, and L. E. R. Volpato, "Agressive osteoblastoma in a seven-year-old girl's mandible: treatment and six-year monitoring," *International Journal of Surgery Case Reports*, vol. 27, no. 27, pp. 5–9, 2016.

[33] D. P. Vinuth, P. Agarwal, D. Gadewar, G. Dube, and R. Dhirawni, "A large multifocal aggressive osteoblastoma of mandible: an immunohistochemistry case study report," *Journal of Dental Research, Dental Clinics, Dental Prospects*, vol. 8, no. 1, pp. 51–55, 2014.

[34] C. Harrington, B. T. Accurso, J. R. Kalmar et al., "Aggressive osteoblastoma of the maxilla : a case report and review of the literature," *Head and Neck Pathology*, vol. 5, no. 2, pp. 165–170, 2011.

[35] A. W. Woźniak, M. Tomasz, K. Osmola, and W. Golusinski, "Malignant transformation of an osteoblastoma of the mandible : case report and review of the literature," *European Archives of Oto-Rhino-Laryngology*, vol. 267, no. 6, pp. 845–849, 2010.

[36] F. Angiero, P. Mellone, A. Baldi, and M. Stefani, "Osteoblastoma of the jaw : report of two cases and review of the literature," *In Vivo*, vol. 20, pp. 665–670, 2006.

[37] A. A. Capelozza, M. G. Dezotti, L. C. Alvares, R. N. Fleury, and E. Sant'Ana, "Osteoblastoma of the mandible : systematic review of the literature and report of a case," *Dentomaxillofacial Radiology*, vol. 34, no. 1, pp. 1–8, 2005.

[38] I. Mohammed, N. A. Jannan, and A. E. Osteoid, "Osteoid osteoma associated with the teeth : unusual presentation," *International Journal of Oral and Maxillofacial Surgery*, vol. 42, no. 2, pp. 298–302, 2013.

[39] S. Thopte, N. Harchandani, S. U. Nisa, and R. Rochani, "Osteoid osteoma of the mandibular condyle : a diagnostic dilemma," *Contemporary Clinical Dentistry*, vol. 9, no. 4, pp. 652–655, 2018.

[40] L. Matthies, T. I. M. Rolvien, T. J. Pakusa et al., "Osteoid osteoma of the mandible – clinical and histological findings," *Anticancer Research*, vol. 39, no. 1, pp. 291–296, 2019.

[41] B. C. Vasconcelos, G. G. Porto, and R. V. Bessa-Nogueira, "Rare benign tumors of the mandibular condyle: report of 2 cases and literature review," *Journal of Oral and Maxillofacial Surgery*, vol. 65, no. 9, pp. 1830–1835, 2007.

[42] P. Infante-Cossio, A. Restoy-Lozano, and F. Espin-Galves, "Mandibular osteoid osteoma," *The Journal of Emergency Medicine*, vol. 52, no. 3, pp. e83–e84, 2017.

[43] T. J. R. Devathambi, W. C. Ambrose, K. Z. T. M. Niazi, and S. Raja, "Osteoid osteoma in anterior border of ramus of mandible: a rare entity," *Journal of Indian Academy of Oral Medicine and Radiology*, vol. 28, no. 4, pp. 449–452, 2016.

[44] I. A. Díaz-Rengifo, A. J. Díaz-caballero, and K. R. Oro, "Painless osteoid osteoma in the maxilla of an elderly female patient," *Journal of Oral and Maxillofacial Pathology*, vol. 23, no. 2, pp. 280–283, 2019.

[45] D. Roscher, M. Belossi, M. Paparella, and F. Stolbizer, "Osteoid osteoma of the maxilla : literature review and case report," *Journal of Dental Applications*, vol. 5, no. 1, pp. 399–402, 2018.

[46] T. Khaitan, P. Ramaswamy, U. Ginjupally, and A. Kabiraj, "A bizarre presentation of osteoid osteoma of maxilla," *Iranian Journal of Pathology*, vol. 11, no. 5, pp. 431–434, 2016.

[47] M. Bajpai and N. Pardhe, "Osteoid osteoma of jaw in a 54-year male," *Journal of the College of Physicians and Surgeons–Pakistan*, vol. 28, no. 6, p. 498, 2018.

12

Angiofibroma of the Mandible: Report of a Rare Case

Mohammed A. AlZayer, [1] **Ali Matouq AlMarzouq**, [1] **Zahrah Hasan Al-Faraj**, [2] **and Eman F. Al-Saleh** [3]

[1] *Dammam Medical Complex, Saudi Arabia*
[2] *Qatif Central Hospital, Saudi Arabia*
[3] *Dammam regional lab and blood bank, Saudi Arabia*

Correspondence should be addressed to Mohammed A. AlZayer; maz1203@hotmail.com

Academic Editor: Darko Macan

Angiofibroma is an uncommon, highly vascular benign lesion that occurs in the head and neck region, typically arising in the nasopharyngeal area, potentially with a locally aggressive course. Angiofibroma with a primary intraoral presentation is extremely rare; few case reports have been published in the literature, with only three cases of angiofibroma in the mandible published to date. In this case, a 37-year-old man presented with swelling at the right mandible and underwent enucleation of the lesion under general anesthesia. After 1-year follow-up, there were no signs of recurrence.

1. Introduction

Angiofibroma is a rare, benign, highly vascularized tumor that commonly presents during male adolescence. Its origin is unknown [1]. It typically arises in the nasopharyngeal area but can develop in extrapharyngeal sites, the most common of which is the maxillary sinus [2]. Although angiofibroma is histologically a benign lesion, it is locally invasive and has a propensity for local extension into adjacent anatomic structures, including the oral cavity [3]. Few cases have been published reporting angiofibroma with a primary intraoral origin [1, 4, 5], with only three cases of angiofibroma in the mandible published to date [4, 6, 7].

2. Presentation of Case

The patient (37 years old; male) presented with swelling of the right posterior mandibular area. He had a clear medical history. He complained of a small, dark blue-colored localized swelling at the area of the attached gingiva between teeth numbers 45 and 46 for 24 days before he went to a general dentist. An antibiotic was prescribed for five days, but his condition did not improve, so the dentist decided to extract tooth number 46. After extraction, the swelling started to gradually increase until it occupied the buccal vestibule. He noted pus and bleeding from the mass. Extraoral examination revealed significant swelling on the right side of the face that extended from the inferior border of the mandible to the level of the zygoma (Figure 1). Swelling was soft and fluctuant; no drainage or change in skin color was noted. All facial nerve branches were functioning well.

The patient had no history of paresthesia related to the inferior alveolar or lingual nerve. Intraorally, a huge mass was found to occupy the right buccal vestibular area. It was firm, measured $5 \times 5 \times 3$ cm, red in color, covered with a whitish film, and pedunculated from the extraction socket, with ulceration noted at the level of the occlusal table due to mastication (Figure 2(a)). Orthopantogram revealed a unilocular radiolucency at the right mandible, periapical to the lower right first and second molar area (3 cm in the

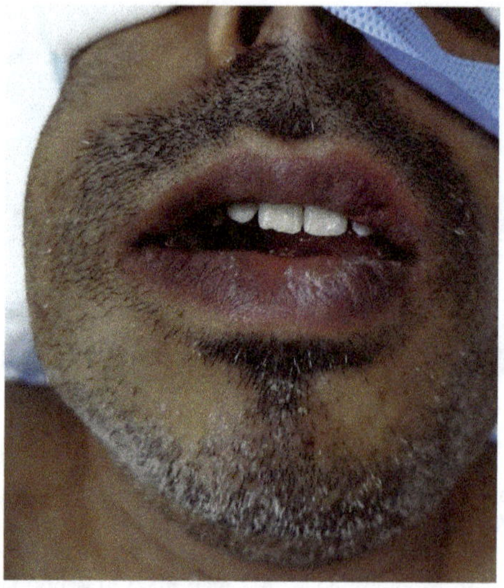

FIGURE 1: Extraoral photograph of the patient showing swelling on right side of the face.

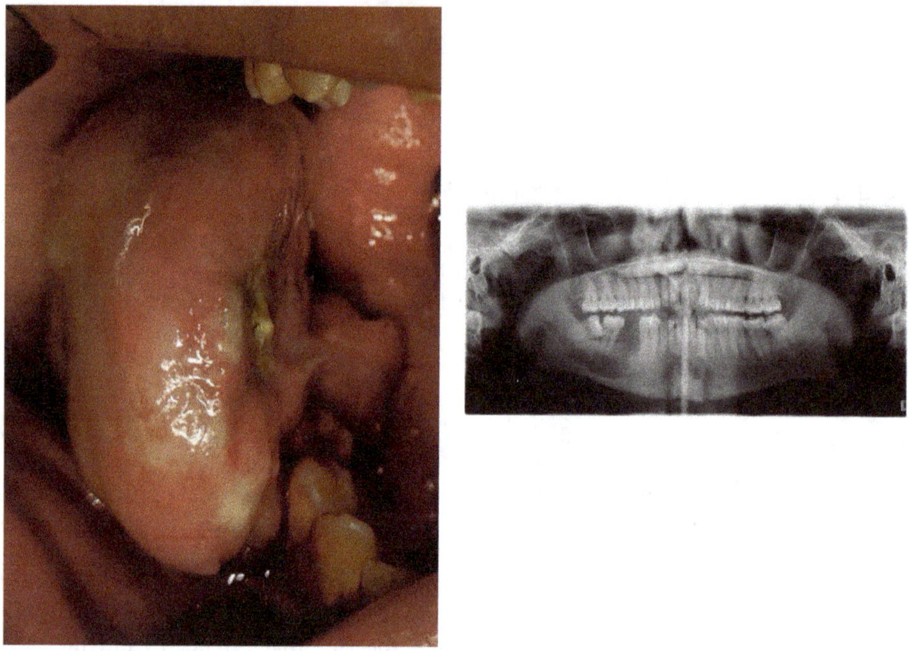

(a) (b)

FIGURE 2: (a) Intraorally, the lesion obliterated the right buccal vestibule. (b) Orthopantogram revealed a unilocular radiolucency at the right mandible.

anterior-posterior dimension) (Figure 2(b)).

Incisional biopsy was performed, and the extraosseous portion was excised and sent for histopathological assessment. Bleeding was encountered during the biopsy, which was controlled by local measures (Surgicel and suture). At the 1-week follow-up visit, the mass had grown again and reached its previous size.

Histopathological findings were suggestive of angiofibroma. Microscopy revealed an ulcerated, markedly inflamed squamous epithelial mucosa with underlying proliferation of fibrous tissue with interspersed abundant vascular channels. The vascular channels had architectural variability from the small capillaries to the sinusoidal ectatic vessels, to the larger vessels of venous type with distinct muscle layer. The fibrous stroma consisted of abundant collagen fibers of variable density and stellate or ovoid spindle cells with a fibroblastic/myofibroblastic appearance (Figure 3).

Computed tomography (CT) angiography was performed to assess lesion vascularity. No obvious large vascular channel supplying the lesion was detected. A large venous tributary in the vicinity of the lesion was observed

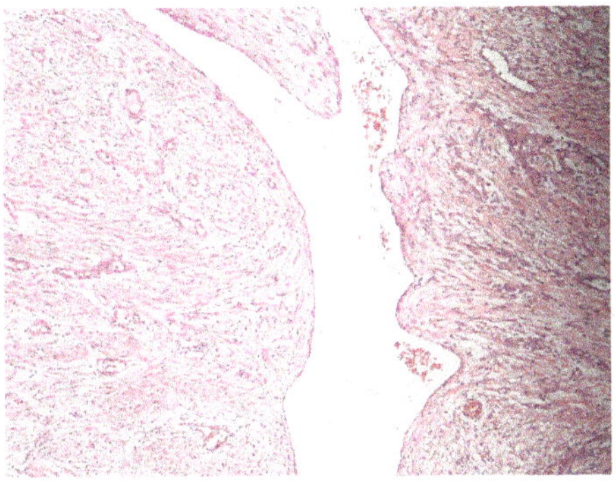

Figure 3: Hematoxylin and eosin stain (H&E) showing the proliferation of fibrous tissue with abundant variably sized vascular channels interspersed among the spindle cells in background, consistent with the diagnosis of angiofibroma (10x).

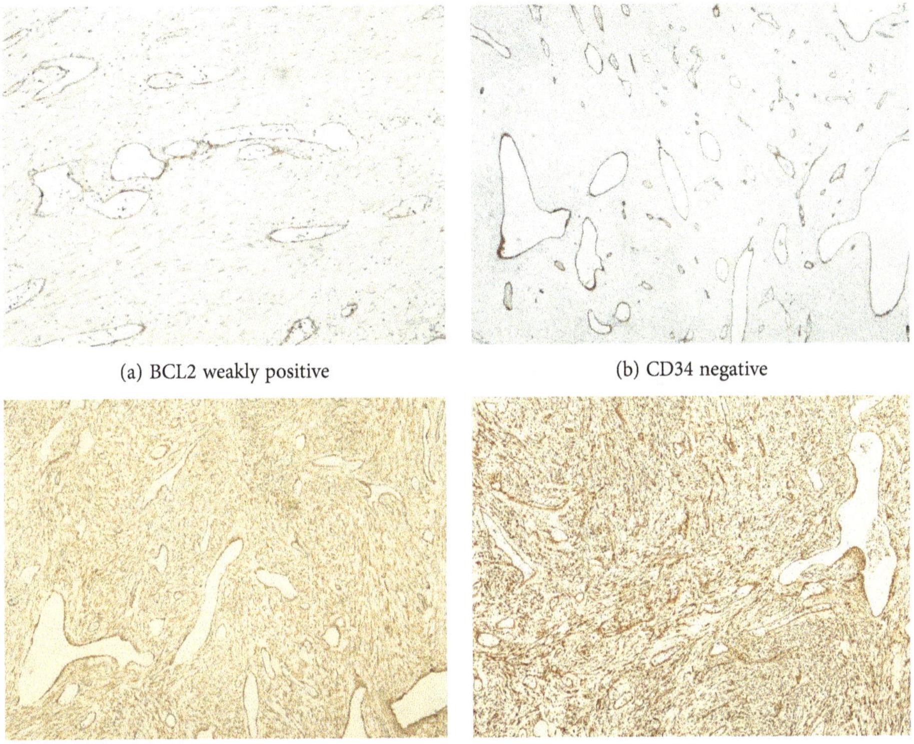

(a) BCL2 weakly positive

(b) CD34 negative

(c) SMA positive

(d) Vimentin positive

Figure 4: Immunohistochemical analysis using different stains.

to be draining into the right external jugular vein. A bony perforation at the lingual side was associated with enhanced soft tissue component.

The decision was made to perform enucleation of the lesion under general anesthesia. The patient was in the supine position during the operation and received oral intubation; hypotensive general anesthesia was applied. Excision of the extraosseous part was performed along with enucleation of the intraosseous lesion. The surgery was uneventful, and the lesion was easily detached from the bone with no adhesion noted. Encountered bleeding was controlled using cautery and bone wax. The wound was closed primarily. The final histopathological report confirmed the presence of angiofibroma and provided the same histopathological description. Immunohistochemical analysis using different stains has been performed to confirm the diagnosis. The lesional cells were positive for vimentin, smooth muscle actin, and Bcl2 and negative for Ck AE1/AE3, desmin, CD34, and S100Prot (Figures 4(a)–4(d)).

The patient received regular follow-up (1 week, 2 weeks, 1 month, 3 months, 6 months, and 1 year). Healing was within normal limits, and no recurrence of overgrowth, swelling, or discharge has been observed (Figure 5).

At 1-year follow-up, CT with contrast and CT angiogram were performed to confirm no recurrence and no arterial or venous regrowth. The report concluded the presence of bone defect with no soft tissue component and no abnormal arterial or venous enhancement. Comparing the

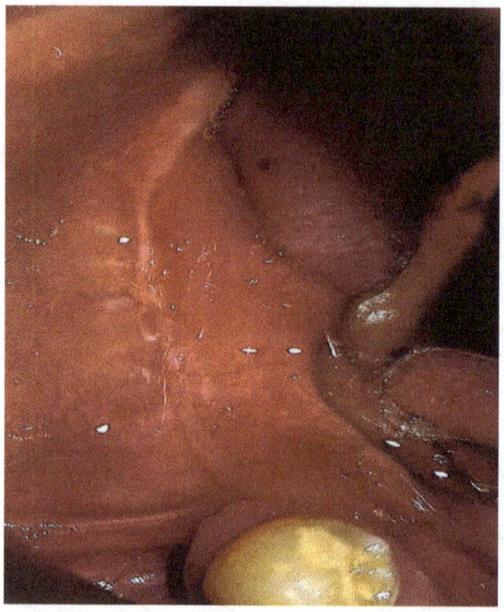

FIGURE 5: One-year postoperative intraoral photograph.

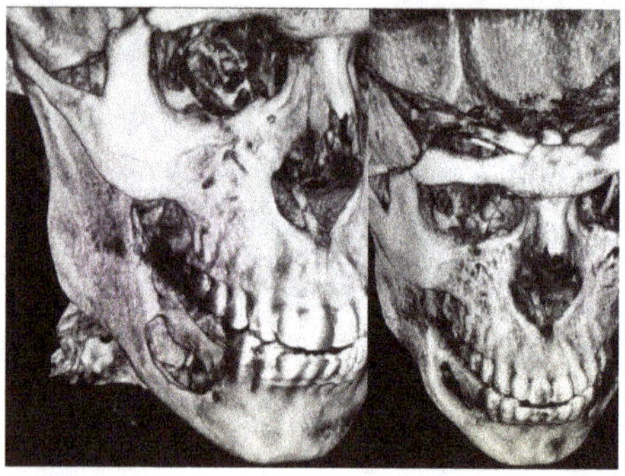

FIGURE 6: Preoperative and one-year postoperative 3D CT scan.

TABLE 1: Comparing the previously published case with our case.

	Ul Khaliq et al. [4]	May et al. [6]	Amini-Salari et al. [7]	Our case
Age	16 years	18 years	23 years	37 years
Gender	Female	Male	Male	Male
Location	Right mandibular first premolar to the right mandibular third molar region	Right condyle	Left mandibular ramus	Right mandibular body
Size	Not mentioned	Not mentioned	1.8 cm × 0.7 cm × 4.1 cm	3 cm × 3 cm
Treatment	Surgical excision	Percutaneous cryoablation	Enucleation	Enucleation
Follow-up	1 year	1 year	6 months	1 year

preoperative CT with the 1-year postoperative CT, bone regeneration was noted, and only a small portion of the inferior border defect remained (Figure 6).

3. Discussion

The significance of this report lies in the rarity of the presence of angiofibroma, which commonly occurs in the nasopharynx, in the mandible.

The etiology of angiofibroma is unclear. Theories about the origin and histogenesis of angiofibroma vary (i.e., developmental, hormonal imbalance, and genetic causes) [8].

Angiofibroma are rare tumors of the maxillofacial region, accounting for 0.05% of head and neck tumors [9]. The presence of angiofibroma in the mandible is extremely rare; only a few cases have been published reporting the presence of angiofibroma in the lower jaw (Table 1) [4, 6, 7].

It is suspected that ectopic tissue may be located farther away from the usual place and may have been the cause of the extranasopharyngeal location [8]. Histologically, tumor has a basic characteristic pattern and is derived from two equally important components: vascular network and connective tissue stroma. Vessels typically vary in size and are irregularly shaped [10].

Nasopharyngeal angiofibromas in the head and neck area usually arise in adolescent males [11]. In their literature review, Ali and Jones compared nasopharyngeal angiofibroma incidence with extrapharyngeal angiofibroma between patients of different sex and age distributions and found that nasopharyngeal angiofibroma is correlated with both age and sex. That is, they found that tumors are seen almost exclusively in males, and their appearance during the second decade of life is one of their most characteristic features. However, they also reported that extranasopharyngeal angiofibromas do not follow the same characteristic age distribution and sex incidence of nasopharyngeal angiofibromas [12]. In 2004, Windfuhr and Remmert evaluated extrapharyngeal angiofibroma incidence and found that patients were older as compared with patient with nasopharyngeal angiofibroma [11].

Depending on the size and location of the angiofibroma, different treatment modalities are available. Most physicians agree that surgery is the primary treatment modality for early-stage disease [13]. Preoperative angiography is the best tool for depicting the vascularization of juvenile angiofibroma, which predominantly receives its vascular supply via the external carotid artery system [14].

In our case, no embolization was planned, as there was no obvious large vascular channel supplying the lesion. No serious bleeding was encountered during the operation. Some authors have reported the successful surgical treatment of juvenile angiofibroma with acceptable blood loss without embolization [3, 5, 14].

Some researchers advised resection to prevent recurrence [5, 8]. Most recurrences produce symptoms within 1 year after treatment, and recurrence is uncommon beyond two years after surgery [15]. No recurrence was noted in our case after 1 year. A similar result has been reported in other studies [4, 6, 7].

Other treatment modalities include radiation therapy, cryotherapy, hormone therapy, embolization, arterial ligation, and sclerosing agent use [16]. May et al. recently reported the use of percutaneous cryoablation for an 18-year-old man who presented with a right condylar angiofibroma with complete recovery and no recurrence after 1-year follow-up [6].

4. Conclusion

The significance of this report lies in the rarity of the presence of angiofibroma, which commonly occurs in the nasopharynx at young age, in the mandible. Although exceedingly rare, angiofibroma should be considered one of the differential diagnoses of a lesion that arises in the mandible.

Consent

Patient provided his consent for the publication of this report.

Acknowledgments

I would like to thank Dr. Ali Al Jishi and Dr. Nawaf Al Mustafa for their kind help and support.

References

[1] T. E. Kabot, M. E. Goldman, S. Bergman, and R. D. Schwartz, "Juvenile nasopharyngeal angiofibroma: an unusual presentation in the oral cavity," *Oral Surgery, Oral Medicine, Oral Pathology*, vol. 59, no. 5, pp. 453–457, 1985.

[2] K. K. Handa, A. Kumar, M. K. Singh, and A. H. Chhabra, "Extranasopharyngeal angiofibroma arising from the nasal septum," *International Journal of Pediatric Otorhinolaryngology*, vol. 58, no. 2, pp. 163–166, 2001.

[3] K. Antoniades, D. Z. Antoniades, and V. Antoniades, "Juvenile angiofibroma: report of a case with intraoral presentation," *Oral Surgery, Oral Medicine, Oral Pathology, Oral Radiology, and Endodontology*, vol. 94, no. 2, pp. 228–232, 2002.

[4] M. I. Ul Khaliq, A. A. Shah, and N. Dar, "A rare case of angiofibroma of the mandible: a case report," *Journal of Oral Biology and Craniofacial Research*, vol. 6, no. 2, pp. 168–170, 2016.

[5] S. Capodiferro, G. Favia, M. G. Lacaita, L. Lo Muzio, and E. Maiorano, "Juvenile angiofibroma: report of a case with primary intra-oral presentation," *Oral Oncology Extra*, vol. 41, no. 1, pp. 1–6, 2005.

[6] L. May, J. Blatter, P. Bize, G. Tsoumakidou, A. Denys, and M. Broome, "Percutaneous cryoablation of benign bony tumours of the mandible," *British Journal of Oral and Maxillofacial Surgery*, vol. 58, pp. 75–78, 2020.

[7] A. Amini-Salari, K. Glomski, D. Ahn, and R. J. Tannyhill 3rd., "Mandibular intraosseous angiofibroma-a rare clinical entity," *Journal of Oral and Maxillofacial Surgery*, vol. 78, pp. 1343–1348, 2020.

[8] Y. Akbas and Y. Anadolu, "Extranasopharyngeal angiofibroma of the head and neck in women," *American Journal of Otolaryngology*, vol. 24, pp. 413–416, 2003.

[9] C. N. Patterson, "Juvenile nasopharyngeal angiofibroma," *Otolaryngologic Clinics of North America*, vol. 6, no. 3, pp. 839–861, 1973.

[10] S. S. Sternberg, "Pathology of juvenile nasopharyngeal angiofibroma; a lesion of adolescent males," *Cancer*, vol. 7, no. 1, pp. 15–28, 1954.

[11] J. P. Windfuhr and S. Remmert, "Extranasopharyngeal angiofibroma: etiology, incidence and management," *Acta Oto-Laryngologica*, vol. 124, pp. 880–889, 2004.

[12] S. Ali and W. I. Jones, "Extranasopharyngeal angiofibromas. Sex incidence and age distribution," *The Journal of Laryngology & Otology*, vol. 96, pp. 559–565, 1982.

[13] J. M. Hodges, A. S. McDevitt, A. I. El-Sayed Ali, and M. E. Sebelik, "Juvenile nasopharyngeal angiofibroma: current treatment modalities and future considerations," *Indian Journal of Otolaryngology and Head & Neck Surgery*, vol. 62, pp. 236–247, 2010.

[14] G. Bertazzoni, A. Schreiber, M. Ferrari, and P. Nicolai, "Contemporary management of juvenile angiofibroma," *Current Opinion in Otolaryngology & Head & Neck Surgery*, vol. 27, pp. 47–53, 2019.

[15] J. G. Batsakis, *Tumors of the Head and Neck: Clinical Pathological Considerations*, Williams & Wilkins Co, Baltimore, 2nd edition, 1979.

[16] B. W. Jafek, A. M. Nahum, R. M. Butler, and P. H. Ward, "Surgical treatment of juvenile nasopharyngeal angiofibroma," *The Laryngoscope*, vol. 83, no. 5, pp. 707–720, 1973.

13

Simultaneous Oral and Umbilical Locations as a First Sign of Pemphigus Vulgaris

Eya Moussaoui, [1,2] Yassine Oueslati, [1,2] Lamia Oualha, [1,2] Mohamed Denguezli, [3] Badreddine Sriha, [4] and Nabiha Douki [1,2]

[1] *Department of Dental Medicine, Sahloul Hospital (Sousse), Dental Faculty of Monastir, University of Monastir, Tunisia*
[2] *Laboratory of Oral Health and Maxillofacial Rehabilitation (LR12ES11), University of Monastir, Tunisia*
[3] *Dermatology Department, Farhat Hached Hospital (Sousse), University of Sousse, Tunisia*
[4] *Cytology and Pathological Anatomy Department, Farhat Hached Hospital (Sousse), University of Sousse, Tunisia*

Correspondence should be addressed to Eya Moussaoui; eyamouss@gmail.com, Yassine Oueslati; oueslati.yassine1991@hotmail.com, Lamia Oualha; lamia.oualha@gmail.com, Mohamed Denguezli; denguezli@yahoo.fr, Badreddine Sriha; badrisriha@gmail.com, and Nabiha Douki; nabiha.douki@gmail.com

Academic Editor: Rui Amaral Mendes

The place of pemphigus vulgaris (PV) among autoimmune bullous diseases (AIBD) is well established. It is an acquired chronic, autoimmune, vesiculobullous disease in which IgG antibodies target desmosomal proteins to produce intraepithelial mucocutaneous blistering. The diagnosis is often challenging for the clinicians. It requires a combination of three major features: clinical, histopathological, and immunological. Clinically, oral lesions are the first manifestations of the disease in 50-90% of the patients with widespread blisters affecting the oral mucosa. On the skin, lesions are characterized by flaccid blisters that rapidly progress into erosions and crust formation. Umbilical lesions as a clinical manifestation of PV are peculiar and have rarely been reported, and they are not yet completely elucidated. Umbilical region involvement in patients with pemphigus was assessed in a limited study totalling just 10 patients. This localisation may be a valuable hint easing the diagnosis at the clinical level for patients with oral mucosal blisters. Dentists must be familiar with the clinical manifestations of PV to make an early diagnosis and start an early treatment which determines the prognosis of the disease. To the best of the authors' knowledge, the coexistence of these lesions with the oral lesions as a first sign of PV in the absence of skin involvement was reported in only one case of pemphigus vegetans (PVe). In this paper, we describe an observation of a female patient that was diagnosed with PV that begun with simultaneous oral and umbilical locations which coexisted for a period of 4 months before the appearance of other cutaneous lesions. We highlight the role of dentists, by being familiar with the clinical manifestations of PV, to make an early diagnosis to start an early treatment which determines the prognosis of the disease and to follow closely the evolution of lesions to change treatment if required. We also discuss the clinical, histological, and immunological features of the disease that enabled the differential diagnosis as well as the appropriate therapeutic management.

1. Introduction

Autoimmune bullous diseases (AIBD) constitute a heterogeneous group of diseases that are at the same time very diverse, infrequent, and of variable prognosis, sometimes pejorative. The place of pemphigus vulgaris (PV) among this group is well established. It is an acquired chronic, autoimmune, vesiculobullous disease in which IgG antibodies target desmosomal proteins (Desmogleins 1 and 3) to produce intraepithelial mucocutaneous blistering [1]. It owes its name to the Greek word "pemphix" which means blister and was first used by Hippocrates in 460-370 B.C. [2]. It is a rare disease with an estimated worldwide annual incidence between 1 and 5 per million [3]. It occurs in all racial and ethnic groups with the highest incidence seen in Ashkenazi Jewish, Mediterranean, Indian, Malaysian, Chinese, and Japanese descent [4]. Occurrence is most common during the fifth and sixth decades of life, although a few cases have been reported in children [5].

Diagnosis of PV is often challenging for the clinicians. It requires a combination of three major features: clinical, histopathological, and immunological, which represent the gold standard for autoimmune blistering diseases [6]. Delay in diagnosis affects the prognosis of the disease and increases the risk of infection and duration of hospitalization and treatment, in addition to reducing the patient's quality of life.

In this report, we describe an observation of a female patient that was diagnosed with PV that begun with simultaneous oral and umbilical locations which coexisted for a period of 4 months before the appearance of other cutaneous lesions. We highlight the role of dentists, by being familiar with the clinical manifestations of PV, to make an early diagnosis to start an early treatment which determines the prognosis of the disease and to follow closely the evolution of lesions to change treatment if required.

We also discuss the clinical, histological, and immunological features of the disease that enabled the differential diagnosis as well as the appropriate therapeutic management.

2. Case Presentation

A 55-year-old woman with no notable medical and family history was referred to our department by her general practitioner following the appearance of multiple lesions of the oral mucosa. The intraoral clinical examination revealed poor oral hygiene, hypersialorrhea, and extensive mucosal damage affecting the entire oral cavity and causing discomfort, pain, and dysphagia. The lesions were located in the internal surfaces of the lips and cheeks, the dorsal and ventral surface of the tongue, and the soft palate mucosa (Figure 1). There were epithelial erosions and postbullous ulcerations with a positive Nikolsky sign indicating acantholysis with dislocation of the epithelial layers (Figure 2). Bulloerosive umbilical involvement was associated with the oral impairment without noting any other cutaneous lesions for four months (Figure 3).

In front of these signs, we conducted an oral biopsy and prescribed topical prednisolone (20 mg; 3 times per day) and chlorhexidine-based (0.12%; 3 times per day) mouthwashes in order to reduce the oral pain awaiting the biopsy result. In a while, her condition worsened (Figure 4). We referred her to the department of dermatology where she was hospitalized and an umbilical biopsy was performed.

On histopathological examinations, the oral biopsy concerned a squamous mucosa lined with a partially visualized coating, with disappearance of the superficial layers and the presence of cells of the basal layer which remain attached to the underlying chorion, drawing a "tapestry nail" appearance, surmounted by a few acantholytic cells. In the chorion, we noted the presence of a polymorphic inflammatory infiltrate rich in eosinophilic polynuclear cells. Direct immunofluorescent examination was negative (Figure 5). As for the umbilical biopsy, the sample received was carried to the deep dermis. It was bordered by the basal layer of the epidermis, drawing the same "tapestry nail" appearance with extensive suprabasal acantholysis and separation of the overlying epidermal layers. The dermis was the site of an inflammatory infiltrate rich in neutrophils and eosinophils of perivascular arrangement with extravasation of red blood cells and without alteration of their wall. Intercellular immunoglobulin G and C3 deposits were observed on direct immunofluorescent examination with a characteristic mesh-like appearance (Figure 6). Based on clinical, histopathological, and immunofluorescence findings, a diagnosis of pemphigus vulgaris (PV) was established.

On laboratory investigations, we found an inflammatory syndrome with increased erythrocyte sedimentation rate (ESR) and C-reactive protein (CRP). Hepatitis (VHB and VHC) and VIH serologies were negative. Mycological direct examination and cultures were negative. On bacteriological culture performed from the umbilicus, *Staphylococcus aureus* growth was observed.

As for the therapeutic management, due to oral pain, a nasoenteral probe was used to feed her. Daily intravenous administration of prednisolone (120 mg/day) and amoxicillin-clavulanic acid (1000 mg thrice a day) was started. The nursing team was instructed to clean the oral cavity and the umbilicus using chlorhexidine (0.12%) mouthwash and ointment. Her condition improved gradually during hospitalization. There was a complete remission of the lesions in the mouth and umbilicus. The patient was advised to continue oral prednisone intake at a dose of 20 mg/day. She underwent monthly follow-ups in dentistry and dermatology departments after discharge from the hospital.

Four months later, the disease recurred. We noticed the appearance of severe cutaneous lesions added to the oral and umbilical ones located in the elbows, forearms, and the periungual area. She was newly hospitalized.

3. Discussion

This report describes a case of pemphigus vulgaris (PV) beginning with simultaneous oral and umbilical locations coexisting for a period of 4 months before the appearance of other cutaneous lesions. Umbilical lesion as a clinical manifestation of pemphigus has been reported very rarely so far and was assessed in a limited study totaling just 10 patients [7]. The reasons why an umbilical lesion may be a presenting feature of pemphigus remain unclear [7].

Recognition of this presentation for patients with PV is relevant; in fact, clinicians generally recall blistering diseases in the navel area only in pregnant and lactating females [8]. It is known that pemphigoid gestationis blisters occur in the umbilical region and later spread to the rest of the body [9]. However, this localisation in mucocutaneous PV is unusual. A possible explanation may be related to antibodies binding to the cadherin superfamily in embryonic remains on the umbilical cord or placenta [7].

In a series of 1209 cases of pemphigus (1111 PV) with involvement of different regions, Chams-Davatchi et al. reported that initial localisation was solely oral in 62./. and umbilical in only 3./. [10]. Very few cases of pemphigus

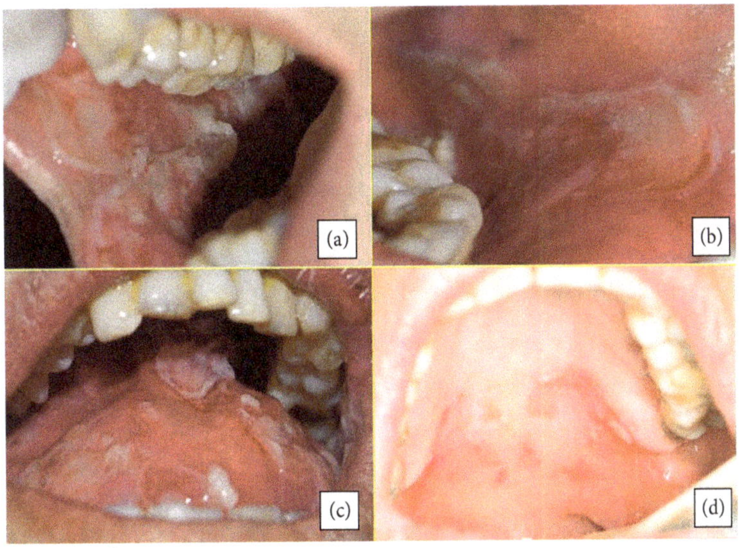

Figure 1: Mucosal damage affecting the entire oral cavity. The lesions were located in the internal surfaces of the lips and cheeks, the dorsal surface of the tongue, and the palatal fibromucosa. There were multiple epithelial erosions and postbullous ulcerations.

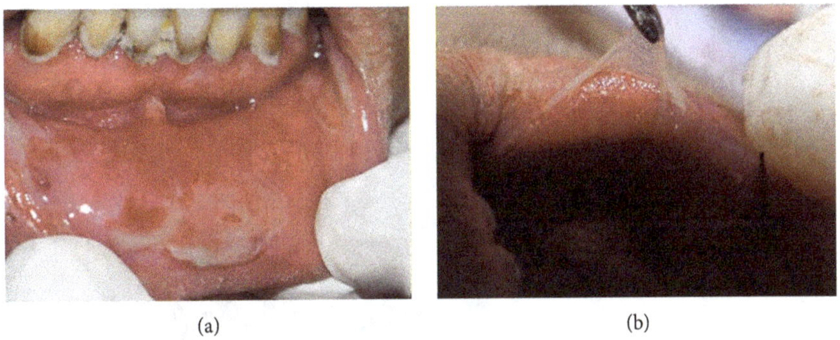

Figure 2: Blisters of the oral mucosa with a positive Nikolsky sign. Presence of poor oral hygiene-associated bullous lesions and ulcerations. Nikolsky sign: epithelial cells are separated from the basement membrane, allowing an assessment of the fragility of epithelial attachment mechanisms (acantholysis).

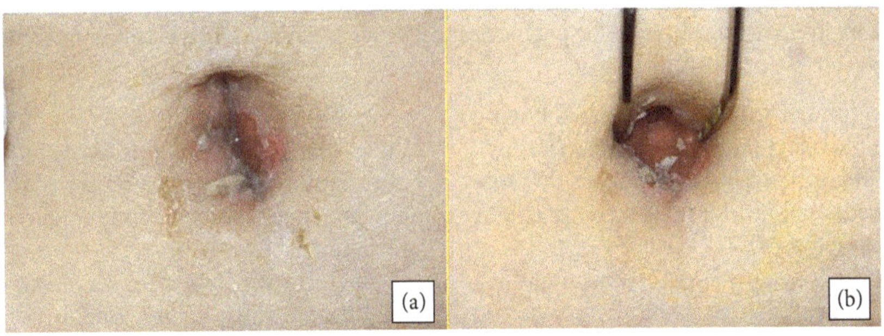

Figure 3: Aspect of the umbilical lesions. Erosions and ulcerations with erythema affecting the umbilical area associated with Staphylococcus aureus growth.

vegetans in the navel area were reported [11, 12]. The coexistence of oral and umbilical lesions as a first sign of PV in the absence of skin involvement was reported in only one case of pemphigus vegetans (PVe). The female patient was followed up for more than one year without appearance of other localisations [12]. For our patient, oral and umbilical lesions were the first sign of PV before the appearance of other cutaneous lesions after four months. Jałowska et al., in a series of 81 PV with nail apparatus involvement and navel area involvement, have found that only females had lesions in the navel area. This correlates with our case reported. Authors speculate therefore that a relationship may exist between the pattern of expression of PV lesions around the umbilicus and the female reproductive system [9], whereas

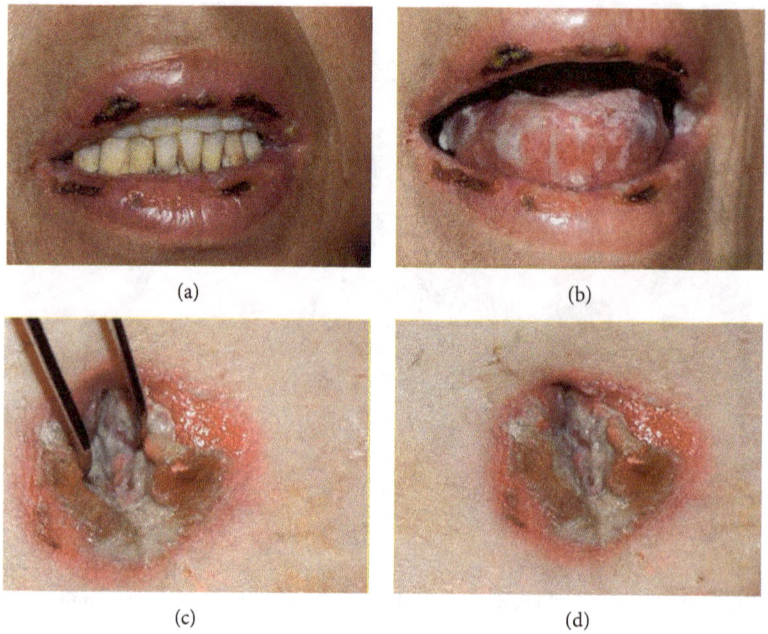

FIGURE 4: Worsening of the lesions 5 days after the first consultation. Extension of the lesions with appearance of multiple crusts in the lips and umbilicus.

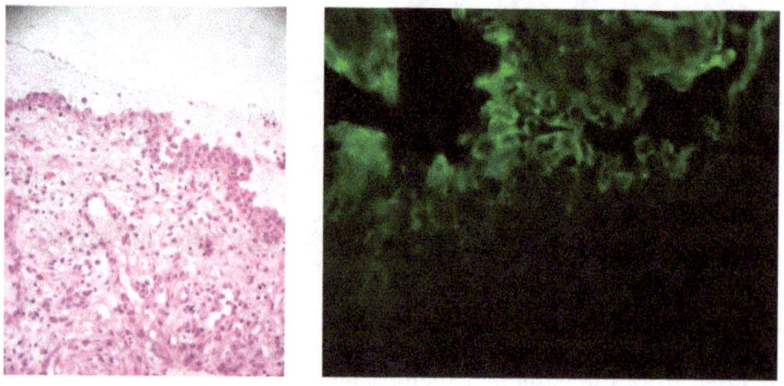

FIGURE 5: Histopathological and IFD of the oral biopsy. The oral biopsy concerned a squamous mucosa lined with a partially visualized coating, with disappearance of the superficial layers and the presence of cells of the basal layer which remain attached to the underlying chorion, drawing a "tapestry nail" appearance, surmounted by a few acantholytic cells. In the chorion, we noted the presence of a polymorphic inflammatory infiltrate rich in eosinophilic polynuclear cells. Direct immunofluorescent examination was negative.

Oliveira Junior et al., in a limited study of 10 patients having pemphigus with umbilical involvement (5 PV, 5 P. foliaceus), showed that between 5 patients with mucocutaneous PV, one was male. In the same series, umbilical lesions were, as in our case, crusts, erosions, and erythema [7].

Diagnosis of the PV is based on identification of clinical manifestations and confirmation by incisional biopsy of the affected perilesional tissue of the skin or mucous membranes [13]. Clinically, oral lesions are the first manifestations of the disease in 50-90% of the patients with widespread blisters affecting the oral mucosa, most commonly in areas subjected to frictional trauma [14]. On the skin, lesions are characterized by flaccid blisters that rapidly progress into erosions and crust formation and occasionally develop opportunistic infections [15]. At the end of the 19th century, a Russian dermatologist, Pyotr Vasiliyevich Nikolsky, first described a clinical sign characterized by blisters spreading upon the application of a horizontal, tangential pressure to the skin and which would subsequently become widely known as "Nikolsky's sign." When this sign tested positive, epithelial cells are separated either from one another or from the basement membrane, allowing an assessment of the fragility of epithelial attachment mechanisms [16].

These features were observed in our patient with extensive blisters affecting the oral mucosa, a positive Nikolsky sign and a bulloerosive umbilical involvement.

Oral mucosal blisters can recall many differential diagnoses making the clinical diagnosis difficult. They include other autoimmune bullous diseases (AIBD), erosive lichen planus, and *Stevens-Johnson* and *Lyell* syndromes, as well as the lesions caused by acute viral infections like *Herpes simplex* and erythema multiforme. Dentists must be familiar with the clinical manifestations of PV [14]. In fact, the oral cavity may be the only site of involvement for many months before the appearance of other localisations, and this may lead to delayed diagnosis and inappropriate treatment of a

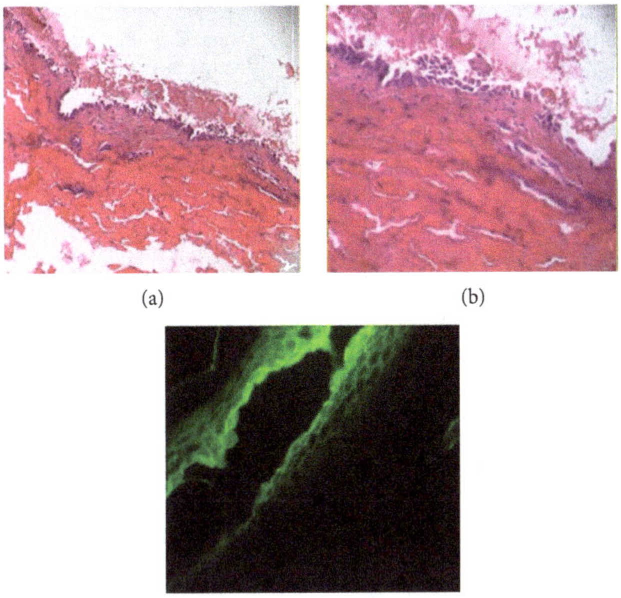

(a) (b) (c)

FIGURE 6: Histopathological and IFD of the skin biopsy. The sample received was carried to the deep dermis. It was bordered by the basal layer of the epidermis, drawing the same "tapestry nail" appearance with extensive suprabasal acantholysis and separation of the overlying epidermal layers. The dermis was the site of an inflammatory infiltrate rich in neutrophils and eosinophils of perivascular arrangement with extravasation of red blood cells and without alteration of their wall. Intercellular immunoglobulin G and C3 deposits were observed on direct immunofluorescent examination with a characteristic mesh-like appearance.

potentially fatal disorder [14]. These lesions may occur anywhere on the oral mucosa, but mostly in the buccal mucosa followed by palatal, lingual, and labial mucosa. The gingiva is the least commonly affected site, and the commonest manifestation is desquamative gingivitis. In this case, oral lesions were located only in nonkeratinized mucosa (internal surfaces of the lips and cheeks, the dorsal surface of the tongue, and the soft palate) [14]. The clinician should be able to distinguish the lesions of PV from those caused by other diseases [14]. For recurrent aphthous stomatitis, oral ulcers (aphthae) are surrounded by an erythematous halo and regular margins with yellowish base [17, 18]. Acute herpetic gingivostomatitis is associated to prodromic symptoms followed by the onset of small yellowish vesicles that rapidly rupture, giving rise to ulcers with an erythematous halo. It affects mostly keratinized mucosa [18]. In cicatricial pemphigoid, skin lesions precede oral lesions, and blisters are smaller with a shorter duration than in PV. Bullous pemphigus is rare on the mucosa and develops on normal or erythematous skin with intense pruritus and symmetric lesions that appear on flexion areas, root of extremities, thighs, and abdomen. For erythema multiform, the presence of target-shaped skin lesions will make the diagnosis. Erosive lesions in erosive lichen planus are charaterised by the presence of Wickham striae [17]. Lyell syndrome and Stevens-Johnson syndrome are severe dermatosis that are mostly caused by medication. They are characterized by toxic epidermal necrolysis in which epidermal detachment affects more than 30% of the body surface area in Lyell syndrome but affecting less than 10% of the body surface area in Stevens-Johnson syndrome. A positive Nikolsky sign and a positive Asboe Hansen sign are confirmatory signs. In these dermatosis, skin involvement usually occurs prior to mucous membrane involvement and the rapid withdrawal of the drug improves prognosis [19, 20].

The association of only oral and umbilical erosive postbullous lesions was not mentioned in the literature with the previous diseases, so it may be a valuable hint easing the diagnosis at the clinical level and recalling PV in patients other than pregnant and lactating females [9].

As for the histopathological features, the oral and the skin biopsy shared the same features with extensive suprabasal acantholysis affecting the epithelium and a "tapestry nail" appearance. As for the direct immunofluorescence, it was negative in the oral biopsy and positive in the skin biopsy. This result is possibly due to the fact that the oral biopsy was carried in an ulcerated area which affected the final result. In fact, blisters in the oral mucosa are short-lived; they have a very thin roof that could be rapidly ulcerated because of the presence of teeth [17]. It is recommended that the incisional biopsy should be done in a perilesional intact or clinically uninvolved tissue of the skin or mucous membranes [16]. In our case, the diagnosis was confirmed by the characteristic deposition of IgG and C3 antibodies that bind to cell surface painting a mesh-like appearance of the umbilical lesion. The navel area involvement can therefore facilitate the performance of DIF in individuals with very painful or seriously damaged oral lesions.

Therapeutic management requires a multidisciplinary approach. Patients with PV need to maintain good oral hygiene, which may be compromised due to pain and blistering. Oral conditions can worsen with an accumulation of dental biofilm, causing gingivitis, or exacerbation of preexisting periodontal disease. Daily use of topical corticosteroids (prednisolone) and chlorhexidine mouthwashes helps to reduce pain and inflammation. As for systemic treatment, corticosteroids are most effective to control disease activity either alone or in combination with other immunosuppressive/immunomodulant drugs such as azathioprine, mycophenolate, and rituximab [21]. Our patient showed a gradual improvement in her condition after systemic corticosteroid intake, but PV lesions rapidly recurred, worsened, and expanded to other skin lesions requiring the addition of immunosuppressive therapy. Apart from the blisters, the risk of infection is always present. We treated a coexisting infection (*Staphylococcus aureus*) with amoxicillin-acid clavulanic.

Before the advent of corticosteroid therapy, pemphigus was fatal, with a mortality rate of up to 75% in the early 1950s [22]. It is still a life-threatening disorder. For every patient, the optimal management requires 3 crucial steps: an accurate diagnosis, a correct evaluation of the spread and severity of the disease, and a comprehensive analysis of his systemic condition (age, comorbidities) and, if present, the side effects of previous therapies [15]. Multidisciplinary teams are extremely important for providing comprehensive patient care, preventing further damage, improving the prognosis and quality of life, and reducing the length of hospital stay. Added to that, regular monitoring is the major rule to detect any recurrence of the disease.

4. Conclusion

This report described the case of a female patient that was diagnosed with mucocutaneous PV which begun with simultaneous oral and umbilical locations coexisting for a period of 4 months before the appearance of other cutaneous lesions. The association of these two localisations may be a valuable hint easing the diagnosis at the clinical level for patients with oral mucosal blisters. Further reports and studies are necessary to achieve a better understanding of the disease in order to give the appropriate care.

Consent

A statement of informed consent was signed to allow the use of her medical and dental records and photos.

Acknowledgments

The authors thank the Laboratory of Research on Oral Health and Facial Rehabilitation (LR12ES11) for their support.

References

[1] M. Cholera and N. Chainani-Wu, “Management of pemphigus vulgaris,” *Advances in Therapy*, vol. 33, no. 6, pp. 910–958, 2016.

[2] S. Z. Burgan, F. A. Sawair, and S. S. Napier, “Case report: oral pemphigus vulgaris with multiple oral polyps in a young patient,” *International Dental Journal*, vol. 53, no. 1, pp. 37–40, 2003.

[3] A. Iamaroon, P. Boonyawong, P. Klanrit, S. Prasongtunskul, and K. Thongprasom, “Characterization of oral pemphigus vulgaris in Thai patients,” *Journal of Oral Science*, vol. 48, no. 1, pp. 43–46, 2006.

[4] I. A. Popescu, L. Statescu, D. Vata et al., “Pemphigus vulgaris - approach and management (Review),” *Experimental and Therapeutic Medicine*, vol. 18, no. 6, pp. 5056–5060, 2019.

[5] A. Ariyawardana, W. M. Tilakaratne, M. Dissanayake et al., “Oral pemphigus vulgaris in children and adolescents: a review of the literature and a case report,” *International Journal of Paediatric Dentistry*, vol. 15, no. 4, pp. 287–293, 2005.

[6] P. S. Aractingi, P. F. Aubin, M. F. Pr et al., “Auteurs et membres du Collège des enseignants en dermatologie de France,” in *Annales de dermatologie et de vénéréologie*, Elsevier, 2008.

[7] J. V. Oliveira Júnior, C. W. Maruta, J. X. Sousa Jr. et al., “Clinical and immunological profile of umbilical involvement in pemphigus vulgaris and pemphigus foliaceus,” *Clinical and Experimental Dermatology: Clinical dermatology*, vol. 38, no. 1, pp. 20–24, 2013.

[8] T. Çetinarslan, A. Ermertcan, P. Temiz, and S. Kurutepe, “Pemphigus vegetans arising in umbilicus: successful clearance with intralesional steroid,” *Indian Journal of Dermatology, Venereology and Leprology*, vol. 84, no. 4, p. 522, 2018.

[9] M. Jałowska, J. Gornowicz-Porowska, A. Seraszek-Jaros, M. Bowszyc-Dmochowska, E. Kaczmarek, and M. Dmochowski, “Clinical significance of umbilical region involvement in pemphigus vulgaris in a series of 81 ethnic Poles: a comparative analysis of the distribution of lesions in two infrequent locations,” *Advances in Dermatology and Allergology*, vol. 38, no. 1, 2021.

[10] C. Chams-Davatchi, M. Valikhani, M. Daneshpazhooh et al., “Pemphigus: analysis of 1209 cases,” *International Journal of Dermatology*, vol. 44, no. 6, pp. 470–476, 2005.

[11] S. Mokni, I. Lahouel, A. Aounallah et al., “Pemphigus à début gravidique: à propos de 4 observations,” in *Annales de Dermatologie et de Vénéréologie*, Elsevier Masson, 2017.

[12] A. Jimenez, P. Hoyer, and M. Wilkerson, “An atypical presentation of pemphigus vegetans in the umbilicus,” *Skin*, vol. 4, no. 5, pp. 452–455, 2020.

[13] K. J. Dal Prá, S. S. S. Assis Tristão, J. B. Franco et al., “Oral management of pemphigus vulgaris in the intensive care unit,” *Special Care in Dentistry*, vol. 40, no. 3, pp. 280–284, 2020.

[14] A. Rai, M. Arora, V. Naikmasur, A. Sattur, and V. Malhotra, “Oral pemphigus vulgaris: case report,” *Ethiopian Journal of Health Sciences*, vol. 25, no. 4, p. 637, 2015.

[15] S. Leuci, E. Ruoppo, D. Adamo, E. Calabria, and M. D. Mignogna, “Oral autoimmune vesicobullous diseases: classification, clinical presentations, molecular mechanisms, diagnostic algorithms, and management,” *Periodontology*, vol. 80, no. 1, pp. 77–88, 2019.

[16] B. Carey, S. Joshi, A. Abdelghani, J. Mee, M. Andiappan, and J. Setterfield, “The optimal oral biopsy site for diagnosis of mucous membrane pemphigoid and pemphigus vulgaris,” *British Journal of Dermatology*, vol. 182, no. 3, pp. 747–753, 2020.

[17] A. Bascones-Martinez, M. Munoz-Corcuera, C. Bascones-Ilundain, and G. Esparza-Gómez, “Oral manifestations of pemphigus vulgaris: clinical presentation, differential diagnosis and management,” *Journal of Clinical & Experimental Dermatology*, vol. 1, p. 112, 2010.

[18] G. T. Lins Filho, N. L. S. Barbosa, E. M. V. de Abreu et al., "Childhood pemphigus vulgaris is a challenging diagnosis," *Autopsy and Case Reports*, vol. 11, article e2021267, 2021.

[19] S. Kourouma, A. Sangaré, M. Kaloga et al., "Stevens-Johnson syndrome and toxic epidermal necrolysis: retrospective study of 185 cases in Abidjan (Côte d'Ivoire)," *Médecine et Santé Tropicales*, vol. 24, no. 1, pp. 94–98, 2014.

[20] J. R. Dowling, K. L. Anderson, and W. W. Huang, "Asboe-Hansen sign in toxic epidermal necrolysis," *Cutis*, vol. 103, no. 4, 2019.

[21] K. Kridin, "Emerging treatment options for the management of pemphigus vulgaris," *Therapeutics and Clinical Risk Management*, vol. Volume 14, pp. 757–778, 2018.

[22] K. E. Harman, S. Albert, and M. M. Black, "Guidelines for the management of pemphigus vulgaris," *British Journal of Dermatology*, vol. 149, no. 5, pp. 926–937, 2003.

14

Airway Management Failure after Delayed Extubation in a Patient with Oral Malignant Melanoma Who Underwent Partial Mandibulectomy and Reconstruction with a Free Flap

Min A. Kwon,[1] Jaegyok Song,[1] Seokkon Kim,[1] Pyeung-wha Oh,[2] and Minji Kang[2]

[1]*Department of Anaesthesiology and Pain Medicine, Dankook University College of Medicine, Cheonan, Republic of Korea*
[2]*Department of Anaesthesiology and Pain Medicine, Dankook University Hospital, Cheonan, Republic of Korea*

Correspondence should be addressed to Jaegyok Song; jaegyoksong@gmail.com

Academic Editor: Gianluigi Caccianiga

Maxillofacial surgery may cause severe complications in perioperative airway management. We report a case of failed airway management in a patient who underwent segmental mandibulectomy, radical neck dissection, and reconstruction with a free flap. The patient was extubated approximately 36 hours after surgery. Approximately 7 hours after extubation, the patient complained of dyspnoea, and respiratory failure followed. Bag-mask ventilation, direct laryngoscopy, video laryngoscopy, and supraglottic airway access were ineffective. The surgical airway was secured with an emergency tracheostomy while performing cardiopulmonary resuscitation. However, the patient experienced permanent hypoxic brain damage. The airway of patients with oral cancer may be compromised postoperatively due to surgical trauma and bulky flap reconstruction. Patients should be closely monitored during the postoperative period to prevent airway failure. Early diagnosis and airway management before airway failure occurs are important. Medical staff should be aware of airway management algorithms, be trained to perform difficult airway management, and have the required equipment readily available.

1. Introduction

Maxillofacial surgery may induce anatomical changes, oedema, and even haematoma formation in the head and neck region, which can cause severe problems with airway management [1–4]. Airway management would be complicated in patients with oral cancer who have undergone invasive surgery, such as reconstruction with a free flap with or without radical neck dissection. Tracheostomy (TT) is used to secure the airway during the perioperative period [5]. However, the rate of TT complications (TT tube dislodgement, loss of the airway, bleeding, pneumothorax, pneumonia, etc.) is as high as 8%–25% [2, 5]. Several studies have reported that compared to TT, delayed extubation (DE) resulted in faster recovery and less time spent in the intensive care unit, without a significant difference in airway-related complications [2, 5, 6].

In this case report, we used a DE strategy. However, there was a failure of airway management 7 hours after DE. We report this case with a brief review of the literature.

2. Case Presentation

We obtained Institutional Review Board (IRB) approval (Dankook University Hospital IRB 2021-02-015) and written informed consent from patient's legal representative for the publication of this report.

A 42-year-old male (American Society of Anaesthesiologists class II; weight, 59 kg; height, 165 cm) with a malignant melanoma in the left side of the oral cavity, gingiva, and buccal mucosa was scheduled for mass excision and reconstruction with a fibular free flap (Figure 1). Preoperative magnetic resonance imaging (MRI) showed an ill-defined mass lesion that was $2.6 \times 2.4 \times 1.8$ cm in size in the left lateral part of

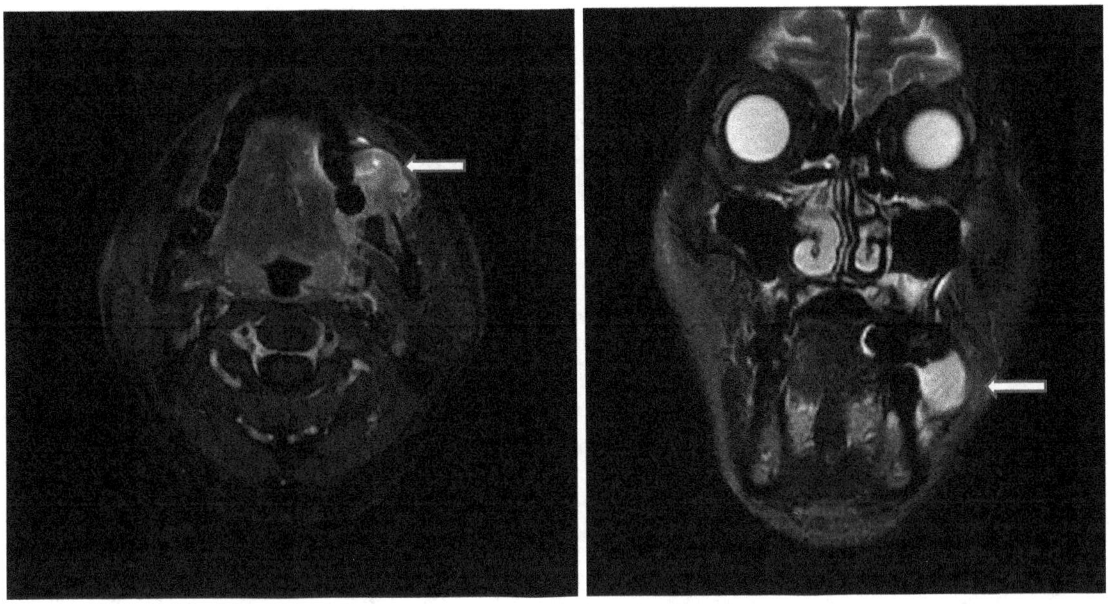

FIGURE 1: A 2.6 × 2.4 × 1.8 cm sized enhancing ovoid mass lesion in the left buccal area and oral cavity.

the oral cavity (Figures 1 and 2, stage III, T2N1). He was previously healthy and had no history of systemic disease or medication. Preoperative evaluations, including laboratory tests, electrocardiography, and chest radiography, were unremarkable.

Patient monitors were instituted, including standard monitors and continuous arterial blood pressure monitoring with radial artery catheter insertion. General anaesthesia was induced with intravenous injections of fentanyl (100 μg), lidocaine (60 mg), propofol (120 mg), and rocuronium (50 mg) and maintained with 7–10 vol% desflurane. After the induction of anaesthesia, nasal packing was performed with cotton swabs moistened with a 0.01% epinephrine solution. Nasotracheal intubation was performed using fibreoptic bronchoscopy (FI-10RBS, Pentax, Japan), and a 6.5 mm reinforced tube was inserted. After intubation, a central venous catheter (CVC, Bio Line, 7 F double lumen catheter, Ewha Biomedics, Republic of Korea) was inserted into the right subclavian vein using the anatomical landmark technique.

Partial mandibulectomy (from # 21 to the mandibular angle), radical neck dissection, and reconstruction with a fibular free flap were performed (Figure 3). The operation time was approximately 13 hours and 25 minutes. The infused volume was crystalloid 7200 ml, colloid 1700 ml, packed red blood cells (pRBC) 5 units, and fresh frozen plasma 5 units. The urine output was 3800 ml, and the estimated blood loss was approximately 1800 ml. The patient was transferred to the intensive care unit and was kept sedated with endotracheal intubation.

The patient recovered from anaesthesia 3 hours after the surgery. Ventilator weaning was initiated at 8 AM on the first postoperative day (POD 1), the ventilator was stopped at 1 PM, and oxygen (5 L/min) was administered via a T-piece. The patient did not complain of respiratory difficulties. The patient was evaluated before extubation, and his mental status was alert, muscle tone was intact, surgical wound condition was visually acceptable, and the endotracheal tube cuff leak test was fair. No bleeding was noted from the surgical wound. Blood pressure was maintained between 110/60 mmHg and 140/90 mmHg. Postoperative pain was treated with an intravenous infusion of patient-controlled analgesia with fentanyl and nefopam. There was no dyspnoea, and arterial oxygen saturation was 100%.

At 8 AM POD 2, the patient was extubated (approximately 36 hours postsurgery), and oxygen (3 L/min) was administered via a nasal prong. Four hours after extubation, his haemoglobin level decreased to 8.9 ml/dl. One unit of pRBC was transfused.

Seven hours after extubation (POD 2, 3 PM), the patient complained of dyspnoea, and arterial oxygen saturation decreased from 100% to 87%. Bag-mask ventilation was initiated but was ineffective. Oral and nasal airway insertion was not sufficient to open the airway. Conventional direct laryngoscopy, video laryngoscopy, and laryngeal mask insertion were not successful because the structures in the oral cavity were severely distorted due to operation site oedema and haematoma. An otolaryngologist performed an emergency TT while performing bag-mask ventilation. During TT, the heart rate decreased from 90 bpm to 42 bpm. Intravenous atropine (0.5 mg) and epinephrine (200 μg) were administered. Ten minutes after the initiation of bag-mask ventilation, cardiopulmonary resuscitation was initiated to treat cardiac arrest, and epinephrine (1 mg) was administered every 5 minutes. The TT tube was secured 28 minutes after the initiation of bag-mask ventilation. Blood pressure was 80/30 mmHg, and dopamine, dobutamine, and norepinephrine infusion (20 μg/kg/min each) were administered. The patient was connected to a ventilator and was sedated with midazolam. On POD 3, midazolam sedation was stopped; however, patient's mental status was semicomatose, and he showed seizure-like movements. A neurology consult was obtained, and postoperative computed tomography showed severe swelling and increased soft tissue density with

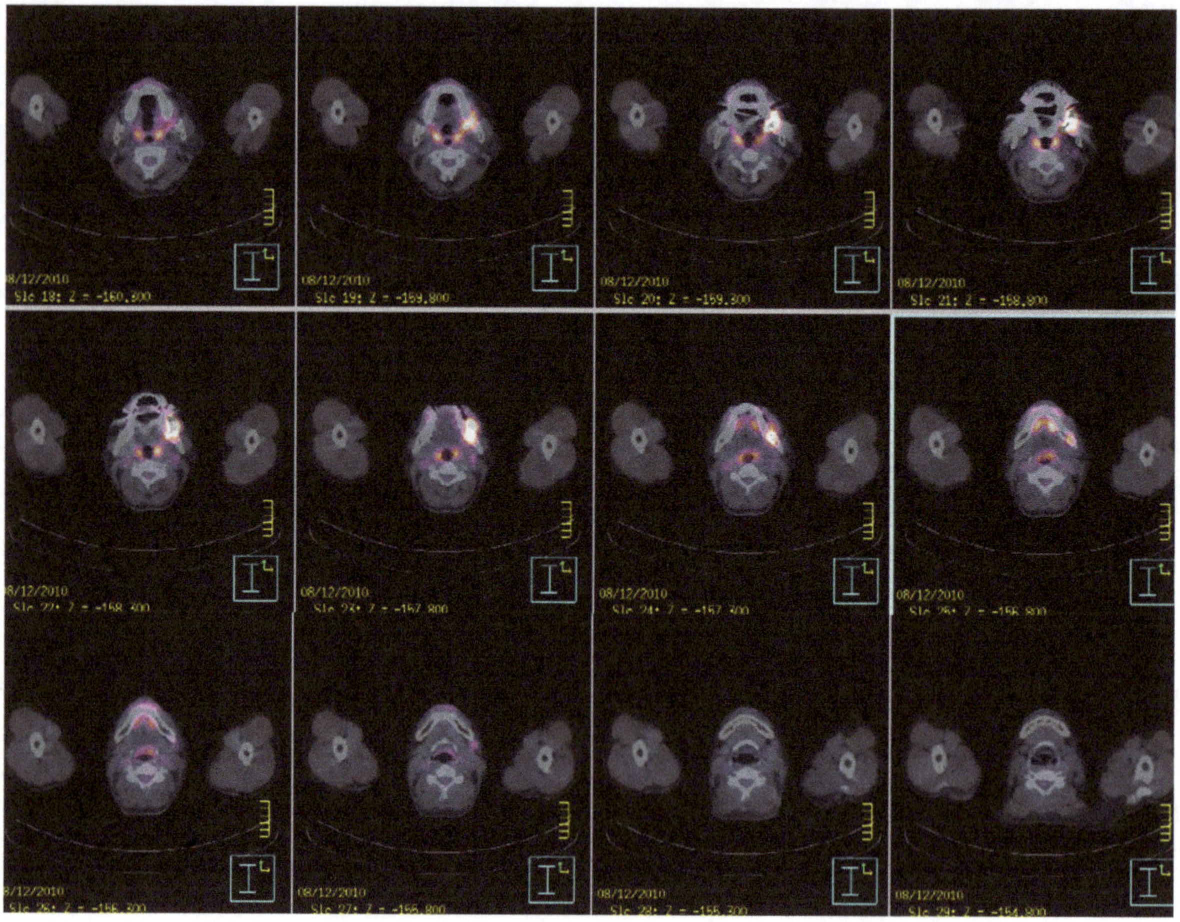

FIGURE 2: A positron emission tomography-computed tomography scan shows a focal hypermetabolic lesion in the left part of the oral cavity and multiple mild hypermetabolic lesions in the left cervical level Ib, II, and V.

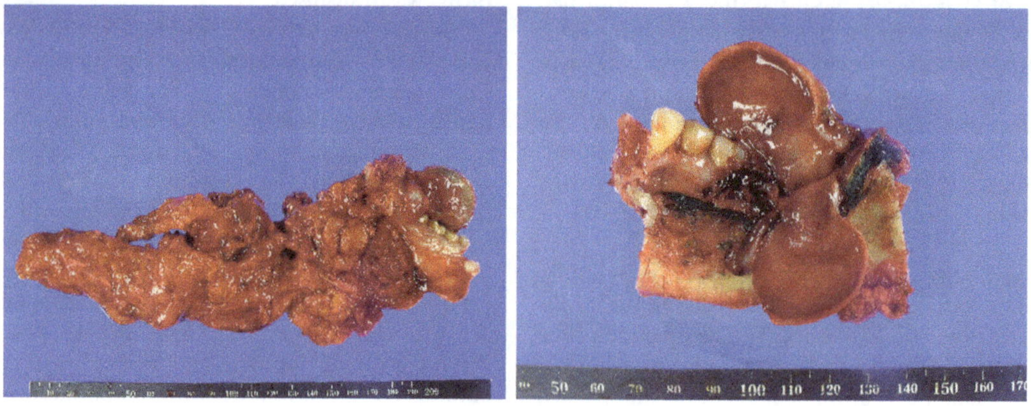

FIGURE 3: The resected tumour and related lymphoid tissue.

airway compression in the left side of the face and neck (Figure 4). On POD 4, a brain MRI showed a diffusely restricted lesion involving the whole cerebral cortex and basal ganglia. The patient received conservative treatment but his mental status did not recover. On POD 67, a recurring tumour was found. Further chemotherapy or radiotherapy was considered; however, it was decided that it would not be beneficial. On POD 103, the patient was transferred to a hospice.

3. Discussion

We report case of postoperative airway management failure in a patient with oral cancer. Our report showed the importance of early recognition and airway management for patients with head and neck cancer. Difficult airway management and subsequent "can't intubate, can't oxygenate" (CICO) emergency is a significant contributor to patient mortality and morbidity, including airway trauma, brain damage, or death [7]. Oral

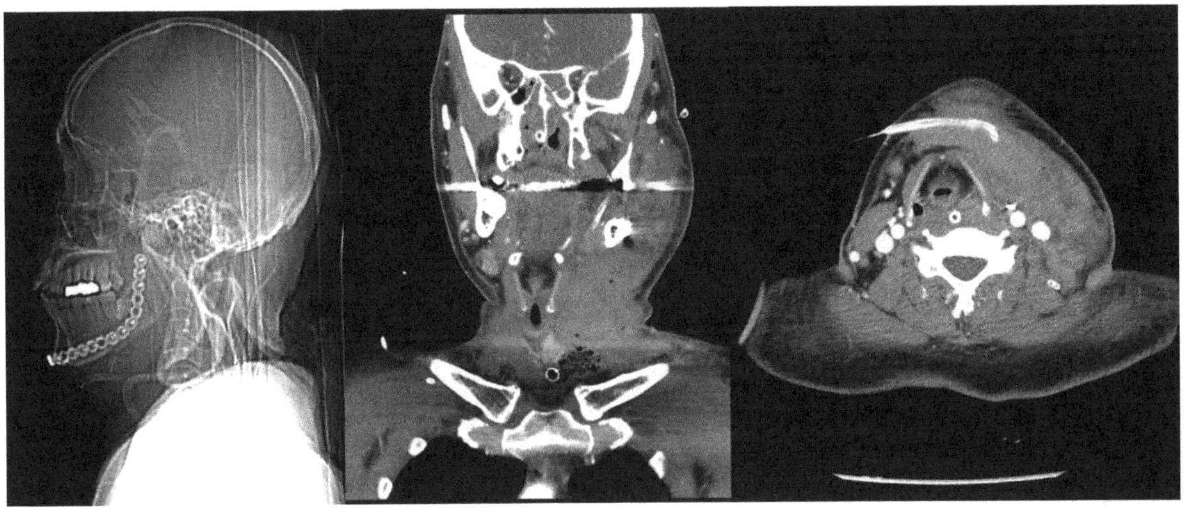

FIGURE 4: Neck computed tomography shows severe swelling and soft tissue density lesion in the left face and neck with airway compression.

cancer surgery, including extensive tumour resection and reconstruction with a bulky flap, wound haematoma, and oedema in the upper airway, may induce upper airway obstruction and related complications [5].

There have been reports comparing TT and DE in oral cancer surgery. DE is considered a safe option and prevents complications related to TT [2, 3]. However, some of these reports were retrospective reviews, and there was a possibility that DE was applied in cases with relatively few risk factors. Singh et al. [2] recommended considering TT for patients with significant risk factors, including obstructive sleep apnoea, obesity, poor lung function, anticipated difficult reintubation, and oral resection with bilateral neck dissection. The study [2] recommended a DE time of 24–48 hours. Several scoring systems have been proposed for deciding between DE and TT [6]. However, these systems criticise the overestimation of the need for TT and could not identify the right indications for it [5, 6]. Recently, Myatra et al. [5] proposed a simple algorithm. In major oral cancer surgery, DE is considered in patients with the following conditions: tumour stages T1 and T2, the absence of extensive surgical resection, primary closure or reconstruction using a fasciocutaneous flap, the absence of preoperative radiotherapy, and no neck dissection. They reported no extubation failure in 417 patients who underwent DE. However, the algorithm is still controversial regarding the choice between DE and TT.

The tracheal reintubation rates after maxillofacial surgery range between 0.7% and 11.1% [8]. A preextubation checklist has been proposed, which significantly decreases the reintubation rate from 7% to 3% [9]. This checklist includes tests for spontaneous breathing, mental status, oxygen saturation (>95%), need for tracheal suction (less than every 2 hours), minimal oral secretions, spontaneous cough, and endotracheal tube cuff leak. However, the cuff leak test cannot identify airway obstruction proximal to the level of the pharynx, which is a potentially important area [1].

Graboyes et al. [1] performed a retrospective review of 15 cases of failed extubation in 129 cases of DE. Postoperative haematoma or haemorrhage was the most common cause of failure (47%), followed by upper airway oedema (33%). Forty-seven percent of failed extubation cases (7/15) occurred within 6 h. Upper airway oedema results in faster failure of extubation (within 6 h) compared to postoperative haematoma (only one case failed within 6 h, median POD 3.5). They assumed that hypertension and tachycardia, which occurred after recovery from sedation and extubation, were the causes of haematoma. Additionally, major vessel ligation (most commonly of the internal jugular vein) may have caused an increase in venous pressure that incited bleeding from small venous collaterals that would not have bled at a low venous pressure.

For this patient, we should have considered the surgical airway early. Joffe et al. [8] reported a closed claim analysis of difficult airway management strategies between 2000 and 2012. Supraglottic airway insertion was successful in only 4 of 23 cases due to upper airway obstruction or pathology, previous neck radiotherapy, multiple intubation attempts before the supraglottic airway, and morbid obesity. Transtracheal jet ventilation resulted in 42% device failure, causing subcutaneous emphysema with or without pneumothorax in 5 of 8 cases, making it difficult to secure surgical airways. They reported that two or more judgement failures occurred in 38% of cases owing to a lack of proper airway management plans, hesitation to utilise a supraglottic airway as a bridge to oxygenation, and delay in attempting a surgical airway during CICO emergency. Although video laryngoscopy has been a good alternative, there are reports that it is not always successful [7, 10, 11]. According to recent guidelines, correct utilization of equipment when faced with difficult airway situations should be rehearsed regularly with the healthcare team [7].

A detailed checklist and airway evaluation should be performed before extubation. Medical staff should be aware that airway-related complications can occur 2–3 days after DE in patients who have undergone head and neck surgery. Early diagnosis and treatment before airway failure can decrease airway-related complications.

In conclusion, we report a case of failed airway management during the postoperative period. Airway compression caused by haematoma and oedema in the oropharyngeal area is thought to be the cause of difficult airway access. DE also carries the risk of causing airway failure after extubation. Medical staff should be aware of this, and close observation and reevaluation of the airway are needed even 24 hours after extubation. Early diagnosis and securing of the airway are essential. Medical staff should be trained to be familiar with difficult airway management algorithms and have the equipment needed available around the clock.

Acknowledgments

This work was financially supported by the Dankook University Hospital.

References

[1] E. M. Graboyes, J. P. Bradley, D. Kallogjeri, L. F. Cavallone, and B. Nussenbaum, "Prognosis and patterns of failure for the extubation of patients who remain intubated after head and neck surgery," *The Annals of Otology, Rhinology, and Laryngology*, vol. 124, pp. 179–186, 2015.

[2] T. Singh, P. Sankla, and G. Smith, "Tracheostomy or delayed extubation after maxillofacial free-flap reconstruction?," *The British Journal of Oral & Maxillofacial Surgery*, vol. 54, pp. 878–882, 2016.

[3] M. Riekert, M. Kreppel, R. Schier, J. E. Zöller, V. Rempel, and V. C. Schick, "Postoperative complications after bimaxillary orthognathic surgery: a retrospective study with focus on postoperative ventilation strategies and posterior airway space (PAS)," *Journal of Cranio-Maxillo-Facial Surgery*, vol. 47, pp. 1848–1854, 2019.

[4] K. E. Hannig, R. W. Hauritz, C. Jessen, and A. M. Grejs, "Acute awake fiberoptic intubation in the ICU in a patient with limited mouth opening and hypoxemic acute respiratory failure," *Case Reports in Anesthesiology*, vol. 2019, Article ID 6421910, 2019.

[5] S. N. Myatra, S. Gupta, A. K. D'Cruz et al., "Identification of patients for a delayed extubation strategy versus elective tracheostomy for postoperative airway management in major oral cancer surgery: a prospective observational study in seven hundred and twenty patients," *Oral Oncology*, vol. 121, 2021.

[6] A. Abe, E. Umemura, H. Hayashi, Y. Ito, and M. Adachi, "Evaluation of scoring systems for airway management after oral cancer surgery: a retrospective study," *The Annals of Otology, Rhinology, and Laryngology*, vol. 130, pp. 873–880, 2021.

[7] N. Sakalihasan, R. Limet, and O. D. Defawe, "Abdominal aortic aneurysm," *The Lancet*, vol. 365, pp. 1577–1589, 2005.

[8] A. M. Joffe, M. F. Aziz, K. L. Posner, L. V. Duggan, S. L. Mincer, and K. B. Domino, "Management of difficult tracheal intubation: a closed claims analysis," *Anesthesiology*, vol. 131, pp. 818–829, 2019.

[9] L. F. Cavallone and A. Vannucci, "Review article: extubation of the difficult airway and extubation failure," *Anesthesia and Analgesia*, vol. 116, pp. 368–383, 2013.

[10] M. Bobbs, M. D. Trust, P. Teixeira et al., "Decreasing failed extubations with the implementation of an extubation checklist," *American Journal of Surgery*, vol. 217, no. 6, pp. 1072–1075, 2019.

[11] A. Gupta and N. Gupta, "Failed videolaryngoscopy in an infant with giant vallecular cyst managed successfully with a 'three-person technique' of fibre-optic intubation," *BML Case Reports*, vol. 12, article e231035, 2019.

15

Recording the Centric Relation in an Edentulous Patient using the Existing Complete Denture Mounted with Gothic Arch Tracer

Xu Wei[1], **X. F. Meng**[1], **Lang Guo**[2], **Xiaoping Luo**[1], and **Wei Han**[1]

[1]*Department of Prosthodontics, Nanjing Stomatological Hospital, Medical School of Nanjing University, Nanjing, China*
[2]*Department of Otolaryngology, Nanjing Stomatological Hospital, Medical School of Nanjing University, Nanjing, China*

Correspondence should be addressed to Xu Wei; weixu982003@163.com

Academic Editor: Rui Amaral Mendes

An 80-year-old man sought treatment at our hospital. He was dissatisfied with his old complete denture due to its poor stability and retention. The old complete denture had been used for about 20 years. The prolonged use of an unsuitable complete denture led the patient to be accustomed to unilateral mastication (UM). Due to the patient long-term habitual mandibular deviation, using the physiological technique to get the centric relation (CR) achieved an incorrect horizontal maxillomandibular record. This clinical report presents a technique using the existing complete denture mounted with a Gothic arch tracer to determine the CR. This technique is an inexpensive, simple, and reliable method that allows fabricating the final impression and obtaining the maxillomandibular relationship record (MMRR) in one step.

1. Introduction

The determination of the correct MMRR is one of the most sensitive and rigorous procedures in complete denture treatment. For some patients, it is difficult to determine the CR due to the habitual mandibular deviation induced by previous inadequate dentures. An inexperienced dentist is prone to obtain an erroneous MMRR in this situation. The Gothic arch tracer has been acknowledged as one of the most reliable and accurate patient-guided methods for obtaining the CR [1]. A method for fabricating the final impression and determining the CR using the existing complete denture mounted with a Gothic arch tracer in one step is described in the present article.

2. Case Report

An 80-year-old man came to our hospital for a new complete denture. His complete denture had been used for about 20 years. He was dissatisfied with the complete denture due to its poor retention, frequent ulcers, and unaesthetic appearance. The old complete denture showed a decreased vertical dimension of occlusion. The extraoral examination revealed the patient's mandible deviated to the right of the old complete denture (Figure 1).

The worn occlusal surface of the maxillary artificial teeth was covered with the wax rim, checking the parallelism of the maxillary horizontal plane with the interpupillary line in the frontal view and the parallelism of the occlusal template with the camper line (nasoauricular plane) in the lateral view. The occlusal vertical dimension (OVD) was determined using the interocclusal rest space method. Softened wax rim was added onto the occlusal surface of the mandibular denture. The patient was asked to swallow once the predetermined OVD had been reached. Checking the existing complete denture bases' extension, the denture bases should be ground away approximately 2 millimeters above the deepest part of the muccobuccal fold. Then placing silicone border molding material (Virtual Heavy, Ivoclar Vivadent AG, Liechtenstein) to the existing maxillary complete denture for border molding, the patient was asked to make three functional movements: saying "woo," saying "eee," and sucking the operator's finger. Using a brush to distribute the high-flow silicone impression material (Virtual Light, Ivoclar Vivadent AG, Liechtenstein) evenly onto the

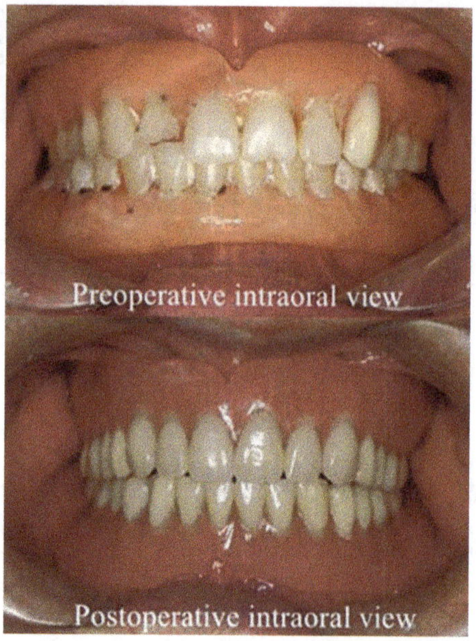

FIGURE 1: Intraoral view of the old complete denture and the new complete denture.

t-
i-

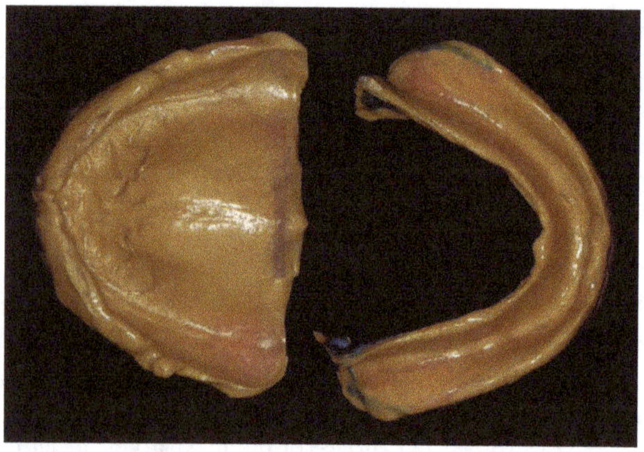

FIGURE 2: The final function impression with the existing complete denture.

ssue surface of the maxillary existing complete denture and

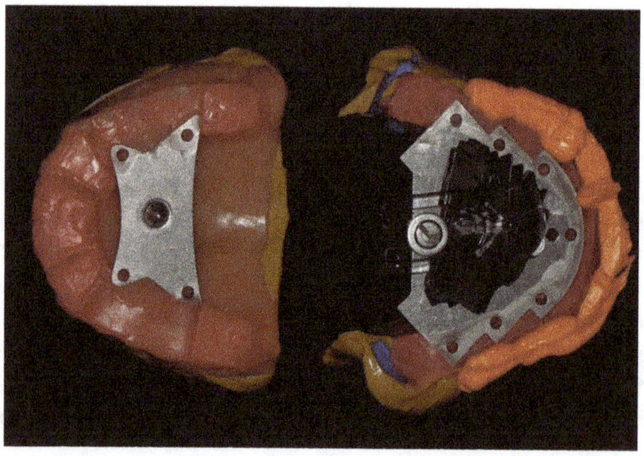

FIGURE 3: Mounting the Gothic arch tracer to the existing complete denture and the Gothic arch apex of the CR was obtained.

inserting the denture into the mouth, the patient was asked to bite gently and repeat making the three functional movements. The mandibular final impression was taken in the same manner. Besides the three maxillary functional movements, the patient should be asked to move the tongue from side to side, push the back of the denture with the tongue, and swallow in a closed-mouth position during manufacturing the mandibular final impression. The final functional impression was obtained using the closed-mouth impression technique (Figure 2).

The Gothic arch tracer (CRS 10, Candulor Registration Set, Ivoclar Vivadent AG, Liechtenstein) was mounted on the existing complete denture. The tracing stylus was set on the maxilla, the tracing recording table was set on the mandible, and the recording table was parallel to the camper's line. Repetitious training was performed for the patient's mandibular protrusion and laterotrusion movements until an accurate arrow point tracing (Gothic arch apex, GoA) was obtained. A fine hole in the plastic cover was placed at the GoA point to engage the stylus in the CR when the interocclusal recording material (O-bite, DMG, Germany) was being made (Figure 3).

The working models were mounted in an articulator (Amann Girbach, Vorarlberg, Austria) with a facebow transfer (Amann Girbach, Vorarlberg, Austria). To confirm the jaw position and aesthetics, wax denture try-in was done and the patient was satisfied with his appearance. Fortunately, the maxillomandibular relation remained stable in maximal intercuspal position. Harmonious occlusion and articulation were achieved. If the patient repeatedly goes into an accustomed position, the patient was treated with a therapeutic complete denture, of which the maxillary premolars and molars were artificial ceramic teeth and mandibular premolar and molar region was just like a splint. A therapeutic complete denture was used to rectify maxillomandibular relation until a stable jaw position is achieved. In a customary manner, a new complete denture was finished. The retention, stability, and occlusion of the complete denture were good. According to the sealing mechanism of a mandibular suction-effective denture [2], we used an electrolaryngoscope to observe the posterior border seal on the tongue and buccal mucosa above the polished surface in the retromolar pad region; the buccal mucosa and tongue side contact point (BTC point) could be seen during mouth closure (Figure 4) [2]. Recall appointments were scheduled 1 month, 3 months, and 6 months; the patient reported improvements in chewing and speaking in addition to his appearance (Figure 1).

3. Discussion

The accuracy of MMRR is essential for an appropriate complete denture [3]. Fenlon et al. has demonstrated a positive correlation between complete denture usage and the accuracy of the MMRR [4]. The Gothic arch tracer is used to obtain the CR for a new complete denture with record base and wax rim [5]. Due to its technique sensitivity of the procedure, the Gothic arch tracer remains a largely underutilized tool. The accurate Gothic arch tracing needs stable and retentive bases to obtain the correct MMRR. Using the existing complete denture can skip the procedure of making

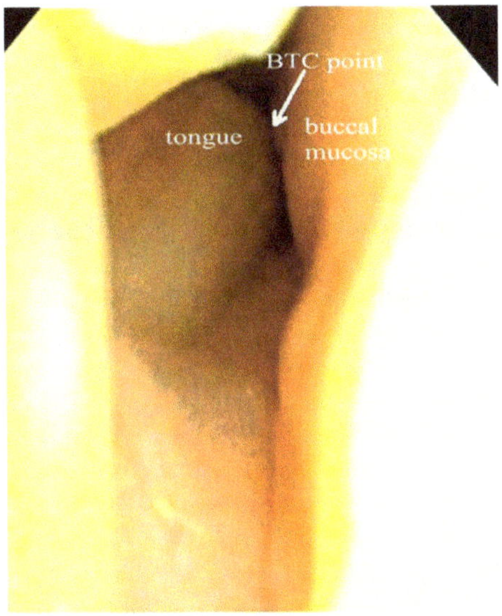

FIGURE 4: Electrolaryngoscope observation of the BTC point during mouth closure.

the temporal record base, and the stability and fitness of the existing complete denture bases with final impressions are better than the temporal record base or wax base. The Biofunctional Prosthetic System (BPS, Ivoclar Vivadent AG, Liechtenstein) for complete dentures uses the "Gnathometer," which consists of custom trays and the Gothic arch tracer, to determine the CR and fabricate the final impression in one step. However, the "Gnathometer" is an expensive and special device. Using the existing complete denture mounted with Gothic arch tracer is an inexpensive, simple, and reliable alternative that can make impression taking and bite registration in one step.

4. Conclusions

Recording the centric relation of edentulous patients using the existing complete denture mounted with Gothic arch tracer is an inexpensive, simple, and reliable method. It can fabricate the final impression and obtain the maxillomandibular relationship record (MMRR) in one step.

Consent

Informed consent was voluntarily obtained from the patient and his family for publication of the photographs in this report.

Acknowledgments

This work was supported by grants from the Medical Science and Technology Development Foundation, Nanjing (YKK16159 and YKK20154), and the Jiangsu Natural Science Foundation (BK20200150).

References

[1] Y. Watanabe, "Observation of horizontal mandibular positions in an edentulous patient using a digital gothic arch tracer: a clinical report," *The Journal of Prosthetic Dentistry*, vol. 91, no. 1, pp. 15–19, 2004.

[2] J. Abe, K. Kokubo, and K. Sato, *Mandibular suction-effective denture and BPS: a complete guide*, Tokyo: Quintessence Publishing Co. Ltd., Tokyo, Japan, 2012.

[3] S. B. Critchlow and J. S. Ellis, "Prognostic indicators for conventional complete denture therapy: a review of the literature," *Journal of Dentistry*, vol. 38, no. 1, pp. 2–9, 2010.

[4] M. R. Fenlon, M. Sherriff, and J. D. Walter, "Association between the accuracy of intermaxillary relations and complete denture usage," *The Journal of Prosthetic Dentistry*, vol. 81, no. 5, pp. 520–525, 1999.

[5] A. R. Mysore and M. A. Aras, "The magic slate as recording medium for Gothic arch tracing," *The Journal of Prosthetic Dentistry*, vol. 108, no. 1, p. 60, 2012.

16

Lymphangioma of the Lower Lip—A Diagnostic Dilemma: Report of a Rare Case with a Brief Literature Review

Shamimul Hasan,[1] **Syed Ansar Ahmad**,[2] **Mandeep Kaur**,[1] **Rajat Panigrahi**,[3] **and Swagatika Panda**[4]

[1]*Department of Oral Medicine and Radiology, Faculty of Dentistry, Jamia Millia Islamia, New Delhi, India*
[2]*Department of Oral and Maxillofacial Surgery, Faculty of Dentistry, Jamia Millia Islamia, New Delhi, India*
[3]*Department of Oral Medicine and Radiology, Institute of Dental Sciences, Siksha 'O' Anusandhan University, Bhubaneswar, Odisha, India*
[4]*Department of Oral and Maxillofacial Pathology, Institute of Dental Sciences, Siksha 'O' Anusandhan University, Bhubaneswar, Odisha, India*

Correspondence should be addressed to Shamimul Hasan; shasan1@jmi.ac.in

Academic Editor: Rui Amaral Mendes

Hamartomas are tumor-like deformities typified by cellular propagation indigenous to the original site, although they display growth arrest without the possibility for further growth. Various hamartomatous oral lesions include hemangiomas, lymphangiomas, nevi, odontomas, Cherubism, etc. Lymphangiomas are benign, developmental hamartomatous entities typified by abnormal proliferation of lymphatic vessels. They are usually congenital, and more than 90% of cases occur by 2 years of age, with a rare occurrence in adults. They have a site affinity for the head and neck, and oral lesions are relatively uncommon. The dorsum of the tongue is the commonest oral site of predilection; however, the lip is a rare site of involvement. Hereby, we present an uncommon case of lymphangioma of the lower lip in a 45-year-old male patient, who reported to our hospital with an asymptomatic lower lip submucosal mass present for the last 3 years. Our case is unique as it occurred on the lower lip of a 45-year-old male. A detailed history and clinical evaluation, ultrasonography, and histopathology confirmed the diagnosis of lymphangioma.

1. Introduction

Hamartoma is described as a benign, unifocal/multifocal, developmental abnormality, encompassing a blend of cytologically normal mature cells and tissues native to the anatomic site, and exhibits a disordered architectural outline with a preponderance of one of the elements [1].

Lymphangioma refers to hamartomatous entities originating from abnormal lymphatics which cease to drain into other lymphatics or veins, thus causing lymph stagnation resulting in the development of large cyst-like dilated lymphatics [2, 3]. Lymphangiomas are typified by aberrant propagation of lymphatic vessels and are considered non-neoplastic developmental anomalies rather than actual tumors [4–6].

Owing to the intimate proximity to the primitive jugular lymphatics, most cases occur in the head and neck region (75%), followed by the clavicle and axillary regions (25%) [7–11]. The oral cavity is an infrequently involved site, with most occurrences seen in the anterior 2/3rd of the dorsal aspect of the tongue. However, occasional cases may involve the palate, cheek, gingiva, lips, and alveolar ridges [4, 7,

9–13]. Infants and children below the age of 2 years are mostly affected, with uncommon occurrences in adults [3, 6, 12, 14].

Hereby, we present an unusual case of lymphangioma of the lower lip in a 45-year-old male patient. Our case is unique in a few aspects as it manifested age and site variation.

2. Case Description

A 45-year-old male patient with no known comorbidities reported to our Outpatient Department with a complaint of a mass in the lower lip region for the past 3 years. The initially smaller mass has shown gradual progression, although the lesion has been static for the past 3-4 months. There was a negative history of similar lesions in any other part of the body. However, there was an occasional factitial habit of lip biting. The extraoral examination was unremarkable. On intraoral examination, a solitary, well-delineated nodular mass was noticeable in the submucosa of the lower lip, 2 × 1.5 cm in diameter, extending anteriorly 3 cm away from the mucocutaneous junction, posteriorly blending and obliterating the vestibule, and mesiodistally extending from right canine to the left lateral incisor region. The overlying mucosa was of the same color as the adjacent mucosa, smooth-surfaced with few interspersed areas exhibiting a granular appearance. Palpatory findings were suggestive of a nontender, nonfluctuant mass, soft to firm in consistency, nonpulsatile, and not fixed to the adjacent tissues. Multiple grainy nodules were also felt on palpation. The lesion did not blanch on pressure, and there was no sensory deficit in the lip region. A solitary, sessile, bluish-white, soft, and nontender swelling, 3.5 × 2.5 mm in diameter, was also seen on the right aspect of the vermilion border with mild hyperkeratinization, features in sync with the factitial lip biting. The patient's oral hygiene was fair and class II was seen with 31 (Figures 1(a) and 1(b)). The tooth fracture occurred around 20 days back while biting on a peanut, and the tooth was nondiscolored and asymptomatic.

3. Differential Diagnosis

Considering the anamnesis and clinical appearance of a localized, slow-progressing, smooth-surfaced, well-defined, asymptomatic, freely movable mass located within the lower lip submucosa, the lesion was considered of benign origin. Entities of minor salivary gland origin (mucocele, salivary duct cysts, and benign and malignant minor salivary gland tumors) and infectious origin (odontogenic/nonodontogenic) and mesenchymal tumors of adipose tissue (lipoma), vascular entities (hemangioma and lymphangioma), smooth muscle lesions (leiomyoma), or neural derivatives (traumatic neuroma, schwannoma, and neurofibroma) were given a place in the list of differential diagnosis.

The lower lip is extremely vulnerable to factitial injury and has a propensity for minor salivary gland tissues; thus, mucocele or salivary duct cysts account for the majority of swellings/lumps in this area. In the present case, the probability of the mass being a mucocele may be negated by its large size (mucoceles larger than 1.5 cm in diameter are extremely infrequent) [10], age of the patient (mucoceles are more likely to occur in children and young adults) [10, 15], chronic duration of 3 years, soft-firm consistency, and covered with normal overlying mucosa. However, a solitary, bluish-white colored, soft, and nontender swelling in the right aspect of the vermillion border with an associated occasional lip biting may be clinically diagnosed as a mucocele.

The possibility of salivary duct cysts is highly unlikely as they characteristically appear as bluish, firm nodular swellings on the floor of the mouth and rarely on the lips [16].

Benign minor salivary gland tumors (primarily pleomorphic adenomas and canalicular adenomas) primarily involve the upper lip, with infrequent occurrence on the lower lip. Moreover, pleomorphic adenoma is usually seen in younger individuals (<40 years), and canalicular adenoma has an elderly female predilection (>60 years) [17]. These features contrast with the present case.

The diagnosis of a malignant minor salivary gland tumor (adenoid cystic carcinoma and acinic cell carcinoma) may be ruled out based on the location, well-circumscribed mass, chronic duration, and lack of fixation [18].

Soft tissue infections of the lip (odontogenic/nonodontogenic) may be negated due to the asymptomatic and chronic duration of the lesion with normal dentition. Soft tissue lip abscess is generally ill-defined and fluctuant and exhibits inflammatory signs (pain and erythema) [19].

Lipoma is a nonneoplastic adipose tissue tumor, with an uncommon (1-4%) occurrence in the oral cavity. Lipomas characteristically manifest as a slow-growing, yellow-colored, soft, asymptomatic submucosal mass, with a typical "slip sign," occurring mostly on the tongue and cheek region [20].

Hemangioma diagnosis may be negated taking into account the patient's age and gender (hemangiomas occur exclusively in infancy and young adults, especially in girls), chronicity of the lesion, noncompressibility, lack of a peculiarly bright red lesion, and a negative diascopy test [16, 19].

Lymphangioma, a benign hamartomatous lesion of the lymphatic system, primarily affects infants and children and involves the tongue, although few lip cases have also been documented [3]. The lip lesions frequently exhibit an asymmetric, asymptomatic, firm, and nodular pattern [19].

Leiomyoma, a benign smooth muscle tumor, infrequently occurs in the oral cavity due to the absence of smooth muscle in the region [21]. The lesion mostly affects individuals in the 3rd decade and manifests as a slow-progressing, asymptomatic mass.

Reactive and neoplastic neural lesions (traumatic neuroma, neurofibroma, and schwannoma) may also be considered in the present case. The oral traumatic neuroma typically manifests as a nodular lesion, in close proximity to the mental foramen, tongue, or lips. However, the lesions are painful on palpation [22].

Schwannomas (neurilemmomas) are benign neural tumors and manifest as discrete, firm, smooth-surfaced nodular lesions of the same color as the adjacent mucosa. They have a site affinity for the head and neck region, although lip involvement is an extremely rare occurrence [17, 23].

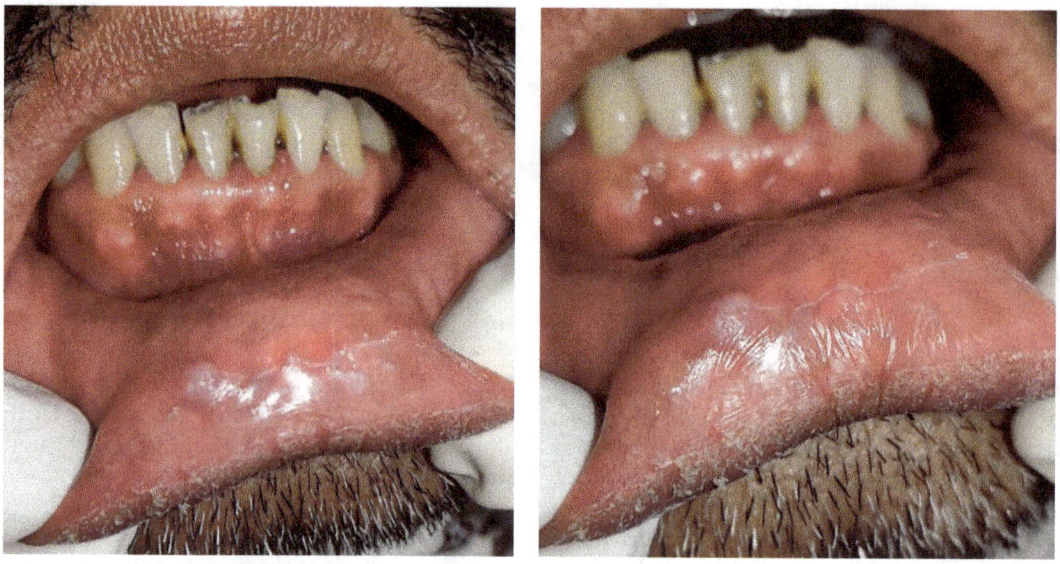

(a) (b)

FIGURE 1: (a, b) Solitary, well-circumscribed submucosal mass in the lower lip, with an adjacent bluish-white swelling depicting a mucocele.

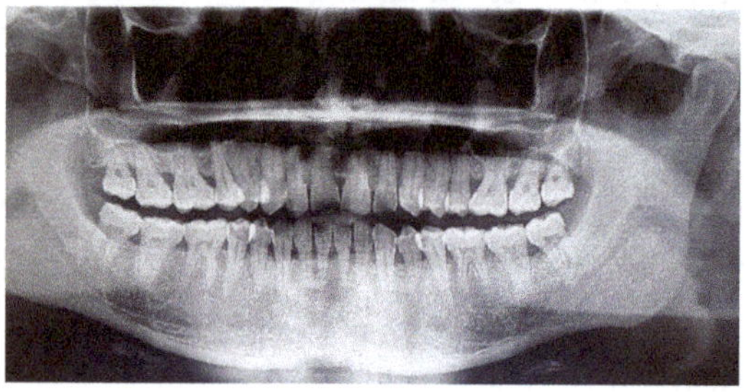

FIGURE 2: OPG demonstrating an ill-defined periapical pathology with #31.

Neurofibroma (NF) is a nerve sheath neoplasm, manifesting as a localized lesion or as a component of the diffuse neurofibromatosis syndrome. However, solitary NF is an extremely unusual occurrence in the oral cavity (6% occurrence) and infrequently affects the lower lip [23].

To summarize, our clinical impression was suggestive of a benign minor salivary gland lesion.

4. Investigations and Treatment Plan

With these differentials in mind, the patient was subjected to further investigations. Negative results were obtained on diascopy with a glass slide and fine-needle aspiration (FNA) of the mass that revealed blood-tinged clear fluid resembling lymphatic fluid. The minimally invasive procedure of FNA not only aids in the initial tissue-based diagnosis of salivary gland lesions but also aids in sorting and contemplating the treatment strategy for the patient [24].

Hematologic evaluation including complete blood count, serum calcium, phosphorus, and parathormone levels was within normal limits. A low platelet count (thrombocytopenia) may indicate a risk of bleeding prior to surgical interventions, with a plethora of bleeding symptoms such as bruising, nosebleeds, and, rarely, grievous or fatal bleeding [25]. Orthopantomogram (OPG) was unremarkable except for the presence of an ill-defined periapical pathology i.r.t #31 (Figure 2).

Ultrasound was done using a linear probe with special 2D enhancement features including compound and speckle reduction imaging (SRI). The study revealed tiny anechoic cystic lesions with internal septa, measuring approximately 1.9×1.0 mm (clinically visible lesion) with adjacent tiny lesions measuring 1.1×0.6 mm and 1.7×1.5 mm (Figure 3(a)). Another similar morphological lesion was apparent on the left side measuring 1.5×0.8 mm (Figure 3(b)). The color Doppler was suggestive of an avascular anechoic lesion (Figure 3(c)). USG serves as a noninvasive aid for the diagnosis of soft tissue lesions, delineation of cystic from solid lesions, and benign from malignant masses. The color Doppler USG may be employed to ascertain the presence or absence of vascular flow in normal tissues and in diseased states [26].

Magnetic resonance imaging (MRI) of the lower lip was advised, but the patient denied the investigation due to financial constraints.

After taking written consent from the patient, an excisional biopsy was done under local anesthesia. The lesion was enucleated via a blunt horizontal incision of the mucosa with no. 15 blades, taking utmost care not to injure the vital structures. Fine-dissecting scissors and artery forceps were used to excise the lesion. 3-0 vicryl was used to suture the muscle bed, and the lip was approximated and sutured with silk. Grossly, the excised specimen was a nodular mass, firm in consistency, and measured 3×2 cm (Figure 4). The enucleated specimen was submitted for histopathological examination.

Histological evaluation of the hematoxylin and eosin-stained sections (10x) reveals an atrophic epithelium beneath which there are numerous dilated lymphatic

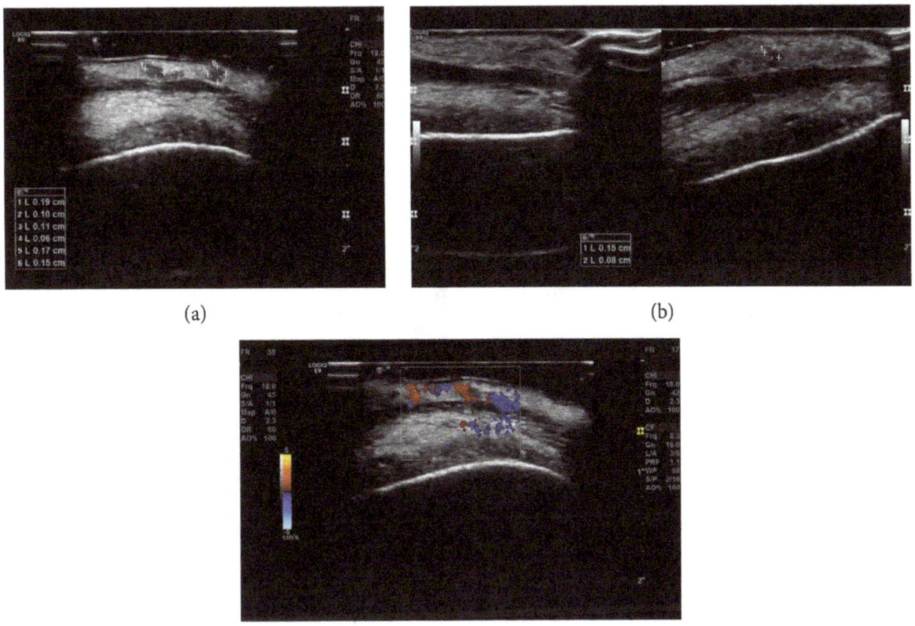

(a) (b) (c)

FIGURE 3: (a, b) Adjacent tiny lesions on the right and left sides of the lip. (c) The color Doppler was suggestive of an avascular anechoic lesion.

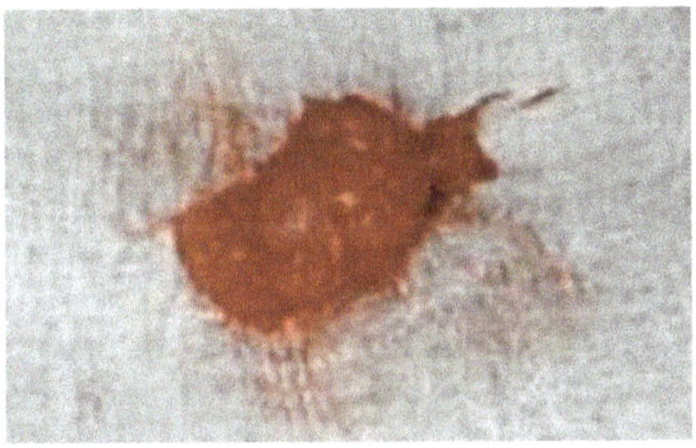

FIGURE 4: Gross excised specimen was suggestive of a firm nodular mass.

channels lined by endothelial cells within the papillary and reticular layers of the lamina propria. The large dilated lymphatics just are filled with lymph and infiltrated with inflammatory cell infiltrates, predominantly lymphocytes, neutrophils, and plasma cells. The histopathological features were in coherence with a diagnosis of lymphangioma (Figure 5). However, the patient was lost for further follow-up.

5. Discussion

There exists a diverse pattern in defining lymphangiomas; however, the nonneoplastic proliferation of lymphatic channels delineating a lymphatic hamartoma represents the classical description of lymphangiomas [27].

Lymphangiomas emanate from the sequestration of primordial lymphatic cells. The lymphatic channels persistently accumulate lymph; however, they fail to join with the larger vessels, causing lymphatic obstruction, thus imparting a cystic appearance [7]. They are rare entities with an incidence of about 1 : 6,000 to 1 : 16,000 live births and are attributed to about 6% of benign, 11% of maxillofacial tumors, and 9% of soft tissue tumors in the pediatric age group [3, 27, 28].

Embryologically, lymphangiomas are mostly congenital (50%); the majority of the lesions (90%) manifest by 2 years of age or in rare cases, which may be acquired [3, 7, 9–12, 28–30]. The probable predisposing factors for acquired lymphangiomas include long-standing trauma, inflammation, and lymphatic blockage due to infection, radiotherapy, or surgery.

Congenital lymphangiomas can also occur in association with hemangiomas, certain chromosomal aberrations (Noonan syndrome, Turner syndrome, and Down syndrome), fetal hydrops, fetal alcohol syndrome, cardiac anomalies, and familial pterygium colli [12, 13, 31]. Lymphangioma in adults is an uncommon occurrence, with only a few documented cases [3, 7, 11, 14, 29–31].

Our patient was a 45-year-old male with an occasional factitial habit of lip biting. The repeated local trauma in the lower lip region could have triggered the proliferation of lymphatic vessels.

The close anatomical proximity to the primordial jugular lymphatic sac probably justifies the lymphangioma site predilection for the head and neck region (90% of cases seen in the head and neck region) [6–11]. The oral cavity is rarely the site of occurrence, and the commonest affected oral site is the anterior 2/3rd of the dorsum of the tongue (often resulting in macroglossia) [9, 12, 13]. Other affected oral sites in decreasing order are the palate, buccal mucosa, gingiva, floor of the mouth, and lips [4, 7, 9–14, 31].

The symptoms of adult-onset lymphangioma are atypical and vary considerably, thus, posing a diagnostic dilemma [32].

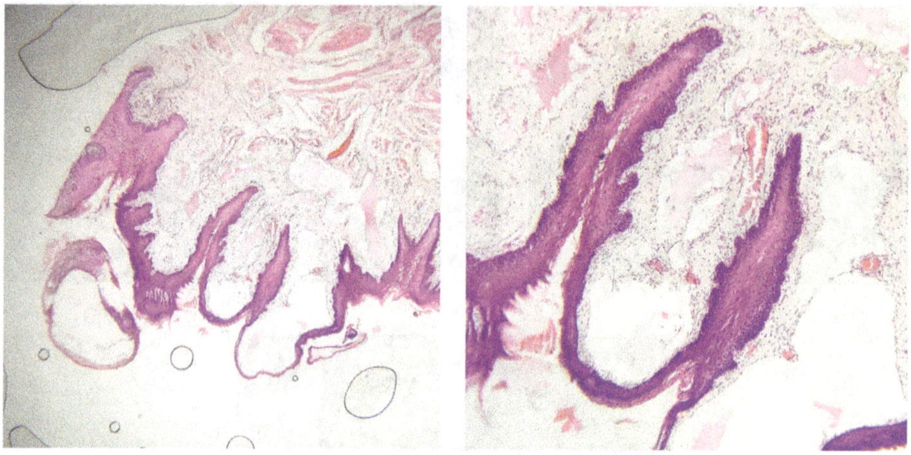

(a) (b)

FIGURE 5: (a) The photomicrograph (10x) reveals the atrophic epithelium beneath which there are numerous dilated lymphatic channels lined by endothelial cells. (b) The photomicrograph (400x) shows large lymphatic channels below the stratified squamous epithelium.

Lymphangiomas of the lower lip are unusual and account for <1% of the lip biopsies. Lip lesions clinically mimic mucocele, thus causing a diagnostic difficulty [10], as seen in the present case. Lip involvement and the associated anomalies are described as macrocheilia [12, 31].

An extensive literature search was carried out on the Google Scholar and PubMed search engines using the following keywords: lymphangioma, lymphatic malformation, oral cavity, lip, and lower lip. Case reports published in the English language up to December 2021 were thoroughly searched. This extensive bibliographic research finally resulted in 16 case reports, after excluding studies that were duplicates, not case reports, and those which were not in the English language.

The parameters extracted from these cases are summarized in Table 1, and they concerned the following: year of occurrence, age and gender, age at the time of initial presentation, location, size, chief complaint, and treatment. Out of the 16 reported cases, 7 cases were seen in males, in the age range of 14 months-69 years, size range from 0.3 cm to 4 cm, and mostly manifesting as swelling/enlargement. Most of the cases were treated by surgical excision, with few cases exhibiting recurrences.

The reported cases of lip lymphangiomas are summarized in Table 1.

The lesion extent directs the clinical appearance of lymphangiomas [3, 4, 11, 14]. They frequently manifest as a long-standing, asymptomatic, progressively expanding soft tissue mass that has been reasonably inactive, with intermittent episodes of exacerbation and remission, eventually remaining as a residual mass [3, 12, 31]. Superficial lymphangiomas typically manifest as pebbly, vesicle-like lesions, with the characteristic "frog-egg" or "tapioca pudding" presentation, although occasionally, the vesicles may appear purplish/bluish-red owing to the secondary hemorrhage into the lymphatic system [3, 10, 13, 14, 27]. However, a soft, diffused nodular submucosal mass with a similar texture and color as the contiguous mucosa depicts the classical description of deep-seated lymphangiomas [3, 12–14].

Our case presented as a solitary, slow-growing, well-circumscribed, asymptomatic, soft-firm, nonblanching, nodular submucosal mass in the lower lip region with normal overlying mucosa, although a few interspersed areas exhibited a granular appearance. A solitary, sessile, bluish-white, soft, and nontender swelling, 3.5x 2.5 mm in diameter, was also seen (in proximity to the mass) on the right aspect of the lip vermilion border with mild keratinization.

Several detrimental effects such as breathing and speech difficulty, pain, tongue protrusion, or jaw anomalies may be seen with deep lesions owing to the impingement on the contiguous anatomical structures [3, 13, 27].

Secondary infection may predispose to Ludwig's angina. The postsurgical sequalae may include bleeding, seroma formation, repeated episodes of cellulitis, and leakage of lymphatic fluid [33].

Several hypotheses have been recommended for the etiopathogenesis of lymphangiomas. The first hypotheses propose that congenital lymphangiomas result from sequestration of primordial lymphatics; however, they fail to connect to the main lymphatic vessels or veins [34]. The second hypothesis states that the failure of the lymphatic vessels to drain into the veins causes lymph accumulation and leads to the formation of large cyst-like dilated lymphatics [27]. According to the third hypothesis, lymphangiomas may develop through aberrant budding of the lymphatic vessels, thus establishing new anomalous divisions. The fourth hypotheses suggest that long-standing inflammation may evoke lesion development by triggering the proliferation of lymphatic channels [29]. The most recent hypotheses document an increased expression of vascular endothelial growth factor-C (VEGF-C) and vascular endothelial growth factor R3 [35].

Histopathologically, lymphangiomas consist of dilated lymphatic vessels with one or two endothelial layers, with

TABLE 1

S. No.	Author and year	Age and gender	Age at the initial presentation	Site	Size (cm)	Chief complaint	Treatment	Recurrence
1.	Nagata (1984)	27/M	5	Right buccal mucosa-lower lip	—	Mass lesion	Excision	Yes
2.	Fukuda M et al. (1989)	14 months/ M	1 month	Right lower lip and buccal mucosa	Thumb-sized tumor	Swelling	Excised several times, cryosurgery treatment many times, vaporized by laser irradiation	Repeated recurrences
3.	Balakrishnan (1991)	4/M	1 week	Neck-submandibular region-bilateral buccal mucosa-right parotid region-both lips-tongue	—	Swelling-difficulty with breathing	Laser therapy	Yes
4.	Park (2002)	69/F	39	Mandible-lower lip	$4 \times 2 \times 1$	Irritation-discoloration	—	—
5.	Ertugul et al. (2008)	23/M	22.5 months	Lower lip	0.6×0.9	Cosmetic concern	Excisional biopsy	No
6.	Nagaoka (2008)	9/F	2	Lower lip	$2.8 \times 1.7 \times 0.1$	Swelling	Excision	—
7.	Jha (2012)	13/M	5	Lower lip	—	Enlargement	Excision	—
8.	Bindu (2013)	13/M	13	Lower lip	1.5×1	Enlargement	Excision	—
9.	de Carvalho (2015)	6/M	—	Lower lip	0.3	Mass	Excision	—
10.	de Carvalho (2015)	4/F	—	Lower lip	1	Mass-difficulty in eating and speaking	Excision	—
11.	Fernandes (2018)	68/F	62	Lower lip	—	Mass	Follow-up	No
12.	Matharu (2019)	4/F	Birth	Lower lip	$0.55 \times 0.17 \times 0.7$	Mass	Cryotherapy	No
13.	Flores (2020)	6/F	6	Lower lip	$0.6 \times 0.5 \times 0.4$	Asymptomatic nodules	Excision	No
14.	Santos et al. (2020)	56/F	48	Lower lip	—	White painless vesiculobullous lesion	Excision	—
15.	Kurude et al. (2020)	10/M	9	Lower lip and buccal mucosa	2–3 mm papules	Asymptomatic lesions on the right buccal mucosa with swelling of the cheek and lips on the right side	Sclerotherapy	—
16.	Ehtisham (2021)	55/M	54	Lower lip	—	Painless growth	Excision	—
17.	Present case	45/M	42	Lower lip	2×1.5	Mass	Surgical excision	—

or without an adventitial layer. Based on the location and contiguous structures, these dilated lymphatic vessels are of variable sizes, thus forming the basis of classification. Cavernous lymphangiomas commonly occur in regions with a rich supply of denser connective tissue and skeletal muscle, causing confined lesions, e.g., oral cavity (dorsal aspect of the tongue, buccal mucosa, and floor of the mouth). This is contrary to cystic hygromas, which develop in loose adipose tissue sites resulting in a diffuse spread and large multicystic lesions [28, 34].

The microscopic findings in our case were incoherent with the published literature.

Most lymphangiomas are diagnosed clinically based on the characteristic manifestations. However, excision and histological assessment, together with diagnostic radiographic aids facilitate the confirmatory diagnosis of lymphangiomas with bizarre clinical characteristics [7, 34].

Ultrasound (USG) is an essential diagnostic aid in assessing the site, shape, size, and extent of lesions. Ultrasound generally exhibits multicystic lesions with internal septations, and the color-flow Doppler depicts the avascular nature of lymphangiomas, thus, not only distinguishing vascular malformations from hemangiomas but also identifying the various vascular patterns of such entities.

In our case, the USG findings were suggestive of multiple anechoic cystic lesions with internal septa on the right and left sides of the lower lip. The color Doppler was suggestive of an avascular anechoic lesion.

However, computed tomography (CT) and magnetic resonance imaging (MRI) are superior to ultrasound in describing the relationship with contiguous anatomical structures and demarcating the lesion extent [27, 29].

Magnetic resonance imaging (MRI) of the lower lip was advised, but the patient denied the investigation due to financial constraints.

Mostly, lymphangiomas are benign in origin; however, they may require surgical treatment due to their infiltrative pattern causing larger lesions to encroach the adjoining vital structures, resulting in cosmetic, functional, and life-threatening sequelae [3, 7].

The treatment strategies should focus on restoring the functions, averting any potential complications (secondary infections/internal hemorrhage), and attaining adequate cosmetic satisfaction [36]. A wide array of proposed management strategies for lymphangiomas are surgical excision, electrocautery, cryotherapy, radiotherapy, intralesional steroids, sclerosing agents (OK432), embolization and ligation, laser treatment with Nd:YAG and carbon dioxide, and radiofrequency tissue ablation technique. However, surgical excision is considered the gold standard of treatment [3, 11–14, 27]. Adult lymphangiomas are mostly encapsulated, thus facilitating the surgical excision [12, 27, 28, 30].

Sclerotherapy with 25% dextrose, hypertonic saline, bleomycin, and picibanil (OK-432) is considered deemed for recurrent, unresectable/surgically demanding lesions [37]. Sclerosing agents have shown superior efficacy in the management of macrocystic lymphangiomas, as compared to the microcystic lyphangiomas [38]. Senthilnathan et al. treated a soft tissue lymphangioma by ultrasonographic-guided bleomycin sclerotherapy. Intralesional bleomycin not only damages the endothelial lining of the lymphangioma but also stimulates the diffusion of the chemical into the cystic spaces, thus, causing thrombosis and fibrosis around the vascular spaces [39].

Recently published reports have also documented the successful management of tongue lymphangiomas by nonablative long-pulsed Nd:Yag lasers and constitutional homoeopathic medicine Tuberculinum, respectively [40, 41].

Surgical extirpation has an accompanying high recurrence rate (10-39%), primarily due to the deeper permeation of the lesion or incomplete surgical removal. Preoperative intralesional administration of sclerosing agents may prove beneficial in such cases [30].

In our case, surgical enucleation of the mass was done using a blunt horizontal incision under local anesthesia.

6. Conclusion

Lymphangiomas are common entities in the pediatric age group and are rarely encountered in adulthood. They may be frequently misdiagnosed owing to the bizarre clinic radiographic manifestations, and histopathologic evaluation provides the confirmatory diagnosis. Lymphangiomas uncommonly involve the oral cavity, with a rare occurrence in the lower lip. Lymphangiomas should always be given a place in the differential diagnosis of a localized submucosal mass of the lower lip.

Consent

The patient was informed about the nature of the disease and treatment protocol. Written informed consent was taken from the patient.

References

[1] S. Patil, R. S. Rao, and B. Majumdar, "Hamartomas of the oral cavity," *Journal of International Society of Preventive and Community Dentistry*, vol. 5, no. 5, pp. 347–353, 2015.

[2] P. S. Joshi, B. Hongal, and A. Sanadi, "Cystic lymphangioma: a differential diagnosis," *Journal of Oral and Maxillofacial Pathology: JOMFP*, vol. 19, no. 3, pp. 393–395, 2015.

[3] H. Bhavya, D. Pavani, T. M. L. Avinash, and P. Geetha, "Oral lymphangioma: a rare case report," *Contemporary Clinical Dentistry*, vol. 6, no. 4, pp. 584–587, 2015.

[4] S. Gupta, P. Ahuja, U. Rehani, and V. Singh, "Lymphangioma of cheek region-an unusual presentation," *Journal of Oral Biology and Craniofacial Research*, vol. 1, no. 1, pp. 47–49, 2011.

[5] J. P. Purohit, P. Tripathi, and I. Singh, "Lymphangioma of tongue," *Indian Journal of Otolaryngology - Head & Neck Surgery*, vol. 58, no. 4, pp. 404-405, 2006.

[6] W. Colangeli, V. Facchini, A. Kapitonov, M. Zappalà, F. Bozza, and R. Becelli, "Cystic lymphangioma in adult: a case report and a review of the literature," *Journal of Surgical Case Reports*, vol. 2020, no. 7, pp. 1–3, 2020.

[7] L. Stănescu, E. F. Georgescu, C. Simionescu, and I. Georgescu, "Lymphangioma of the oral cavity," *Rom J Morphol Embryol*, vol. 47, no. 4, pp. 373–377, 2006.

[8] T. Park, H. S. Lee, E. J. Jung et al., "Concomitant breast and axillary lymphangioma in an adult: a case report and a review of the literature," *Medicine*, vol. 97, no. 45, p. 12946, 2018.

[9] P. R. Bindhu, J. Mathew, P. Thomas, P. Jayanthi, and R. Krishnapillai, "Cavernous lymphangioma of lower lip," *Health Sciences*, vol. 2, pp. 1–7, 2013.

[10] F. K. de Carvalho, T. N. Pinheiro, R. A. B. da Silva, A. M. de Queiroz, L. A. B. da Silva, and P. Nelson-Filho, "Lymphangioma mimicking mucocele in children," *Journal of Dentistry for Children*, vol. 82, no. 3, pp. 10–13, 2015.

[11] S. Ertugrul, G. Ertugrul, A. Aktas, A. Aktümen, and H. Erol, "A case of oral lymphangioma mimicking mucocele," *Journal of*

the Turkish Academy of Dermatology, vol. 11, no. 4, p. 1711411, 2017.

[12] F. Ugurlu, A. Kaya, E. T. Akdogan, V. Olgac, and A. Sipahi, "Oral lymphangioma of the alveolar ridge - a report of a rare case," *Hamdan Medical Journal*, vol. 9, pp. 247–250, 2016.

[13] V. Usha, T. Sivasankari, S. Jeelani, G. S. Asokan, and J. Parthiban, "Lymphangioma of the tongue- a case report and review of literature," *Journal of clinical and diagnostic research: JCDR*, vol. 8, no. 9, pp. 12–14, 2014.

[14] S. Sunil, D. Gopakumar, and B. S. Sreenivasan, "Oral lymphangioma-case reports and review of literature," *Contemporary Clinical Dentistry*, vol. 3, pp. 116–118, 2012.

[15] L. S. Magalhaes, M. N. B. Calazans, A. L. S. Cota, M. A. Nemezio, and M. A. Brêda Junior, "Diagnosis and treatment of mucocele in a pediatric patient: case report," *RGO-Revista Gaúcha de Odontologia*, vol. 68, pp. 1–5, 2020.

[16] N. J. D'Silva, R. Benian, A. Flint, and K. G. Cordell, "Soft tissue swelling of the upper lip," *Oral Surg Oral Med Oral Pathol Oral Radiol Endod*, vol. 5, pp. 271–273, 2008.

[17] B. W. Neville, D. Damm, C. M. Allen, and J. E. Bouquot, *Oral and Maxillofacial Pathology*, Philadelphia: Saunders, 2nd edition, 2002.

[18] G. Ellis, P. L. Auclair, and D. R. Gnepp, *Surgical Pathology of the Salivary Glands: Major Problems in Pathology*, Philadelphia: Saunders, 1991.

[19] B. Krishnan, D. Basu, and J. M. Daniel, "A discrete swelling of the upper lip: a diagnostic and clinical stepladder," *Journal of Maxillofacial and Oral Surgery*, vol. 13, no. 3, pp. 300–304, 2014.

[20] A. T. Hoseini, S. M. Razavi, and A. Khabazian, "Lipoma in oral mucosa: two case reports," *Dental Research Journal*, vol. 7, no. 1, pp. 41–43, 2010.

[21] G. Orsini, M. Fioroni, C. Rubicini, and A. Piattelli, "Leiomyoma of the lip: report of a case," *Journal of Oral and Maxillofacial Surgery*, vol. 59, pp. 80–83, 2001.

[22] K. Subhashraj, S. Balanand, and S. Pajiniammalle, "Ancient schwannoma arising from the mental nerve. A case report and review," *Med Oral Patol Oral Cir Buccal*, vol. 14, pp. 12–14, 2009.

[23] E. Chrysomali, S. I. Papanicolaou, N. P. Dekker, and J. A. Regezi, "Benign neural tumors of the oral cavity," *Oral Surgery, Oral Medicine, Oral Pathology, Oral Radiology, and Endodontology*, vol. 84, pp. 381–390, 1997.

[24] R. N. Satarkar, A. Sangwaiya, P. Singh, S. Kalhan, and N. S. Puja, "Fine needle aspiration cytology-based spectrum of salivary gland lesions at a teaching institute in north India," *Pathology Update: Tropical Journal of Pathology & Microbiology*, vol. 5, no. 12, pp. 976–982, 2019.

[25] L. J. Estcourt, R. Malouf, C. Doree, M. Trivella, S. Hopewell, and J. Birchall, "Prophylactic platelet transfusions prior to surgery for people with a low platelet count," *Cochrane Database of Systematic Reviews*, vol. 2017, no. 9, p. CD012779, 2017.

[26] P. S. Joshi, J. Pol, and A. S. Sudesh, "Ultrasonography - A diagnostic modality for oral and maxillofacial diseases," *Contemporary Clinical Dentistry*, vol. 5, no. 3, pp. 345–351, 2014.

[27] J. Matharu and V. Patel, "Cryotherapy for the management of a lip lymphangioma - a case report and literature review," *Oral Surgery*, vol. 12, pp. 230–237, 2019.

[28] E. L. H. Omar-Amir, E. A. M. Ali, and M. A. K. Osman, "Clinical profile of lymphatic malformation from one oral and maxillofacial center in Sudan," *Open Journal of Stomatology*, vol. 7, pp. 345–352, 2017.

[29] C. Ramashankar, N. K. S. Prabhakar, and G. Giraddi, "Lymphatic malformations: a dilemma in diagnosis and management," *Contemporary Clinical Dentistry,*, vol. 5, no. 1, pp. 119–122, 2014.

[30] M. Gupta, "Lymphangioma of the tongue presenting as macroglossia," *Indian Journal of Paediatric Dermatology*, vol. 18, pp. 132-133, 2017.

[31] S. S. Yoganna, R. Gowda, R. Prasad, and B. Sekar, "Oral lymphangioma of the buccal mucosa- a rare case report," *Journal of Pharmacy & Bioallied Sciences*, vol. 6, no. 1, pp. 188–191, 2014.

[32] H. Hou-Kuang, H. Hua-Hsin, T. C.-J. Chun-Hung, T. Da-Tian, and S. L.-S. Ming-Hsui, "Adult lymphangioma of the oropharynx: a case report," *Anticancer Research*, vol. 40, pp. 1631–1636, 2020.

[33] A. AlGhamdi and M. AlBaqami, "Lymphangioma of the tongue in a pediatric patient," *Journal of Pediatric Surgery Case Reports*, vol. 75, pp. 1–6, 2021.

[34] M. Kaur, V. Gombra, R. V. Subramanyam, and S. Hasan, "Lymphangioma of the buccal mucosa – a case report and review of literature," *Journal of Oral Medicine, Oral Surgery, Oral Pathology and Oral Radiology*, vol. 1, no. 3, pp. 123–125, 2015.

[35] A. Tayefeh, A. Asadollahi, and M. V. Saatloo, "A rare case report of oral lymphangioma in buccal mucosa," *Ann Clin Case Stud*, vol. 2, no. 4, pp. 31–42, 2020.

[36] N. Khanum, J. D. Smitha, and S. Kanwar, "Microcystic lymphatic malformation of tongue-a case report," *SVOA Dentistry*, vol. 2, no. 2, pp. 67–70, 2021.

[37] A. A. Kurude, M. M. Phiske, K. K. Kolekar, and C. S. Nayak, "Lymphangiomas: rare presentations in oral cavity and scrotum in pediatric age group," *Indian Journal of Dermatology, Venereology and Leprology*, vol. 86, p. 230, 2020.

[38] X. Liu, C. Cheng, K. Chen, Y. Wu, and Z. Wu, "Recent progress in lymphangioma," *Frontiers in Pediatrics*, vol. 15, no. 9, p. 735832, 2021.

[39] N. Senthilnathan, M. Narayanan, K. Appusamy, K. R. Mohan, S. Gokul-Raj, and R. Thangave, "An unusual clinical appearance of lymphangioma in the cheek in a 52-year-old female - a rare case report," *Journal of Evolution of Medical and Dental Sciences*, vol. 10, no. 28, pp. 2134–2138, 2021.

[40] S. Mozafarpoor, A. Asilian, A. Goodarzi, Z. Ebrahimi, F. Mokhtari, and Z. R. Moqaddam, "Treatment of tongue lymphangioma circumscriptum with non-ablative long-pulsed Nd:YAG laser: a case report and review of literature," *Iranian Journal of Dermatology*, vol. 24, pp. 242–248, 2021.

[41] S. Parveen and S. K. Mahasin-Ali, "A child with lymphangioma of tongue treated with constitutional homoeopathy medicine- a rare case report," *Homœopathic Links*, vol. 34, no. 1, pp. 62–69, 2021.

17

Complete Spontaneous Bone Regeneration following Surgical Enucleation of a Mandibular Cemento-Ossifying Fibroma

Saeed Shirafkan,[1] Mehdi Gholamian,[1] Ali Rohani,[1] Sadaf Sadat Mahmoudinezhad,[1] Mahshid Razavi,[2] and Kooshan Moradi[1]

[1]*Department of Oral and Maxillofacial Surgery, School of Dentistry, Ahvaz Jundishapur University of Medical Sciences, Ahvaz, Iran*
[2]*Department of Oral and Maxillofacial Radiology, School of Dentistry, Ahvaz Jundishapur University of Medical Sciences, Ahvaz, Iran*

Correspondence should be addressed to Sadaf Sadat Mahmoudinezhad; sadafmahmoudinezhad@gmail.com

Academic Editor: Darko Macan

Background. Cemento-ossifying fibroma (COF) is a type of benign fibro-osseous tumor that mainly occurs in the maxillofacial region. Bone reconstruction after the surgery is often performed with bone transplantation. However, the present case report describes the accurate diagnosis and successful surgical resection of a COF with periosteum preservation, after which the defect was completely and spontaneously filled with the newly formed bone through a natural process. *Case Presentation.* A 32-year-old Iranian female patient presented with a history of gradual development of painful swelling, spontaneous pain, and lower lip and chin hypoesthesia in the lower third of the left side of her face. The dome-shaped swelling was tender. The patient was suffering from renal infection and urethral prolapse and was taking folic acid. She also mentioned a positive family history of similar swellings in her mother and uncle. Intraoral examination indicated a lesion in buccal and lingual vestibules extending from the first premolar to the third molar teeth. It had a firm consistency, and the covering mucosa was normal in terms of color and texture. The aspiration test was negative. The lesion had caused severe mobility of the second premolar and first and second molar teeth. Panoramic radiography revealed an extensive well-defined unilocular radiolucency. Significant knife-edge resorption of the first and second molar roots at the involved site and thinning of the alveolar crest and inferior border of the mandible were also clear. Cone-beam computed tomography showed severe expansion in the buccal and moderate expansion in the lingual aspect, causing thinning of both the buccal and lingual cortical plates. Histopathological analysis revealed neoplastic tissue mixed with fibrous connective tissue and several round and oval-shaped calcification foci. Immunohistochemical analysis confirmed the final diagnosis (COF) with the presence of SMA-8. The lesion was removed by enucleation and curettage, while the periosteum was carefully preserved. Fixation with screw and plate was also performed. *Conclusions.* Correct diagnosis of COF and precise implementation of the periosteal osteogenesis technique, in this case, resulted in entirely and spontaneously bone regeneration, which was a rare and favorable outcome with minimum cost and complications for the patient.

1. Background

Cemento-ossifying fibroma (COF) is a benign fibro-osseous tumor that mainly involves the maxillofacial region [1]. This neoplastic lesion has a capsule and is almost well defined. It contains a mixture of fibrous tissue and different amounts of calcified tissues resembling bone, cementum, or both [2, 3]. COF was first categorized as a fibro-osseous neoplasm by the World Health Organization [4]. It often occurs in the second to fourth decades of life and is more common in females [3]. It does not involve the long bones; instead, it commonly occurs in the tooth-bearing areas of the jaws [5]. The mandible, particularly at the molar–premolar region, is the most common location for the occurrence of COF [6]. It originates from the mesenchymal cells, which are found in the periodontal ligament and capable of forming fibrous tissue, cementum, bone, or a combination of all [2, 7]. Most COF lesions have a slow growth pattern and often remain undetected by the patient

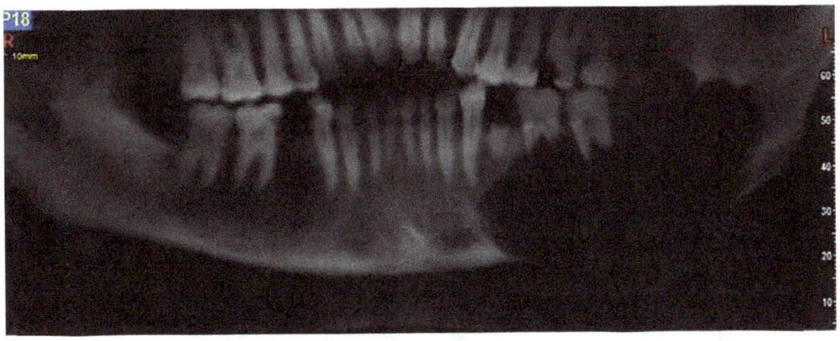

Figure 1: Panoramic view upon presentation.

until swelling of the face becomes prominent. However, in rare cases, COF may grow rapidly and cause clinical symptoms [2]. The incorrect surgical technique could lead to relapse. Thus, correct diagnosis and treatment plan can lead to optimal predictable results in the management of COF [8]. Herein, we report the diagnostic workup (which included radiographic, histopathological, and immunohistochemical assessments), and successful surgical resection of a COF. Following surgery, the bone defect was completely filled with the newly formed bone through a spontaneous natural process.

2. Case Presentation

This retrospective study was approved by the ethics committee. The study was performed in accordance with the ethical standards as laid down in the 1964 Declaration of Helsinki. The patient gave her informed consent prior to use of her medical reports and images in the present case report study. The present manuscript is written following CARE guidelines.

A 32-year-old female patient presented to a dental clinician complaining of gradual development of painful swelling in the lower third of the left side of her face. After the initial examination, the dental clinician referred her to the Oral and Maxillofacial Surgery Department.

2.1. Extraoral Examination. Extraoral examination revealed a dome-shaped swelling in the lower third of the left side of the face. The skin over the involved site had normal color and texture. The lesion was tender on palpation, and the patient reported spontaneous pain and hypoesthesia of the lower lip and chin toward the left side. The patient also declared suffering from renal infection and urethral prolapse and was taking folic acid. She also mentioned a positive family history for such lesions (in her mother and uncle).

2.2. Intraoral Examination. Intraoral examination indicated a lesion in the mandibular left side buccal and lingual vestibules extending from the first premolar to the third molar teeth. It had a firm consistency, and the covering mucosa was normal in terms of color and texture. The aspiration test was negative. The lesion had caused severe mobility of the second premolar and the first and second molar teeth.

2.3. Imaging Findings. Panoramic radiography revealed an extensive well-defined unilocular radiolucency in the body of the mandible at the left side, extending from the apex of

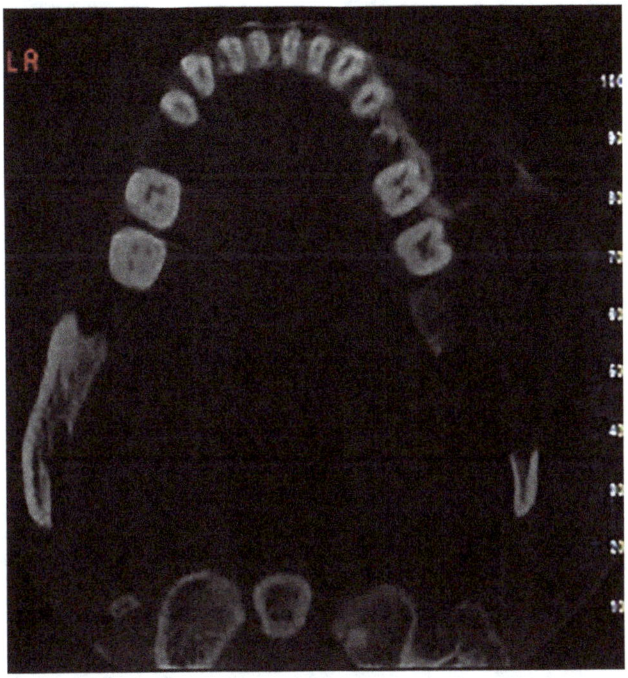

Figure 2: Axial CBCT section upon presentation.

the first premolar of the same side to the upper third of the mandibular ramus horizontally, and from the alveolar crest to the inferior border of the mandible vertically. It had caused severe expansion toward the mandible's inferior border and the alveolar crest (Figure 1). Significant knife-edge resorption of the first and second molar roots at the involved site and thinning of the mandible's alveolar crest and inferior border were also evident.

Cone-beam computed tomography was then performed. The axial and cross-sectional views indicated severe expansion in the buccal and moderate expansion in the lingual aspect, causing thinning of both the buccal and lingual cortical plates (Figures 2 and 3). Labiolingual and superoinferior lesion sizes on the cross-sectional CBCT section were 37.2 mm and 42.9 mm, respectively (Figure 4). Also, the anteroposterior size of the lesion in the axial CBCT section was 63.8 mm (Figure 5). Some calcification foci were also noted in the radiolucent lesion. According to the radiographic findings, the list of differential diagnoses included ossifying fibroma, central giant cell granuloma, and aneurysmal bone cyst.

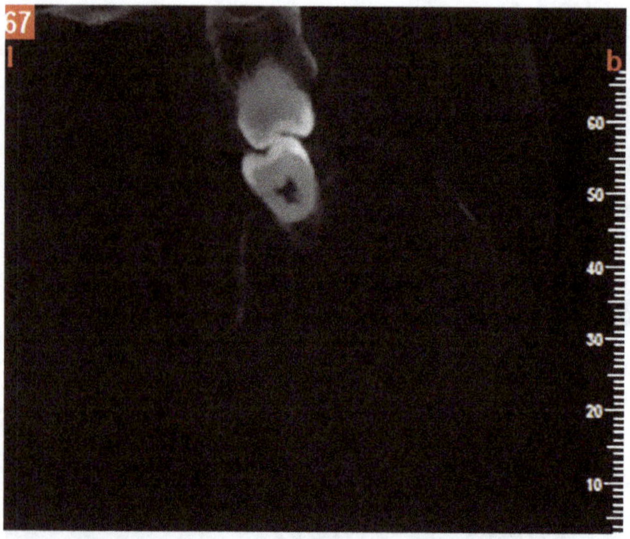

Figure 3: Cross-sectional CBCT image upon presentation.

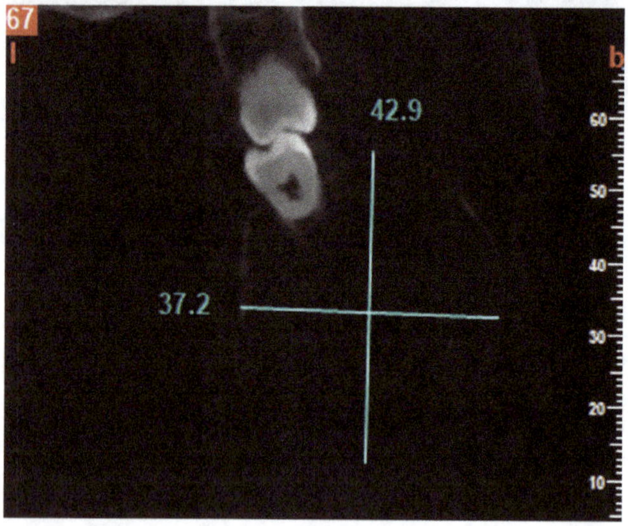

Figure 4: Labiolingual and superoinferior size of the lesion on cross-sectional CBCT section. (labiolingual size = 37.2 mm, superoinferior size = 42.9 mm).

2.4. Histopathological Findings. Histopathological analysis of the enucleated lesion was performed by an oral and maxillofacial pathologist. The pathology report disclosed a lesion with cream color and firm consistency measuring 3 × 4 × 5 cm, which was associated with 3 teeth. Microscopic assessments revealed neoplastic tissue mixed with fibrous connective tissue and several round and oval-shaped calcification foci. The primary diagnosis by the pathologist was spindle cell neoplasm, which is a malignancy in the list of differential diagnoses with many other benign and malignant lesions. Since the radiographic findings indicated that the inferior border of the mandible had not been invaded or perforated, and was only displaced due to severe expansion of the lesion, the pathological diagnosis of spindle cell neoplasm was questioned by the surgeon, because malignancies often invade the border and cause destruction of cortical bone. Thus,

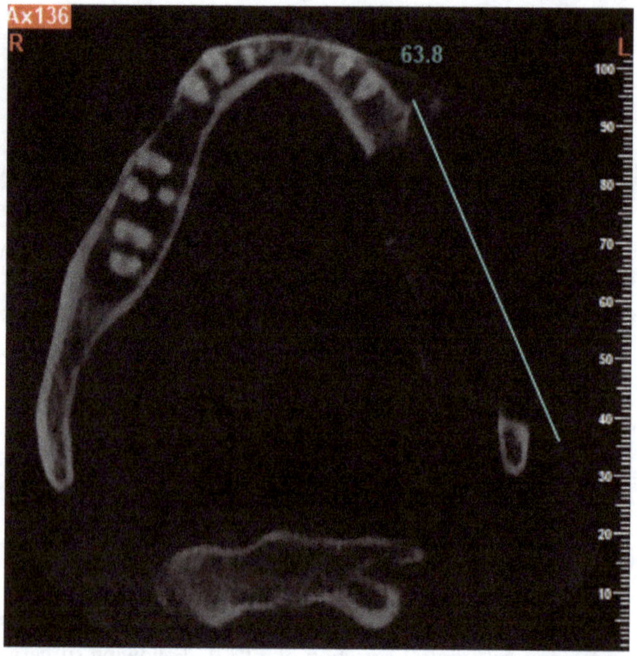

Figure 5: Anteroposterior size of the lesion in axial CBCT section.

immunohistochemical analysis was requested, which was positive for smooth muscle actin (SMA-8). The presence of this marker led to a definite diagnosis of COF.

2.5. Surgical Procedure. Surgical enucleation was performed 9 months after the development of the lesion. Precise diagnostic workup revealed the benign nature of the lesion. Thus, to adopt the most conservative approach for minimal removal of intact bone and also to benefit from the inherent regenerative potential of the periosteum, it was decided to perform enucleation and curettage. Accordingly, the submandibular or Risdon approach was adopted to access the lesion after disinfecting with chlorhexidine and povidone-iodine [9]. First, a mark was made on the skin 3 cm below the inferior border of the mandible to preserve the marginal mandibular nerve. The local anesthetic agent was then administered. After gentle and careful elevation of the periosteum (to preserve and protect it), the tumor was resected subperiosteally with 1 cm of safe margin both anteriorly and posteriorly (considering its benign nature and also for maximum preservation of healthy bone tissue) (Figures 6–8). A reconstruction plate was then adapted and installed to reinstate the occlusion. After enucleation of the tumor and curettage, the area was copiously irrigated. The incision was then sutured after approximation of the dissected layers. Arch bar and elastics were then placed. The follow-up sessions were scheduled at 1 week, 3 months, 6 months, 1 year, and 3 years postoperatively (Figures 9–12). After 1 year from surgery, which was the time for bone grafting, a panoramic radiograph was requested, which revealed complete bone fill of the defect. Also, 3 years after the surgery, cross-sectional CBCT images revealed complete bone regeneration and no recurrence of the COF (Figure 12). The histopathological evaluation of the regenerated bone was also assessed. An incisional biopsy was obtained during plate removal, and

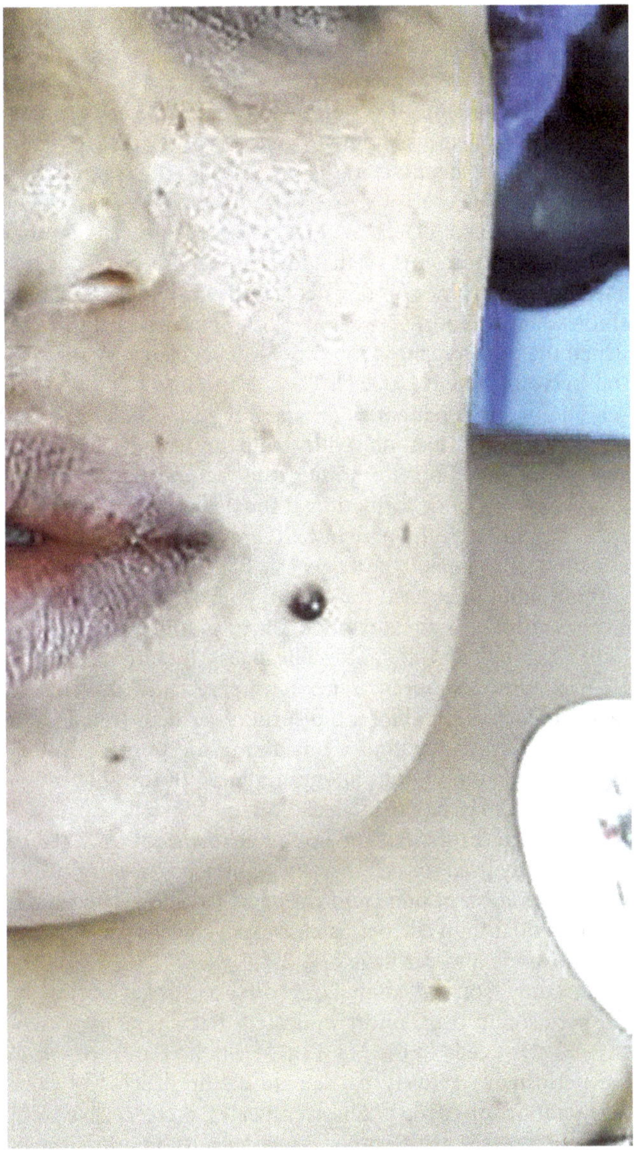

FIGURE 6: Extraoral preoperative view.

the sections were stained with hematoxylin and eosin. Figure 13 shows a well-shaped trabecular bone and bone marrow space filled with dense fibrous connective tissue, which indicates spongy bone histology.

The skin of the lip corner, chin, and face of the involved side was also carefully examined, which revealed paresthesia. After ensuring complete spontaneous bone fill of the defect, the plate was removed in another surgical procedure.

3. Discussion

Oral and maxillofacial surgeons are searching for ways to functionally and esthetically reconstruct the mandibular bone defects caused by the resection of lesions. However, the available approaches for the reconstruction of mandibular bone defects are complex and challenging. Recently, oral and maxillofacial surgeons have been more interested in benefiting the spontaneous bone regeneration capacity of the bone, which is likely to happen with the preservation of the periosteum after mandibulectomy. To reinstate the normal morphology and function of the lost or injured tissue, it would be ideal to benefit from the inherent healing and regenerative potentials of the human body in reconstructive procedures. Therefore, this topic has gained increasing popularity in regenerative medicine. This approach has numerous advantages for reconstruction of mandibular bone defects such as reduction of costs and postoperative complications. However, such advantages should be weighed against the possibility of shortcomings such as unpredictability of the amount of formed bone in some cases [10–12].

To induce spontaneous bone regeneration, the periosteum should remain intact to serve as a natural source of viable bone cells and provide the necessary vascular support. Also, the periosteum should be able to serve as a barrier against the migration of soft tissue into the defect to allow osteogenesis [13–17], which was precisely performed in the present case.

Assessment of more than 600 cases over 20 years in a retrospective study revealed that following regional resection of the mandible, the possibility of spontaneous bone regeneration

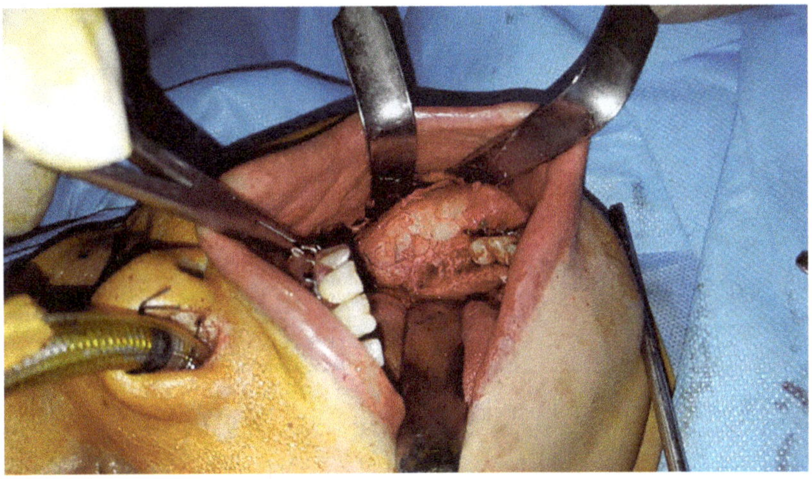

FIGURE 7: Intraoral intraoperative view.

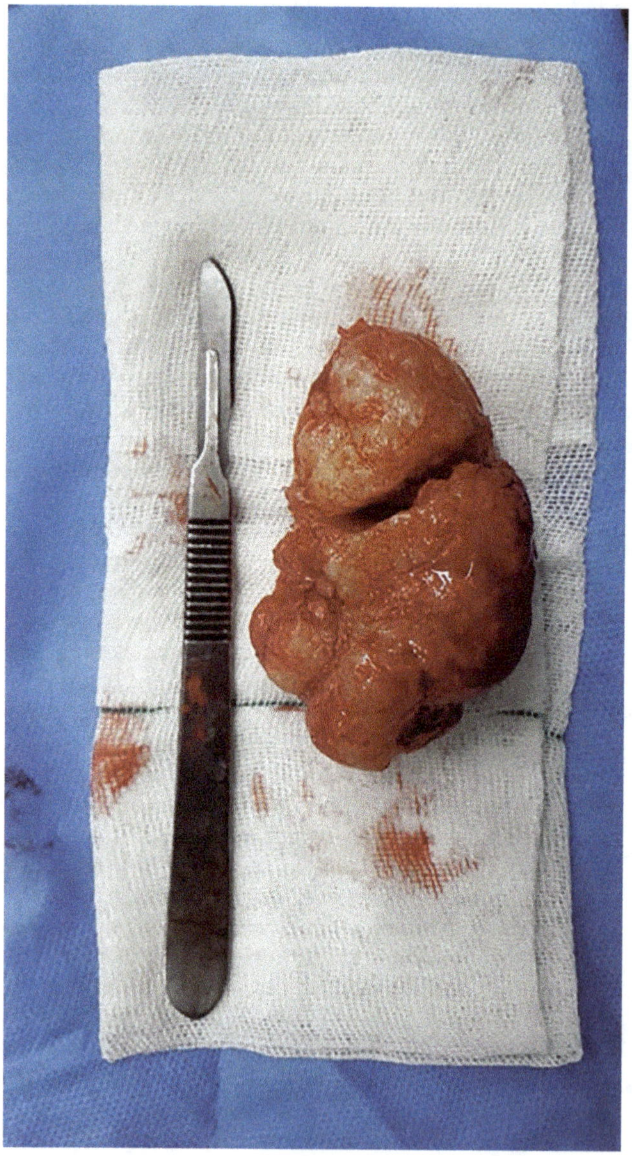

Figure 8: Enucleated lesion.

would only be 2%. The present case was among the aforementioned 2% fraction in whom spontaneous bone regeneration resulted in complete bone fill of the defect [13, 18].

The mechanism of action of the periosteal osteogenesis involves angiogenesis and neurogenesis [10, 19, 20]. The reason behind angiogenesis in the process of bone regeneration is obvious. However, with regard to neurogenesis, particularly in the maxillofacial region, it has been discussed that the expression of genes related to neurogenesis has a positive effect on the promotion of osteogenesis in this region. Some studies have reported a controlling mechanism through which the bone regeneration process is regulated by the central nervous system [10, 21].

The younger patient's age, stability of the defective segment following fixation with plate and screw, and the absence of infection are among the factors that affect the process of new bone formation at the defect site. In the present case, although the patient had a positive history of renal infection, spontaneous osteogenesis happened appropriately without additional need for a bone graft [13, 17, 22].

According to the textbook of *Oral and Maxillofacial Pathology* by Neville and colleagues, mutations in the HRPT2 tumor suppressor gene were recently detected in two patients with different disorders such as renal cysts and COF of the jawbone. Considering the positive history of renal infection in our patient, mutation of the abovementioned gene may be postulated [23].

Evidence shows that the bone marrow stem cells, which are currently used for cell therapy approaches in orthopedics for regeneration of bone and cartilage, have lower regenerative potential than the periosteum-derived cells for regeneration of bone and cartilage [24, 25].

A study conducted in 2020 on bone regeneration by the periosteum progenitors indicated that a type of mesenchymal stem cells known as $Prx1^+$ cells that are present in the periosteum actively participate in the process of bone regeneration of defects. The number of these cells significantly decreases with aging, which results in impairment of the regenerative potential of bone over time. Also, they

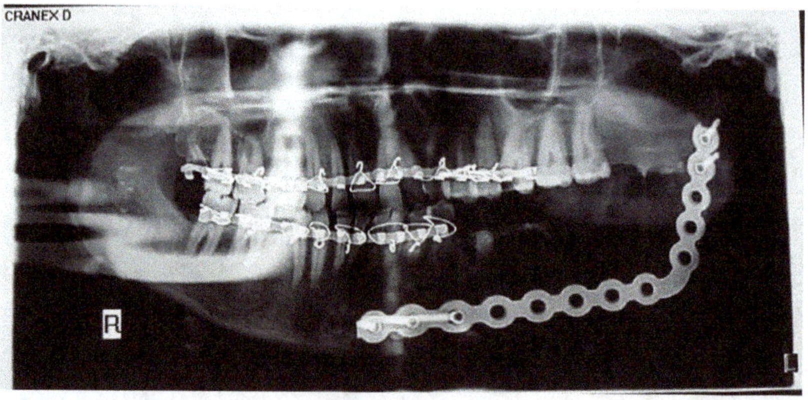

Figure 9: Panoramic view at 1 week postoperatively.

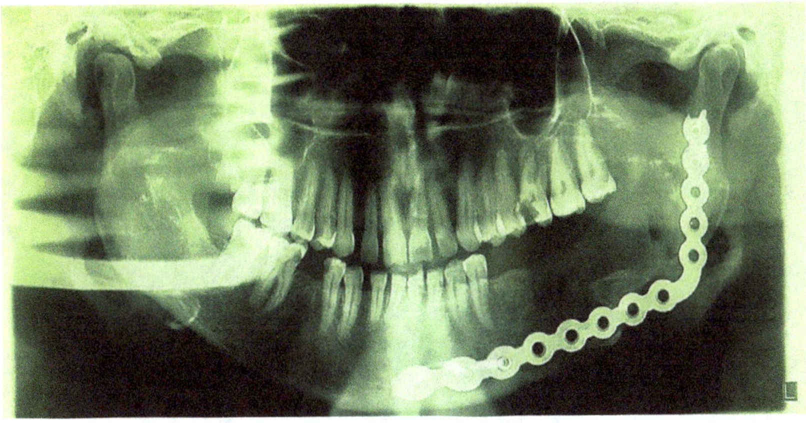

FIGURE 10: Panoramic view at 1 year postoperatively, indicating spontaneous bone fill of the defect.

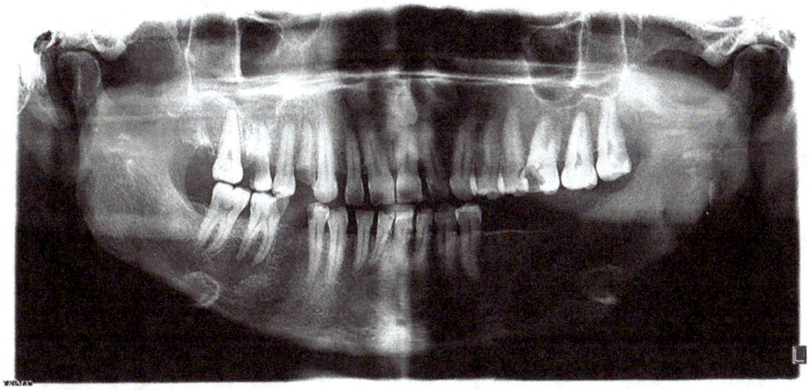

FIGURE 11: Panoramic view at 3 years postoperatively, indicating spontaneous bone fill of the defect.

confirmed that $Prx1^+$ mesenchymal stem cells can enhance early healing of bone defects [24]. Moreover, some other studies have documented that periosteum-derived $Nestin^+$ and $LepR^+$ cells located in the outer layer of the periosteum are capable of regeneration and chemotaxis of bone progenitor cells [26, 27]. Unlike the $Prx1^+$ cells that are exclusively found in the skeletal system, the $Nestin^+$ and $LepR^+$ cells are present in other tissues as well [24, 28, 29]. Furthermore, it has been discussed that the bone morphogenetic protein 2 (BMP2) also serves as an initial regulator of periosteal bone regeneration. The BMP2 is famous for its role in skeletal growth and development and is believed to have an inherent potential to induce bone regeneration. The target cells of BMP2 are located in the periosteum. Also, it has been claimed that maximum therapeutic efficacy can be achieved by benefitting from the recombinant form of BMP2 to increase the density of the newly formed bone in the process of periosteal bone regeneration [30–32].

Recently, a protein known as periostin was discovered, which is synthesized in response to mechanical stress, injuries, and pathological conditions [25, 33–35]. In different cancer types, particularly the common high-risk cancers such as the lung cancer, elevated levels of periostin are associated with poor prognosis and metastasis [36]. In addition, a considerable increase in the level of periostin in periosteal cells has been reported in skeletal injuries, highlighting its role in optimal regeneration of the injured bone [25].

Review of the recently published articles indicates the occurrence of periosteal osteogenesis not only in the maxillofacial region but also in other parts of the human skeleton. In 2020, Rajak et al. [37] reported a case of an aneurysmal bone cyst in the clavicle. They reported bone regeneration induced by the intact periosteum after marginal resection of the lesion on the first follow-up.

In 2020, Colangeli et al. [38] reported a 12-year-old boy with Ewing's sarcoma in the ulnar diaphysis. The patient underwent an extensive resection of the ulnar diaphysis, and then an ipsilateral fibula graft was harvested as an autologous non-vascularized graft. The periosteum was carefully preserved in the process of bone harvesting. Radiographic examinations of the donor site performed in the first six months after surgery indicated complete bone regrowth and regeneration at the graft harvesting site. Some studies have discussed that chemotherapy may damage the periosteum and impair its bone regenerative potential. However, in their case, despite the conduction of chemotherapy, the periosteum preserved its regenerative capacity. According to the literature, younger age and the presence of a thicker periosteum increase the possibility of faster and more extensive bone regeneration [38–41].

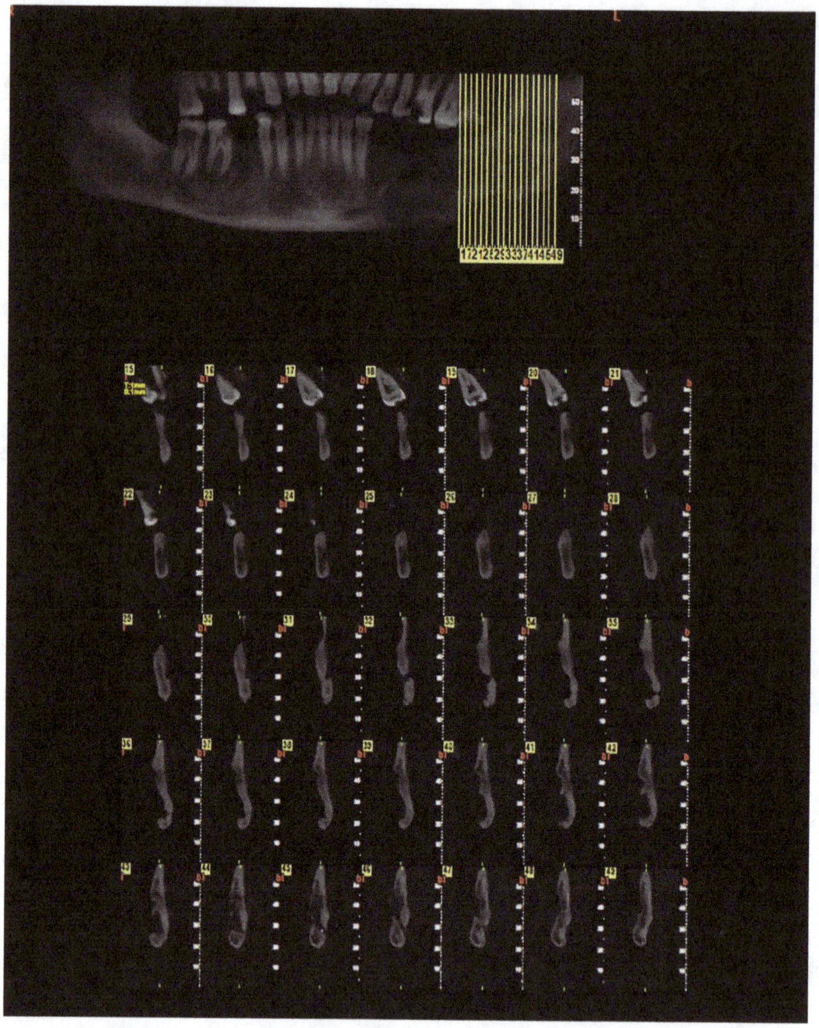

FIGURE 12: Cross-sectional CBCT images at 3 years postoperatively, indicating spontaneous bone fill of the defect (after ensuring complete spontaneous bone fill of the defect, the plate was removed in another surgical procedure).

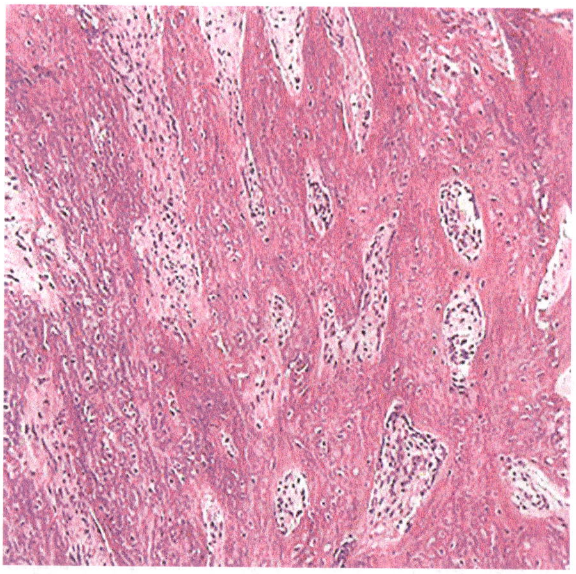

FIGURE 13: Well-shaped trabecular bone and bone marrow space filled with dense fibrous connective tissue.

COF may manifest different radiographic patterns depending on its degree of mineralization. Initially, it manifests as a radiolucent lesion. The calcified foci gradually increase as the lesion matures until a completely radiopaque appearance is created [6, 42, 43]. The main characteristic feature of COF is its eccentric growth pattern, which results in its expansion in all directions and eventual formation of a prominent spherical mass, which is easily differentiable from the adjacent tissues [3, 43]. Titinchi and Morkel [34] showed that in approximately 50% of the cases, COF is radiopaque. It manifests as a combined radiolucent–radiopaque lesion in 35%, and purely radiolucent lesion in only 15% of the cases; our case was categorized in the latter group.

According to the existing literature on this topic, clinically, COF is often painless and appears as a slow-growing mass in the jaw with tooth displacement as its first symptom. Moreover, the teeth at the site remain vital, and root resorption rarely occurs [44, 45]. However, in the present case, the lesion had caused root resorption without causing tooth displacement. Root resorption was reported in 12% of the cases in the study by Titinchi and Morkel and the majority of

COFs causing root resorption were multilocular, and occurred in young patients. However, the lesion in our patient was unilocular and caused root resorption of the teeth at the site [46].

The well-defined margin of COF aids in its differentiation from invasive sarcomas and carcinomas. Accordingly, the attending surgeon of the present case suspected the accuracy of the initial pathological diagnosis regarding the lesion being a spindle cell neoplasm and requested immunohistochemical analysis [47, 48]. COF often expands without perforating the surrounding cortical bone and forms a distinct spherical shape [47].

Since COF can be clearly differentiated from the adjacent bone, it can be resected conservatively. The suggested treatment plans include enucleation for small lesions, curettage for the lesions with no distinct radiolucency around them, and en bloc resection along with bone regeneration for large lesions close to the inferior border of the mandible [46].

Due to resistance to radiation, radiotherapy of COF would be complicated. It has a good prognosis although the risk of relapse in the maxilla is much higher than that in the mandible due to greater complexity of the surgical procedure in the maxilla particularly for large lesions [49]. Complete and precise surgical resection of the lesion at the earliest time possible has been widely advocated [46].

4. Conclusions

Finally, it should be noted that precise diagnosis of the lesion in the present case and correct adoption of periosteal bone regeneration approach resulted in complete bone regeneration, which was a rare and favorable outcome with minimum cost and complications for the patient.

Abbreviations

COF: Cemento-ossifying fibroma
SMA: Smooth muscle actin

Consent

The patient signed the consent form before participation. Written informed consent was obtained from the patient for publication of this case report and any accompanying images. A copy of the written consent is available for review by the Editor-in-Chief of this journal.

Authors' Contributions

All authors contributed to the study conception and design. Material preparation, data collection and analysis were performed by SS, MG, AR, SM, KM, and MR. The first draft of the manuscript was written by SM and all authors commented on previous versions of the manuscript. All authors read and approved the final manuscript.

References

[1] W. Sc and M. Pharoah, *Oral Radiology: Principles and Interpretation*, Mosby Elsevier, St Louis, MO, 2009.

[2] R. Ram, A. Singhal, and P. Singhal, "Cemento-ossifying fibroma," *Contemporary Clinical Dentistry*, vol. 3, no. 1, pp. 83–85, 2012.

[3] A. H. M. Ong and C. H. Siar, "Cemento-ossifying fibroma with mandibular fracture. Case report in a young patient," *Australian Dental Journal*, vol. 43, no. 4, pp. 229–233, 1998.

[4] M. Gonçalves, R. Píspico, F. A. Alves, C. E. B. Lugão, and A. Gonçalves, "Clinical, radiographic, biochemical and histological findings of florid cemento-osseous dysplasia and report of a case," *Brazilian Dental Journal*, vol. 16, no. 3, pp. 247–250, 2005.

[5] S. A. Khan, N. K. Sharma, V. Raj, and T. Sethi, "Ossifying fibroma of maxilla in a male child: report of a case and review of the literature," *National Journal of Maxillofacial Surgery*, vol. 2, no. 1, pp. 73–79, 2011.

[6] C. A. Waldron, "Fibro-osseous lesions of the jaws," *Journal of Oral and Maxillofacial Surgery*, vol. 51, no. 8, pp. 828–835, 1993.

[7] Y. Liu, H. Wang, M. You et al., "Ossifying fibromas of the jaw bone: 20 cases," *Dento Maxillo Facial Radiology*, vol. 39, no. 1, pp. 57–63, 2010.

[8] D. B. Kamadjaja, "Cemento-ossifying fibroma of the jaw," *Dental Journal (Majalah Kedokteran Gigi)*, vol. 42, no. 4, pp. 164–171, 2015.

[9] N. Dorestan, N. Ostadian, S. S. Mahmoudinezhad, A. Farajzadeh Sheikh, and K. Moradi, "Comparative efficacy of 0.2% chlorhexidine and 10% Betadine for perioral skin disinfection prior to oral surgical procedures: a clinical trial," *Irish Journal of Medical Science*, p. 2021, 2021.

[10] Z. Li, J. Pan, J. Ma, Z. Zhang, and Y. Bai, "Microarray gene expression of periosteum in spontaneous bone regeneration of mandibular segmental defects," *Scientific Reports*, vol. 7, p. 1, 2017.

[11] P. Sharma, R. Williams, and A. Monaghan, "Spontaneous mandibular regeneration: another option for mandibular reconstruction in children?," *British Journal of Oral and Maxillofacial Surgery*, vol. 51, no. 5, pp. e63–e66, 2013.

[12] O. Ahmad and G. Omami, "Self-regeneration of the mandible following hemimandibulectomy for ameloblastoma: a case report and review of literature," *Journal of Maxillofacial and Oral Surgery*, vol. 14, no. S1, pp. 245–250, 2015.

[13] S. Rai, V. Rattan, S. S. Jolly, V. K. Sharma, and M. M. Mubashir, "Spontaneous regeneration of bone in segmental mandibular defect," *Journal of Maxillofacial and Oral Surgery*, vol. 18, no. 2, pp. 224–228, 2019.

[14] P. J. Boyne, "The restoration of resected mandibles in children without the use of bone grafts," *Head & Neck Surgery*, vol. 6, no. 2, pp. 626–631, 1983.

[15] S. Shuker, "Spontaneous regeneration of the mandible in a child a sequel to partial avulsion as a result of a war injury," *Journal of Maxillofacial Surgery*, vol. 13, no. 2, pp. 70–73, 1985.

[16] M. O. Ogunlewe, J. A. Akinwande, A. L. Ladeinde, and W. L. Adeyemo, "Spontaneous regeneration of whole mandible after total mandibulectomy in a sickle cell patient," *Journal of Oral and Maxillofacial Surgery*, vol. 64, no. 6, pp. 981–984, 2006.

[17] S. A. Espinosa, J. Villanueva, H. Hampel, and D. Reyes, "Spontaneous regeneration after juvenile ossifying fibroma resection: a case report," *Oral Surgery, Oral Medicine, Oral Pathology, Oral Radiology, and Endodontology*, vol. 102, no. 5, pp. e32–e35, 2006.

[18] A. Bataineh, "Spontaneous bone regeneration of the mandible: in a case of osteosarcoma and literature review," *Austin Journal of Dentistry*, vol. 3, no. 1, p. 1031, 2016.

[19] S. Ivanovski, S. Hamlet, M. Retzepi, I. Wall, and N. Donos, "Transcriptional profiling of "guided bone regeneration" in a critical-size calvarial defect," *Clinical Oral Implants Research*, vol. 22, no. 4, pp. 382–389, 2011.

[20] R. Al-Kattan, M. Retzepi, E. Calciolari, and N. Donos, "Microarray gene expression during early healing of GBR-treated calvarial critical size defects," *Clinical Oral Implants Research*, vol. 28, no. 10, pp. 1248–1257, 2017.

[21] S. Takeda and G. Karsenty, "Molecular bases of the sympathetic regulation of bone mass," *Bone*, vol. 42, no. 5, pp. 837–840, 2008.

[22] O. Güven, "Formation of condyle-like structure after treatment of temporomandibular joint ankylosis: literature review and long-term follow-up of two patients," *Case Reports in Medicine*, vol. 2017, 7 pages, 2017.

[23] B. W. Neville, D. D. Damm, C. Allen, and A. C. Chi, "Oral and maxillofacial pathology," *Elsevier Health Sciences*, 2015.

[24] H. Xiao, L. Wang, T. Zhang et al., "Periosteum progenitors could stimulate bone regeneration in aged murine bone defect model," *Journal of Cellular and Molecular Medicine*, vol. 24, no. 20, pp. 12199–12210, 2020.

[25] O. Duchamp de Lageneste, A. Julien, R. Abou-Khalil et al., "Periosteum contains skeletal stem cells with high bone regenerative potential controlled by periostin," *Nature Communications*, vol. 9, no. 1, pp. 1–15, 2018.

[26] B. Gao, R. Deng, Y. Chai et al., "Macrophage-lineage TRAP+ cells recruit periosteum-derived cells for periosteal osteogenesis and regeneration," *The Journal of Clinical Investigation*, vol. 129, no. 6, pp. 2578–2594, 2019.

[27] G. Tournaire, S. Stegen, G. Giacomini et al., "Nestin-GFP transgene labels skeletal progenitors in the periosteum," *Bone*, vol. 133, article 115259, 2020.

[28] A. Bernal and L. Arranz, "Nestin-expressing progenitor cells: function, identity and therapeutic implications," *Cellular and Molecular Life Sciences*, vol. 75, no. 12, pp. 2177–2195, 2018.

[29] B. O. Zhou, R. Yue, M. M. Murphy, J. G. Peyer, and S. J. Morrison, "Leptin-receptor-expressing mesenchymal stromal cells represent the main source of bone formed by adult bone marrow," *Cell Stem Cell*, vol. 15, no. 2, pp. 154–168, 2014.

[30] K. Tsuji et al., BMP2 activity, although dispensable for bone formation, is required for the initiation of fracture healing," *Nature Genetics*, vol. 38, pp. 1424–1429, 2006.

[31] J. W. Lowery, D. Pazin, G. Intini et al., "The role of BMP2 signaling in the skeleton," *Critical Reviews in Eukaryotic Gene Expression*, vol. 21, no. 2, pp. 177–185, 2011.

[32] S. Minear, P. Leucht, J. Jiang et al., "Wnt proteins promote bone regeneration," *Science Translational Medicine*, vol. 2, no. 29, article 29ra30, 2010.

[33] N. Bonnet, K. N. Standley, E. N. Bianchi et al., "The matricellular protein periostin is required for sost inhibition and the anabolic response to mechanical loading and physical activity," *The Journal of Biological Chemistry*, vol. 284, no. 51, pp. 35939–35950, 2009.

[34] F. Titinchi and J. Morkel, "Ossifying fibroma: analysis of treatment methods and recurrence patterns," *Journal of Oral and Maxillofacial Surgery*, vol. 74, no. 12, pp. 2409–2419, 2016.

[35] N. Bonnet, E. Gineyts, P. Ammann, S. J. Conway, P. Garnero, and S. Ferrari, "Periostin deficiency increases bone damage and impairs injury response to fatigue loading in adult mice," *PLoS One*, vol. 8, no. 10, article e78347, 2013.

[36] I. Malanchi, A. Santamaria-Martínez, E. Susanto et al., "Interactions between cancer stem cells and their niche govern metastatic colonization," *Nature*, vol. 481, no. 7379, pp. 85–89, 2011.

[37] A. Rajak, A. Sethia, A. Limbu, and R. P. S. Kalawar, "Aneurysmal bone cyst of the clavicle: a case report," *Journal of Orthopaedic Case Reports*, vol. 9, no. 6, pp. 3–5, 2020.

[38] M. Colangeli, P. Spinnato, and M. Manfrini, "Periosteum preservation in bone regeneration," *Canadian Medical Association Journal*, vol. 192, no. 32, p. E920, 2020.

[39] A. Agarwal and A. Kumar, "Fibula regeneration following non-vascularized graft harvest in children," *International Orthopaedics*, vol. 40, no. 10, pp. 2191–2197, 2016.

[40] P. Virolainen, N. Inoue, M. Nagao, F. J. Frassica, and E. Y. Chao, "The effect of a doxorubicin, cisplatin and ifosfamide combination chemotherapy on bone turnover," *Anticancer Research*, vol. 22, no. 4, pp. 1971–1975, 2002.

[41] C. N. Steiger, P. Journeau, and P. Lascombes, "The role of the periosteal sleeve in the reconstruction of bone defects using a non-vascularised fibula graft in the pediatric population," *Orthopaedics & Traumatology, Surgery & Research*, vol. 103, no. 7, pp. 1115–1120, 2017.

[42] J. Silvestre-Rangil, F. J. Silvestre, and J. Requeni-Bernal, "Cemento-ossifying fibroma of the mandible: presentation of a case and review of the literature," *Journal of Clinical and Experimental Dentistry*, vol. 3, no. 1, pp. e66–e69, 2011.

[43] S. Jayachandran and S. Sachdeva, "Cemento-ossifying fibroma of mandible: report of two cases," *Journal of Indian Academy of Oral Medicine and Radiology*, vol. 22, no. 1, pp. 53–56, 2010.

[44] H. Sarwar, M. Jindal, and S. Ahmad, "Cemento-ossifying fibroma-a rare case," *Journal of the Indian Society of Pedodontics and Preventive Dentistry*, vol. 26, no. 3, pp. 128–131, 2008.

[45] T. Akcam, H. A. Altug, O. Karakoc et al., "Synchronous ossifying fibromas of the jaws: a review," *Oral Surgery, Oral Medicine, Oral Pathology, Oral Radiology*, vol. 114, no. 5, pp. S120–S125, 2012.

[46] F. Titinchi and J. Morkel, "Ossifying fibroma: analysis of treatment methods and recurrence patterns," *Journal of Oral and Maxillofacial Surgery*, vol. 74, no. 12, pp. 2409–2419, 2016.

[47] A. J. Kuta, C. Worley, and G. E. Kaugars, "Central cementoossifying fibroma of the maxillary sinus: a review of six cases," *American Journal of Neuroradiology*, vol. 16, no. 6, pp. 1282–1286, 1995.

[48] R. Mithra, P. Baskaran, and M. Sathyakumar, "Imaging in the diagnosis of cemento-ossifying fibroma: a case Series," *Science*, vol. 2, p. 52, 2012.

[49] B. Bertrand, P. Eloy, J. P. Cornelis, S. Gosseye, J. Clotuche, and C. Gilliard, "Juvenile aggressive cemento-ossifying fibroma: case report and review of the literature," *The Laryngoscope*, vol. 103, no. 12, pp. 1385–1390, 1993.

18

Broken File Retrieval in the Lower Right First Molar using an Ultrasonic Instrument and Endodontic Micro Forceps

Ratna Meidyawati, Endang Suprastiwi, and Hasti Dwi Setiati

Department of Conservative Dentistry, Faculty of Dentistry, Universitas Indonesia, Indonesia

Correspondence should be addressed to Endang Suprastiwi; esuprastiwi@yahoo.co.id

Academic Editor: Daniel Torres-Lagares

Broken files affect cleaning, shaping, and filling processes of the root canal, thereby causing maintenance failure. *Objective.* This report explains how to remove broken files using ultrasonic instruments and endodontic micro forceps. *Case Report.* A 25-year-old female patient had incomplete root canal treatment at the lower right first molar 1 week ago. There were radiolucency in the bifurcation and apical root and the presence of broken files in the 1/3 coronal mesiolingual root. The retrieval started by making a staging platform with an ET20 ultrasonic tip. Endodontic micro forceps were used including a screw wedge that works by clamping the file fragments through a mechanical lock and pulling them to the coronal. *Conclusion.* It is possible to successfully remove broken files from the root canal using ultrasonic instruments and endodontic micro forceps.

1. Introduction

The success of root canal treatment depends on the results of the cleaning and shaping process. However, there is a risk of broken files because its presence inhibits the process of cleaning, shaping, and filling, thereby leading to treatment failure [1]. A broken file often occurs in the molar teeth, especially at the lower jaw because of poor access, small diameter, and sharp curvature of the root canal. Both hand instruments and machine root canal instruments are mostly made of stainless steel and nickel titanium; therefore, there is a potential that they might break. It has been recorded that the incidence of broken files is 0.25% for hand instruments and 1.68%-2.4% for rotary instruments [2].

There are several alternative treatments for this occurrence, and they include taking the broken file fragment and bypassing it while inside the root canal [1]. However, there are several factors considered in managing these cases, and they include visibility, the location of broken file teeth, and the structure of the remaining tooth tissue [1]. Furthermore, this treatment often requires special assistance because of the risk of complications such as pushing the file apically, extruding fragments outside the apex, risk of tooth fracture due to dentin uptake excess, root perforation, and the occurrence of a ledge [3].

Technological advancement has made it possible to have several tools for file retrieval, including ultrasonic, microtube, and plier devices, with the assistance of a microscope to facilitate visibility and minimize the extraction of root canal dentine [1]. Therefore, this report discussed the management of broken file cases in the mandibular molars by using an ultrasonic device and endodontic micro forceps with the assistance of a microscope.

2. Case Report

A 25-year-old female patient complained that her lower right back teeth are not comfortable with chewing; therefore, root canal treatment was conducted one week ago after one year of spontaneous pain. On intraoral examination, caries reached the pulp in the lower right first molars, with negative vitality and positive percussion. Radiographic examination showed radiolucent images in the bifurcation area and apical

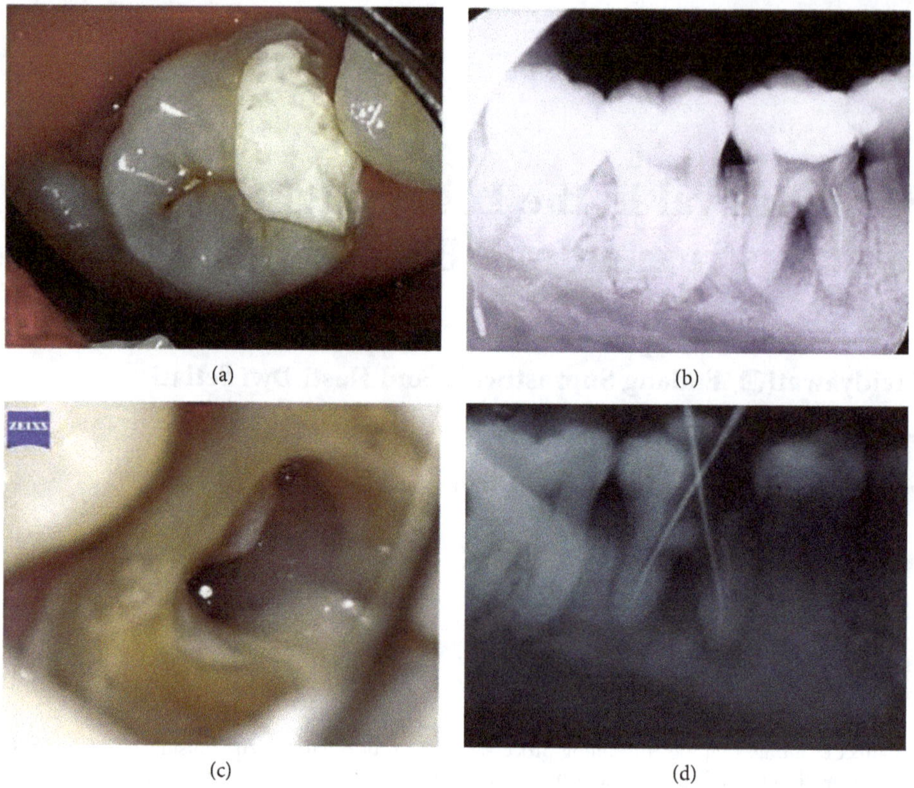

FIGURE 1: (a) Preoperative clinical feature. (b) Preoperative radiograph with a broken file in the mesiolingual canal. (c) Broken file was seen inside the canal (dental microscope magnification). (d) Ensuring the position of the file with an instrument.

mesial and distal roots and a broken file from the orifice to the middle of the mesiolingual root (Figures 1(a) and 1(b)).

Based on the subjective, objective, and radiographic examination, the diagnosis of the right mandibular first molar is symptomatic apical periodontitis, accompanied by a broken file on the mesiolingual root. The treatment conducted was for the nonvital root canals with Ceramage (Shofu Inc., Japan) onlay restoration.

The tooth was prepared to obtain adequate coronal access with 2.5% NaOCl as an irrigant to remove debris. The working length was measured through the use of an electronic apex locator (Root ZX II, Morita). The root canal was prepared in the mesiobuccal and distal roots through the use of ProTaper Next (Dentsply Maillefer, Switzerland) until the master apical file was obtained at X3/16.5 mm mesiobuccal root and X3/17.5 mm distal root. Irrigation was conducted, and the orifices of both root canals were closed with a paper point and cotton to prevent the entry of file fragments. In the mesial root canal, the retrieval started by making a staging platform with a Satelec ET20 (Satelec Acteon, France) ultrasonic tip until 2 to 3 mm of the broken file was exposed. This was aimed at loosening the file from the root canal wall of the dentin and providing a space for the device. The staging platform is the space between the tip of the exposed file and the root canal wall which was further circulated around the file in an anticlockwise direction to give the effect of unscrewing force. This helps in retrieving files with a clockwise cutting action. The energy applied can help loosen the file and provide a space between it and the root canal wall. The Satelec ET25 (Satelec Acteon, France) ultrasonic tip could then be used to loosen those on the part of the wall.

Irrigation was conducted by using 2.5% NaOCl and 17% EDTA, and activation was done through an EndoActivator (Dentsply Maillefer, Switzerland). Since the direct application of ultrasonic devices does not have the ability required to remove the file, endodontic micro forceps (Broken Instrument Removal Kit, Zumax, China) were used including a screw wedge that works by clamping the file fragments through a mechanical lock and pulling them to the coronal (Figure 2(a)). After the file fragment has been successfully lifted (Figure 2(b)), it was confirmed with a photo of the radiograph.

The mesiolingual root canal was prepared through the ProTaper Next (Dentsply Maillefer, Switzerland) up to X3/16.5 mm and the master gutta-percha cone confirmed by radiographic photographs.

It was medicated with calcium hydroxide paste (Calcipex®, Nippon Shika-Yakuhin, Shimonoseki, Japan) and restored temporarily.

Two weeks after the first visit, the root canal was filled with continuous wave compaction through gutta-percha (ProTaper Next® Gutta Percha, Dentsply Tulsa Dental, Switzerland) with an MTA Fillapex sealer and closed with RMGIC (Fuji II LC, GC, Japan) and temporary restoration (Caviton, GC Corporation, Japan).

One week after obturation, the preparations were completed to make Ceramage® onlay (Shofu Inc., Japan). Two weeks after onlay preparation, onlay was cemented using

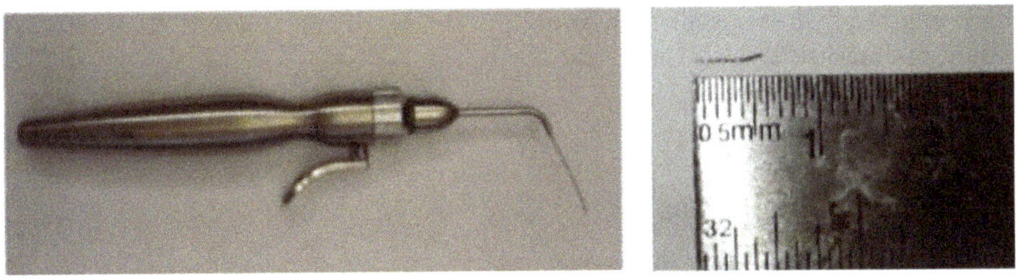

(a) (b)

FIGURE 2: (a) Endodontic micro forceps. (b) Broken file was successfully retrieved.

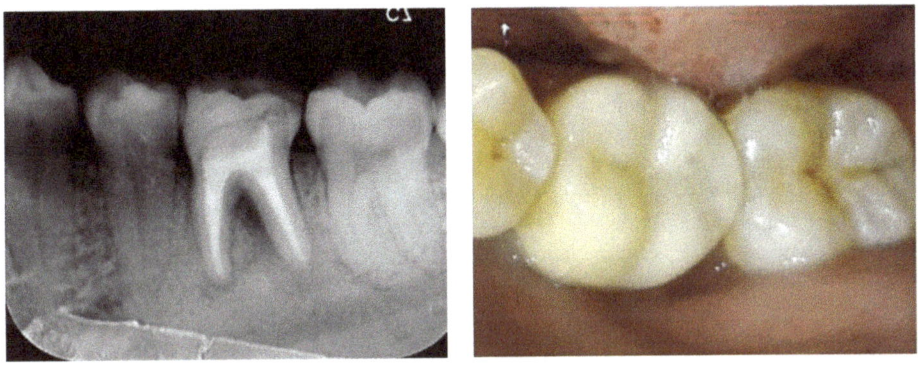

(a) (b)

FIGURE 3: One-month postoperative evaluation: (a) postoperative radiograph; (b) Ceramage® onlay for restoration.

resin cement (Figure 3(b)). The evaluation after one month showed negative on subjective examination and the percussion and palpation test. The radiograph showed bifurcation, and apical radiolucency was reduced.

3. Discussion

The use of an ultrasonic instrument assisted by a microscope is a conservative method of handling a broken file compared to other alternatives [4, 5]. It can erode the structure of the dentine conservatively and is less likely to damage the root structure and periodontal tissue [5]. However, its application was unable to loosen the file until it reached the coronal; therefore, a tool was needed to clamp the file and draw its fragments in the coronal direction through a microtube with either a screw wedge or a loop device (DentalCadre, Seattle, WA) [2]. This is common in broken files longer than 4.5 mm or visible under ultrasonic activation but could not be retrieved by the device [2].

Removal of broken files can be conducted in dry or wet conditions [2]. Dry conditions provide better visibility with a microscope, thus preventing procedural errors [2]. However, heat generated from ultrasonic vibrations is unavoidable, and the temperature has the possibility to increase to more than 10°C on the external root surface causing damage to the periodontal tissue [2]. The files are also susceptible to secondary heat if the ultrasonic tip is in contact with the file [2]. Therefore, EDTA irrigation was conducted when the ultrasonic tip was activated at the lowest power setting [2]. This improved the cleanliness of the root canal wall [2].

The tips used were ET20 and ET25 from the Endo Success™ Retreatment Kit (Satelec Acteon, France), made from titanium niobium alloy and coated with diamond, making them abrasive. The ET20 was moved counterclockwise in 1/3 coronal and ET25 in the middle 1/3 of the root canal to give the file an unscrewing force effect [2].

The root canal was filled with a continuous wave compaction technique and through the use of an MTA Fillapex (Angelus, Brazil) sealer which is good for dentin because of its ability to harden. They also possess good density, thus preventing leakage in the periapical region and closing communication between pulp and periodontal tissue. The MTA content in the sealer supports healing and hard tissue formation in the lesion.

MTA Fillapex has several advantages such as the stimulation of new tissue formation, rapid tissue repair without causing inflammatory reactions, high radio-opacity, provision of good visualization on the radiograph, release of calcium ions to induce rapid tissue regeneration in areas with periapical lesions and microbial activity, making insertion and handling easier, having adequate working time, and being easy to remove (on retreatment, especially if used with gutta-percha) [6, 7]. It can also be used for antimicrobial activity against *M. luteus*, *S. aureus*, *E. coli*, *P. aeruginosa*, *C. albicans*, and *E. faecalis* because of its alkaline pH [7, 8].

In this case, the mandibular right first molars with symptomatic apical periodontitis with a broken file on the orifice to the middle of the mesiolingual root canal were retrieved with a combination of ultrasonic tips and endodontic micro forceps, accompanied by a microscope to increase visibility. The treatment was successful because a broken instrument was completely removed followed by loss of subjective complaints. The radiograph also revealed diminished apical radiolucency.

References

[1] A. Shenoy, P. Mandava, N. Bolla, and S. Vemuri, "A novel technique for removal of broken instrument from root canal in mandibular second molar," *Indian Journal of Dental Research*, vol. 25, no. 1, pp. 107–110, 2014.

[2] S. Cohen and K. Hargreaves, *Pathway's of the Pulp*, Elsevier, Kansas, MO, USA, 11th edition, 2016.

[3] T. Lambrianidis, *Management of Fractured Endodontic Instruments*, Springer, Cham, Switzerland, 2018.

[4] M. B. McGuigan, C. Louca, and H. F. Duncan, "Clinical decision-making after endodontic instrument fracture," *British Dental Journal*, vol. 214, no. 8, pp. 395–400, 2013.

[5] A. H. Gluskin, C. J. Ruddle, and E. J. Zinman, "Thermal injury through intraradicular heat transfer using ultrasonic devices: precautions and practical preventive strategies," *The Journal of the American Dental Association*, vol. 136, no. 9, pp. 1286–1293, 2005.

[6] S. Banerjee, "Bypassing a broken instrument in a severely curved root canal: a case report," *Indian Journal of Conservative and Endodontics*, vol. 2, no. 3, pp. 115–118, 2017.

[7] E. Radeva, "Bypassing a broken instruments (clinical cases)," *Internation Journal of Science and Research*, vol. 6, no. 2, pp. 2015–2017, 2017.

[8] P. Parashos, "Prognosis of root canal treatment with retained instrument fragment(s)," in *Management of Fractured Endodontic Instruments*, T. Lambrianidis, Ed., Springer, 2018.

Rosuvastatin-Induced Oral Ulcer: A Case Report and Review of Literature

Metab Algeffari[1] **and Mansour Alsharidah**[2]

[1]*Department of Family and Community Medicine, College of Medicine, Qassim University, Saudi Arabia*
[2]*Department of Physiology, College of Medicine, Qassim University, Saudi Arabia*

Correspondence should be addressed to Metab Algeffari; m.geffari@qu.edu.sa

Academic Editor: Ronald S. Brown

Background. The benefits of prescribing statins are well published in the treatment of hypercholesterolemia. With such widespread usage of statins, physicians may be ignoring or misdiagnosing the association of oral side effects with these medications. *Case Summary.* A 54-year-old man presented with a painful ulceration on the dorsum of his tongue that had been recurring for 10 months. Originally, he experienced a burning sensation on his tongue, and as the lesion advanced, the pain became more intense specially when consuming spicy or acidic foods. He is on rosuvastatin for the treatment of hypercholesterolemia for over five years. Several months prior to the lesion forming, his physician increased his daily dosage of rosuvastatin from 10 mg to 20 mg. Four weeks later at a follow-up appointment, all workup did not show any significant findings, the examination revealed a new ulcer on the dorsum of the tongue, and he reported no improvement after antifungal lozenges, nor when administered a short one-week treatment with oral steroids. After eight weeks of statin discontinued, the patient showed improvement with no episodes of ulceration. *Conclusion.* Physicians do note that statins affect multiple immunological pathways, which could explain some adverse cutaneous reactions. More research is needed in discovering the link of statins and oral disorders.

1. Introduction

The benefits of prescribing statins are well published in the treatment of hypercholesterolemia [1]. The American Heart Association reports that prescriptions for statins have increased during the past 10 years to 64.9 percent, with prescriptions increasing to 221 million from 134 million, especially in elderly patients [2]. Statins work to lower lipids through inhibition of 3-hydroxy-3-methylglutaryl coenzyme-A (HMG-CoA) reductase [3, 4]. While such widespread usage of cholesterol-lowering drugs has been documented as beneficial, physicians may be ignoring or misdiagnosing the association of oral side effects with these medications.

We present in this report a case of a patient with long-term therapeutic use of rosuvastatin who incurred unusual oral ulcers after an increase in the dosage of rosuvastatin.

2. Case Presentation

In our clinic, a 54-year-old man recently presented with a painful ulceration on the dorsum of his tongue that had been recurring for 10 months. Originally, he experienced a burning sensation on his tongue, and as the lesion advanced, the pain became more intense, especially when consuming spicy or acidic foods. He reported no improvement after antifungal lozenges were prescribed or when administered a short one-week treatment with oral steroids (20 mg/once per day).

The patient did not have an alcoholism or smoking history. His personal and family history showed no evidence of atopic dermatitis or psoriasis, and no new contact exposures, such as new detergents or other similar substances, had been introduced recently. No new supplements or medications were being taken and thus were ruled out as the cause.

The medications he took daily were as follows: aspirin (81 mg), hydrochlorothiazide (25 mg), rosuvastatin (20 mg), coenzyme A reductase and a cholesterol-lowering agent," *Proceedings of the National Academy of Sciences of the United States of America*, vol. 77, no. 7, pp. 3957–3961, 1980.

[4] R. Hajar, "Statins: past and present," *Heart Views: the Official Journal of the Gulf Heart Association*, vol. 12, no. 3, pp. 121–127, 2011.

[5] S. Tahamtan, F. Shirban, M. Bagherniya, T. P. Johnston, and A. Sahebkar, "The effects of statins on dental and oral health: a review of preclinical and clinical studies," *Journal of Translational Medicine*, vol. 18, no. 1, p. 155, 2020.

[6] A. Yuan and S.-B. Woo, "Adverse drug events in the oral cavity," *Oral Surgery, Oral Medicine, Oral Pathology and Oral Radiology*, vol. 119, no. 1, pp. 35–47, 2015.

[7] M. A. Silva, A. C. Swanson, P. J. Gandhi, and G. R. Tataronis, "Statin-related adverse events: a meta-analysis," *Clinical Therapeutics*, vol. 28, no. 1, pp. 26–35, 2006.

[8] W. C. Yuet, H. Khine, and Z. Ahmad, "Statin-associated adverse events," *Clinical Medicine Insights: Therapeutics*, vol. 7, 2015.

[9] M. Pascual Cruz, E. Chimenos Küstner, J. A. García Vicente, X. Mezquiriz Ferrero, E. Borrell Thio, and J. López López, "Adverse side effects of statins in the oral cavity," *Medicina Oral, Patología Oral y Cirugía Bucal*, vol. 13, no. 2, pp. E98–E101, 2008.

[10] D. J. Smith, M. Dillon, J. Russell, and A. Kanatas, "Statins and oral ulceration," *British Dental Journal*, vol. 220, no. 2, pp. 45-46, 2016.

[11] B. Sebök, M. Tóth, B. Anga, F. Harangi, and I. Schneider, "Lichenoid drug eruption with HMG-CoA reductase inhibitors (fluvastatin and lovastatin)," *Acta Dermato-Venereologica*, vol. 84, no. 3, pp. 229-230, 2004.

20

Special Needs Dental Management of the Class 3 Obese Patient

Zanab Malik

Registrar Special Needs Dentistry, Department of Oral Medicine, Oral Pathology and Special Needs Dentistry, Level 3 Westmead Centre for Oral Health, Westmead, NSW, Australia

Correspondence should be addressed to Zanab Malik; zanab.malik@health.nsw.gov.au

Academic Editor: Mark Darling

Obesity, classified as a chronic disease by the World Health Organisation (WHO), is a worldwide public health problem. Obesity has links with numerous systemic diseases which may complicate dental management and as such, patients with obesity and concomitant medical comorbidities are commonly managed by Special Needs Dentistry specialist departments in Australia. The sparsity of available evidence on the dental status in this group is likely due to significant access issues experienced by the class 3 obese, who often weigh >140 kg and therefore are unable to be examined or treated in conventional dental chairs. "Bariatric" is a term used to refer to a specific branch of medicine dealing with causes, prevention, and treatment of obesity. It is used widely in the literature to refer to obese patients; however, dentistry for this cohort ("bariatric dentistry") is less well defined and represents less frequently used terminology. This case report is of a 58-year-old female, with class 3 obesity, who presented in May 2018 for outpatient consult to the Special Needs Unit/Medically Complex Dental Clinic at Westmead Centre for Oral Health, Sydney, Australia, with a compromised and neglected dentition and requiring full dental clearance. The case highlights many of the significant access issues and considerations for safe and effective delivery of dental management. As we move into the future, dental professionals need to become more aware of the growing challenge obesity presents and understand how medical complexities influence dental management. Facilities need to be able to meet this growing need and the specific requirements for a functional and safe bariatric dental service; dependent on both appropriate infrastructure and training.

1. Introduction

WHO defines obesity as "abnormal or excessive fat accumulation that may impair health" [1] and is commonly measured at the population level for adults using the body mass index (BMI). BMI is defined as weight in kilograms divided by the square of the height in metres. Although a clinically useful measure, BMI is limited in not accounting for differences in muscle mass, bone mass, and genetic makeup [2]. Obesity is determined by a BMI of greater than or equal to 30 kg/m^2 with cut-off points adopted for use internationally by the WHO and based on associations between BMI, chronic disease, and mortality. The highest class of obesity, obese class 3, is defined as a BMI of equal to or greater than 40 kg/m^2 with a very severe risk of comorbidities [1].

Limited current evidence recognises an association between obesity (not specific to class 3 obesity) and oral disease, namely, caries and periodontal disease, largely based on cross-sectional prevalence data [3, 4]. However, there are currently no evidence-based clinical guidelines for the dental management of patients with obesity. For those individuals who do not fall within the dental chair safe weight working limits, this necessitates the use of a modified dental chair and possible treatment planning modifications. These management considerations must therefore be extrapolated from case reports or series and expert opinion, identifying a need for further research in this area.

This case report will endeavour to provide further guidance for dental practitioners relating to the management (pre-, peri-, and post-operative) of patients with class 3 obesity. It will highlight the focus on comprehensive medical history taking and understanding the influence of medical comorbidities on dental treatment planning.

2. Patient Case

This is the case study of Mrs. D, a 58-year-old female who presented for outpatient consult to the Special Needs

Unit/Medically Complex Dental Clinic at Westmead Centre for Oral Health, Sydney, Australia, referred by her general medical practitioner for specialist dental management. Her chief complaint was of multiple broken teeth and generalised discomfort from her teeth. She reported a history of right-sided facial swelling a few weeks prior, which had since settled with a self-administered course of antibiotics and increased dosage of her regular pain medications. The patient also reported her dentition was limiting her diet consistency to soft foods and significantly limited her social interactions. She expressed a desire for a "normal" appearance of her teeth and for denture rehabilitation in the future.

2.1. Comorbidities. Mrs. D's medical history was significant for class 3 obesity (BMI of 65 kg/m^2). She was known to the local community obesity service since January 2018 which had resulted in successful weight loss of nearly 20 kg over the previous five months. She had metabolic syndrome and a plan was recommended by her endocrinologist for gastric banding surgery scheduled for November 2018. Mrs. D had moderate obstructive sleep apnoea (OSA) (confirmed via sleep study with no REM sleep in 2014, intolerant of CPAP machine) and reported considerable difficulty with sleep, requiring an upright posture. Remaining systemic history included borderline personality disorder (Abilify, Epilim), depression with a history of self-harm, and subsequent hospitalisation for suicide watch in 2005 (currently managed with Efexor, however, without psychology input). Mrs. D had well-controlled hypertension (Inderal, Frusemide), a history of iron deficiency anaemia (no current iron supplementation) and she experienced occasional migraines with aura, resulting in reduced vision/hearing and headaches (Aspirin prn on migraine onset).

Additionally, Mrs. D had subclinical hypothyroidism (Oroxine), gastro-oesophageal reflux disease (GORD) (Somac) with diverticular disease, urinary incontinence (managed with use of a bariatric commode), and chronic constipation (Coloxyl with Senna, Movicol prn). There was a history of non-alcoholic steatohepatitis (diet control) and renal impairment which was improving. She had osteoarthritis affecting both knees requiring total knee replacements; however, she was deemed unsuitable for surgical intervention due to her current weight (Targin, Panadol Osteo, Vitamin D). There were infected bilateral leg ulcers severely limiting Mrs. D's mobility, requiring use of a walker to mobilise. Her most recent hospitalisation was for emergency surgery following gall stone rupture in 2010. Mrs. D had no known drug allergies.

2.2. Social, Diet and Dental History. Mrs. D had no smoking history and did not imbibe any alcohol. She lived in Sydney in her family home with her husband and dog. She was engaged in employment as a tutor for secondary level mathematics. Her diet consisted of flavoured yoghurt and calorie-restricted meals/shakes. She had recently commenced drinking 600 ml of diet soft drink per day. Due to the nature of her dentition, Mrs. D had already transitioned to a soft diet. She had not engaged in oral hygiene for the last two years due to significant dental pain. Mrs. D had not had any dental intervention for many years as she was unaware of how to access a service with appropriate bariatric facilities and was embarrassed about her dentition. She subsequently avoided interaction with others and her only external engagement outside of her home for the last three years was for medical appointments.

2.3. Clinical Examination. Extra-oral examination at the time of consultation revealed no regional lymphadenopathy, trismus, facial swelling/asymmetry or TMJ pathology. A loss of occlusal vertical dimension was apparent. Baseline observations showed a blood pressure within normal range and oxygen saturation of 97% with Mrs. D seated upright. Clinical and radiographic intra-oral examination revealed generalised dry mucosa secondary to medication-related salivary gland hypofunction and buccal abscesses adjacent to mandibular right central and left lateral incisor retained roots (41, 32). Hard tissue examination revealed a grossly carious mandibular right canine tooth (43) with the remaining teeth evident as retained roots with hopeless prognosis (see Figure 1). Radiographic examination with OPG X-ray confirmed the clinical findings and showed evidence of unerupted maxillary right and left third molar teeth (18, 28) and multiple retained roots with associated periapical pathology (see Figure 2).

Clinical examination and dental treatment was performed in a bariatric dental chair (see Figure 3).

2.4. Treatment Options. There was extensive discussion with Mrs. D regarding the available treatment options which included full dental clearance under local anaesthetic and construction of full maxillary and mandibular dentures following complete gingival healing post-operatively. We discussed realistic expectations surrounding prosthetic rehabilitation given no previous denture history for Mrs. D and reinforced continued soft diet in the interim. Mrs. D was agreeable to this treatment option.

The option of no treatment was discussed with ongoing risk of pain, swelling, and infection. Due to Mrs. D's high BMI and obstructive sleep apnoea, she presented a very high risk for management under sedation or general anaesthesia and a high risk of a medical emergency.

A preventive care plan was instituted by our oral health therapist, which included an antibacterial chlorhexidine gel and saliva substitutes (dry mouth gels) to reduce biofilm burden, stabilise dental disease risk, and assist in future denture use. Diet advice was also reinforced as part of healthy weight intervention.

2.5. Management of This Patient. Pre-operatively, blood tests were ordered to check coagulation studies and Mrs. D's bleeding risk on the background of hepatic dysfunction. They were within normal range to proceed with surgical dental intervention. A STOP-Bang score (scale to determine risk of OSA) of 6/8 confirmed Mrs. D's high risk of OSA consistent with her diagnosis. Mrs. D's baseline blood sugar level and blood pressure was also checked prior to commencing treatment. All appointment times for dental extractions were

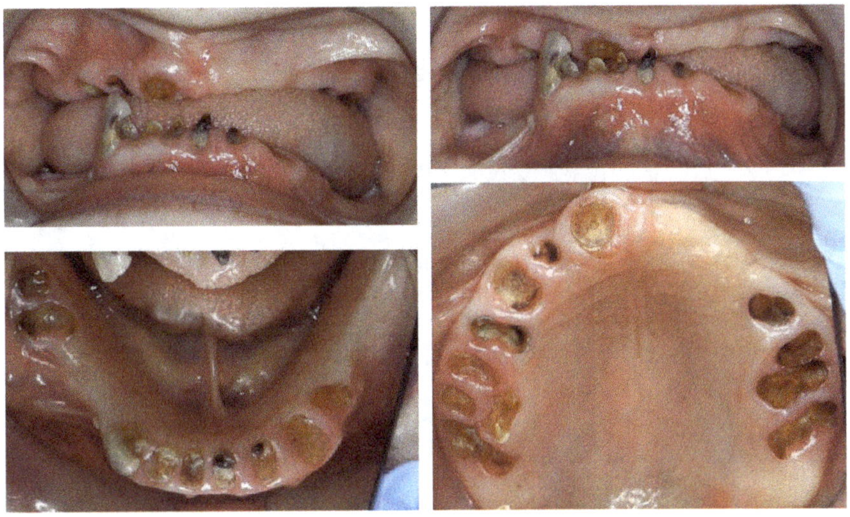

FIGURE 1: Intraoral photographs at time of consult. Buccal abscess adjacent to teeth 41 and 32 retained roots.

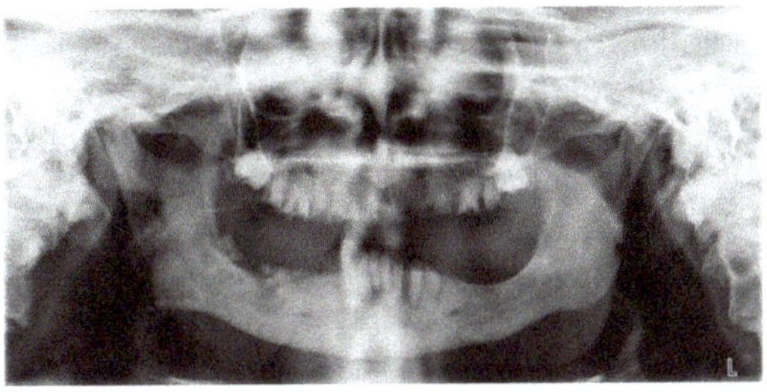

FIGURE 2: Orthopantomogram (OPG) July 2018 showing grossly carious retained roots and associated periapical pathology. Unerupted maxillary right and left third molars are also evident (18, 28).

scheduled in the morning to allow for sufficient time to manage any potential complications.

Peri-operatively, mobilising Mrs. D into the facility, where the bariatric chair was located, required the use of a bariatric wheelchair. Mrs. D was reclined to a semi-supine position during treatment. Patient positioning was also assisted with cushions to help ease discomfort from lower limb pressure ulcers. Hoist facilities were readily available in case of a fall or medical emergency. Non-pharmacological behavioural management was used to alleviate anxiety and help reduce the risk of migraine. Registered nurse support was present for regular monitoring of vital signs especially pulse oximetry to monitor closely for desaturation. Full dental clearance (extraction of remaining 19 erupted teeth) under local anaesthesia over multiple visits was carried out uneventfully in chair. Mrs. D awaits full maxillary and mandibular denture construction at time of publication.

Post-operatively, it was imperative Mrs. D was discharged into the care of a responsible support person (her husband), who attended appointments with her. Appropriate analgesia therapy was recommended for post-operative pain management.

Although Mrs. D coped well with treatment under local anaesthesia, for many patients, given similarly extensive burden of treatment needs and presence of medical comorbidities, this may have necessitated dental treatment under intravenous sedation or general anaesthesia with specialist anaesthetist support, especially if in a setting of confounding dental phobia. In order to reduce anaesthetic risk, medical optimisation prior to surgery would be required. This could be via liaison with the specialist medical obesity service for pre-operative weight loss, the use of CPAP machine pre- and post-operatively on the background of OSA, and likely overnight admission and close monitoring for post-operative complications such as apnoea.

3. Discussion

This case report highlights several considerations in the dental management of patients with class 3 obesity like Mrs. D, who have many medical comorbidities that may require modifications to dental treatment planning.

With regards to cardiac and respiratory function, generalised obesity alters the total blood volume and cardiac function, whereas the distribution of fat around the thoracic cage and abdomen restricts respiratory function [4]. As such, sleep breathing disorders are common amongst obese individuals. OSA may be associated with thick, short necks and increased soft tissue presence surrounding the uvula [5]. A patent airway and satisfactory neck extension can be maintained via correct head positioning, as was ensured for Mrs. D, with regular monitoring of her oxygen saturation levels throughout treatment. However semi-supine positioning resulted in challenges for clinician and dental assistant positioning during aspects of treatment. It has been suggested to carry out a pre-operative assessment of OSA using a screening tool, such as the STOP-Bang score, prior to any treatment and especially prior to sedation or general anaesthetic for the obese patient [5]. Peri-operatively under general anaesthesia or conscious sedation, the presence of OSA complicates airway management and almost doubles the risk of the procedure for developing serious airway problems than the non-obese patient [5].

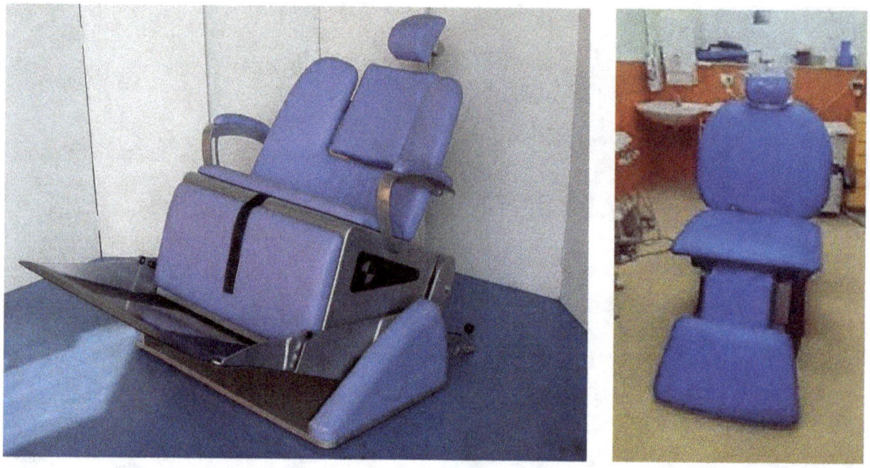

(a) (b)

FIGURE 3: Differing styles of bariatric dental chairs, suitable for all patient groups up to 1000 lbs (454 kg) (image of "Barico" dental chair at Westmead Centre for Oral Health (a) and "bariatric bench" from Design Specific (b) https://www.designspecific.co.uk/html/b_bench_home.html).

Other links with class 3 obesity include GORD due to the impaired communication between the lower oesophageal sphincter and the stomach [2]. There is a dose-dependent association between increasing BMI and GORD [6] and may present a risk of aspiration of gastric contents if treatment is performed under general anaesthesia. Mrs. D had metabolic syndrome increasing her risk of diabetes and cardiovascular disease. There is evidence for intra-abdominal fat deposits as a major contributor to the development of hypertension, elevated plasma insulin concentrations, insulin resistance, diabetes mellitus, and hyperlipidaemia [2, 7]. Ensuring satisfactory blood pressure and blood sugar levels prior to commencing invasive dental treatment such as dental extractions is crucial. Further control may be facilitated through diet and weight management, and the dental team is in an ideal position to provide preventive advice [8].

Excess weight and load on joints predispose patients with obesity to osteoarthritis [9]. The literature suggests that chronic pain and obesity are linked comorbidities [10], adversely impacting each other [9]. Obesity appears to be a risk factor for developing various pain diagnoses including headaches, lower back pain, fibromyalgia, abdominal pain, pelvic pain, and neuropathic pain [9]. Weight loss for obese pain patients appears to be an important aspect of overall pain rehabilitation, although more research is needed to determine strategies to maintain long-term benefits [9].

The association between obesity and mental illness is complicated and bi-directional. Obesity is linked to an increased risk of a psychiatric diagnosis, and in turn, mental illness (or its pharmacological management) may precipitate and perpetuate weight gain and obesity [11]. Some evidence has indicated that the relationship between weight and mental illness is dose dependent [11]. Further compounding Mrs. D's caries risk, many antidepressant and antipsychotic medications have anticholinergic properties which likely contributed to the evident salivary gland hypofunction.

In addition, obesity is unfortunately often associated with negative social consequences. Weight-related stigma, both by others and self-imposed, and internalized anti-obesity attitudes have been found to be associated with emotional distress including symptoms of anxiety and depression [12]. Mrs. D voiced extreme anxiety regarding access and attendance for dental services and her oral health became neglected as a result.

Similarly, one can hypothesise that there are higher levels of oral health problems in the class 3 obese population. However, data supporting this hypothesis is currently lacking. As a result, there may be considerable impact on quality of life [13] which can be further compounded by the loss of teeth [14]. Qualitative research in the emotional effects of complete tooth loss has revealed a wide range of reactions such as bereavement, loss of self-confidence, concerns about appearance and self-image, and a lack of preparation for the loss of teeth [14]. For Mrs. D, this needed to be considered in the context of her long-standing history of anxiety and depression. A post-operative support network and pain management plan is required to minimise these effects, as in the case of Mrs. D. It has been shown consistently that obesity can negatively impact important aspects of health-related quality of life with higher degrees of obesity associated with greater impairment [12]. As demonstrated in the case of Mrs. D, there is a suggested implication that quality of life related to oral health may also deteriorate [15], although this has never been quantitatively measured in a population with obesity.

4. Conclusion

Dental professionals need to develop an understanding of the growing challenges that patients, particularly those with class 3 obesity, present for comprehensive dental management, taking into account their medical complexities. Patients should be referred in a timely manner to appropriate facilities where bariatric dental chairs are available. Patients and their corresponding specialist medical obesity services should be educated about available facilities and funding increased to ensure growing demand can be met. Multidisciplinary holistic management for these patients may necessitate specialist Special Needs Dentistry input for the safe delivery of dental treatment. The paucity of literature related to obesity and dental disease highlights a need for further research in this population.

Acknowledgments

The author would like to thank Mrs. D for kindly consenting to this case report, the staff in the Department of Oral Medicine/Special Needs Dentistry, Level 3 Westmead Centre for Oral Health, Westmead NSW, in particular, Dr. Suma Sukumar (Staff Specialist, Oral Medicine), Dr. Avanti Karve (Staff Specialist, Special Needs Dentistry) and Ms. Cheryl Bedford (Oral Health Therapist) for their assistance with this case.

References

[1] World Health Organisation (WHO), *Obesity: preventing and managing the global epidemic: A report of a WHO consultation*, WHO technical report series: 894, World Health Organisation, Geneva, 2000.

[2] D. Reilly, C. A. Boyle, and D. C. Craig, "Obesity and dentistry: a growing problem," *British Dental Journal*, vol. 207, no. 4, pp. 171–175, 2009.

[3] C. S. Barbosa, G. S. Barbério, V. R. Marques, V. O. Baldo, M. A. R. Buzalaf, and A. C. Magalhães, "Dental manifestations in bariatric patients - review of literature," *Journal of Applied Oral Science*, vol. 17, spe, pp. 1–4, 2009.

[4] R. Levine, "Obesity and oral disease – a challenge for dentistry," *British Dental Journal*, vol. 213, no. 9, pp. 453–456, 2012.

[5] H. Abed and D. Reilly, "Bariatric dentistry: managing the plus-size patient," *Journal of the Irish Dental Association*, vol. 63, no. 6, pp. 333–335, 2017.

[6] J. Lagergren, "Body measures in relation to gastro-oesophageal reflux," *Gut*, vol. 56, no. 6, pp. 741-742, 2007.

[7] J. B. Dixon, "The effect of obesity on health outcomes," *Molecular and Cellular Endocrinology*, vol. 316, no. 2, pp. 104–108, 2010.

[8] A. E. Curran, D. J. Caplan, J. Y. Lee et al., "Dentists' attitudes about their role in addressing obesity in patients a national survey," *Journal of the American Dental Association (Chicago, IL)*, vol. 141, no. 11, pp. 1307–1316, 2010.

[9] A. Okifuji and B. D. Hare, "The association between chronic pain and obesity," *Journal of Pain Research*, vol. 8, pp. 399–408, 2015.

[10] D. A. Marcus, "Obesity and the impact of chronic pain," *The Clinical Journal of Pain*, vol. 20, no. 3, pp. 186–191, 2004.

[11] C. Avila, A. C. Holloway, M. K. Hahn et al., "An overview of links between obesity and mental health," *Current Obesity Reports*, vol. 4, no. 3, pp. 303–310, 2015.

[12] K. R. Fontaine and I. Barofsky, "Obesity and health-related quality of life," *Obesity Reviews*, vol. 2, no. 3, pp. 173–182, 2001.

[13] V. H. Taylor, M. Forhan, S. N. Vigod, R. S. McIntyre, and K. M. Morrison, "The impact of obesity on quality of life," *Best Practice & Research Clinical Endocrinology & Metabolism*, vol. 27, no. 2, pp. 139–146, 2013.

[14] D. M. Davis, J. Fiske, B. Scott, and D. R. D. Davis, "The emotional effects of tooth loss: a preliminary quantitative study," *British Dental Journal*, vol. 188, no. 9, pp. 503–506, 2000.

[15] A. Sheiham, "Oral health, general health and quality of life," *Bulletin of the World Health Organization*, vol. 83, no. 9, pp. 644-645, 2005.

21

Lip Epidermoid Cyst Caused by a Piercing: A Report of a Rare Case

Takashi Ito, Satoshi Fukuzawa, Kenji Yamagata, Shohei Takaoka, Makiko Ohkubo-Sato, Fumihiko Uchida, Naomi Ishibashi-Kanno, and Hiroki Bukawa

Department of Oral and Maxillofacial Surgery, Faculty of Medicine, University of Tsukuba, Tennodai 1-1-1, Tsukuba, Ibaraki 305-8575, Japan

Correspondence should be addressed to Satoshi Fukuzawa; sfukuzawa3104@yahoo.co.jp

Academic Editor: Rui Amaral Mendes

We report the case of a lip epidermoid cyst, caused by piercing in a 23-year-old Japanese woman. She had an exophytic lesion in the lower lip associated with the piercing which was initially diagnosed as a mucous retention cyst. The lesion was resected under local anesthesia, and pathological examination revealed an epidermoid cyst, likely caused by piercings. Piercing-induced epidermoid cysts frequently occur in the tragus. There have been no reports of piercing-induced epidermoid cysts developing in the oral cavity. To our knowledge, this is the first report of a lip epidermal cyst caused by piercings. Six months have passed since the operation, and it has not recurred.

1. Introduction

Body piercings have emerged as a component of recent fashion trends. They are worn on the ears and oral region, specifically the tongue and lips [1]. Epidermoid cysts are encountered in all parts of the body and occur 1.6% of times in the oral cavity [2]. There are also rare reports that it has become malignant [3]. However, to our knowledge, lip epidermal cysts caused by piercings have not been reported. We report the case of an epidermoid lip cyst caused by piercings.

2. Case Report

The patient was a 23-year-old Japanese woman with unremarkable medical and family histories. Five years prior, she had her lower lip pierced, such that it penetrated the left side of the lip and the skin. She stopped wearing her piercings after a few months, and the piercing holes closed spontaneously. Wound indurated or swelling was not noted.

When she was 22 years old, she had her left lower lip pierced again. The earrings were inserted twice. However, the pierced hole from the first set of piercings had been occluded. A mass appeared on the lower lip two months later, and the patient reported to our department due to its persistence.

Intraoral examination revealed a palpable mass, measuring approximately 4 × 4 mm, on the left lower lip. The piercing was in contact with the mass and penetrated the skin and mucosa of the lower-left lip (Figures 1 and 2).

She was clinically diagnosed with a mucous retention cyst of the lower lip. She was instructed to stop using her piercings two weeks before undergoing the lesion resection.

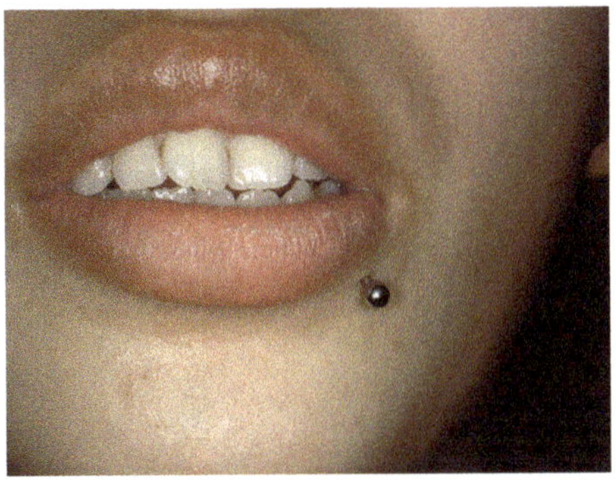

FIGURE 1: Extraoral findings.

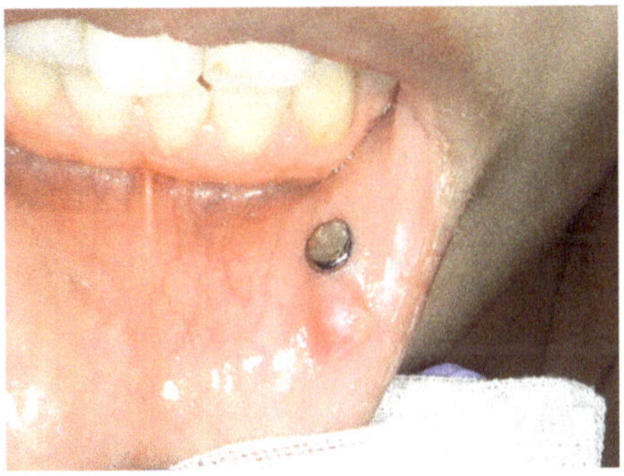

FIGURE 2: Intraoral finding. Tumor formation on the lip mucosa on the mesial side of the lip piercing.

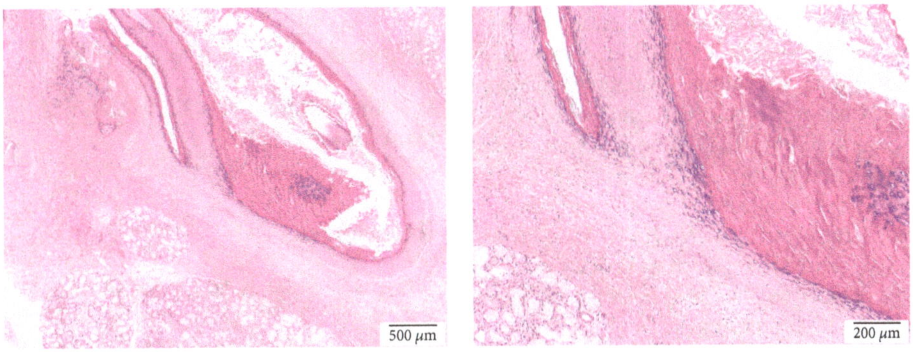

(a) (b)

FIGURE 3: Histopathological findings of the lip cyst. (a) Hematoxylin and eosin stain ×4. (b) Hematoxylin and eosin stain ×100. A cyst covered with keratinized stratified squamous epithelium. Keratin is stored in the cyst.

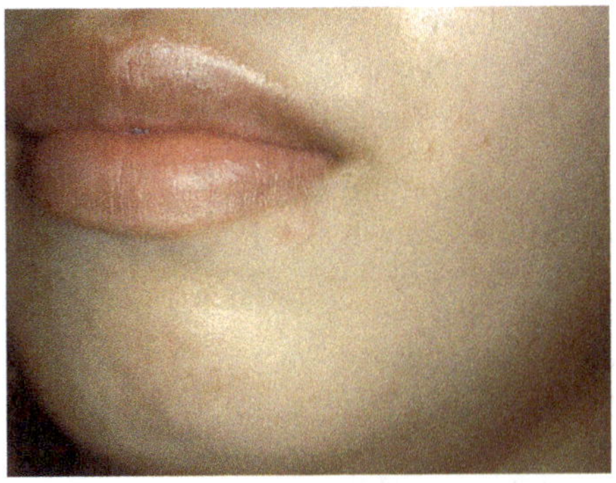

FIGURE 4: Extraoral finding 10 months after the surgery.

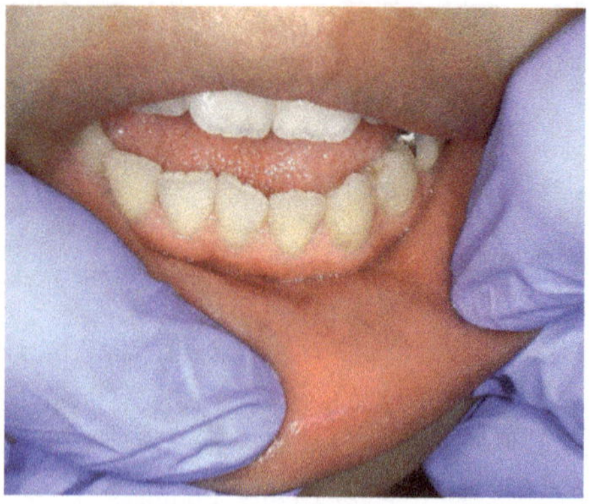

FIGURE 5: Intraoral finding 10 months after the surgery. The wound 10 months after surgery. No recurrence was noted.

The pierced hole was closed intraoperatively. The lesion and the scar on the pierced hole were resected under local anesthesia. Histopathological examination revealed a keratin-containing cyst covered with keratinized stratified squamous epithelium. Therefore, the patient was pathologically diagnosed with an epidermoid cyst (Figure 3).

One year has passed since the operation, and the wound has resolved without infection or recurrence (Figures 4 and 5).

3. Discussion

Piercings has been often applied to the tragus. Piercing complications in the tragus reportedly occur in 35% [4]. Piercings have main complications including infections, allergic reactions, keloid formation, and traumatic lacerations.

Epidermal cysts are soft tissue cysts that commonly develop in the head and neck regions. Congenital causes are associated with invasion and residual embryonic ectoderm. These causes acquired epithelial tissue invasion, such as trauma and inflammation [5].

Kim et al. reported that 14 out of 132 people with tragus piercing complications have experienced epidermoid cysts [6]. Epidermoid cysts, caused by piercings, occur during infection or bleeding. Epidermoid cysts reportedly develop when patients stop using their piercings [7].

Epidermoid cysts are attributed to epithelial invasion and remnants at the ectodermic fusion in the congenital and to the implantation of keratinized epithelium by trauma in the acquired cases [5, 8]. Epidermoid cysts on the lip due to trauma have also been reported due to denture irritation [9].

Chen et al. were the first to report the complications of oral piercings in 1992, and several cases have been reported after that [10]. The major complications of oral piercing are gingival recession and tooth fractures [11–13]. However, epidermoid cysts have not been reported, as complications associated with lip piercings. To the extent of our knowledge, this was the first case report on the occurrence of lip epidermoid cysts with such causality. In our case, the piercings were inserted twice. However, the pierced hole from the first set of piercings had occluded. The epidermoid cyst formation possibly occurred during that time. Alternatively, the epithelium might have invaded under the lip membrane after the second insertion, forming an epidermoid cyst. According to the patient, the cyst developed two months after she had gotten her second set of piercing. However, she did not notice the cyst during the second insertion. Based on this, the second insertion likely caused epithelial invagination.

The process of receiving piercings is invasive, but the publicity materials on its complications have been few.

Since piercings have emerged as a component of the recent fashion trends, cases like the present case may become more common in the future. Thus, dentists and oral surgeons should consider this a differential diagnosis. Moreover, people should be informed regarding the potential complications and risks associated with oral piercings.

Consent

Informed consent has been obtained from the patient for this publication.

References

[1] R. J. G. Moor, A. M. J. C. De Witte, K. I. M. Delmé, M. A. A. De Bruyne, G. M. G. Hommez, and D. Goyvaerts, "Dental and oral complications of lip and tongue piercings," *British Dental Journal*, vol. 199, no. 8, pp. 506–509, 2005.

[2] S. Mahalakshmi, S. Reddy, T. K. Ramamurthy, and B. Shilpa, "Rare locations of epidermoid cyst: case reports and review," *Ethiopian Journal of Health Sciences*, vol. 26, no. 6, pp. 595–601, 2016.

[3] V. Bhatt, M. Evans, and T. J. Malins, "Squamous cell carcinoma arising in the lining of an epidermoid cyst within the sublingual gland - a case report," *The British Journal of Oral & Maxillofacial Surgery*, vol. 46, no. 8, pp. 683–685, 2008.

[4] T. C. Simplot and H. T. Hoffman, "Comparison between cartilage and soft tissue ear piercing complications," *American Journal of Otolaryngology*, vol. 19, no. 5, pp. 305–310, 1998.

[5] R. L. Ettinger and R. D. Manderson, "Implantation keratinizing epidermoid cysts: A review and case history," *Oral Surgery*, vol. 36, no. 2, pp. 225–230, 1973.

[6] M. S. Kim, I. G. Song, K. C. Choi, and B. S. Shin, "Study of complications of ear piercing," *Korean Journal of Dermatology*, vol. 49, no. 1, pp. 20–27, 2011.

[7] M. Kurokawa and Y. Ishii, "Treatment for epidermal cyst following ear piercing," *J JSAPS*, vol. 21, no. 2, pp. 101–105, 1999.

[8] F. S. De Ponte, A. Brunelli, E. Marchetti, and D. J. Bottini, "Sublingual epidermoid cyst," *The Journal of Craniofacial Surgery*, vol. 13, pp. 308–310, 2002.

[9] J. C. Kim and I. P. Hong, "Rare Giant upper lip epidermal cyst in a patient wearing a denture," *Archives of Craniofacial Surgery*, vol. 17, no. 4, pp. 222–224, 2016.

[10] M. Chen and C. Scully, "Tongue piercing: a new fad in body art," *British Dental Journal*, vol. 172, no. 3, pp. 87–895, 1992.

[11] E. W. King, E. Brewer, and P. Brown, "Oral piercings and their complications - how confident are we as a profession?," *British Dental Journal*, vol. 224, no. 11, pp. 887–895, 2018.

[12] P. López Jornet, C. Navarro-Guardiola, F. Camacho-Alonso, V. Vicente-Ortega, and J. Yánez-Gascon, "Oral and facial piercings: a case series and review of the literature," *International Journal of Dermatology*, vol. 45, no. 7, pp. 805–809, 2006.

[13] A. Plessas and E. Pepelassi, "Dental and periodontal complications of lip and tongue piercing: prevalence and influencing factors," *Australian Dental Journal*, vol. 57, no. 1, pp. 71–78, 2012.

22

Clinical, Histological and Radiological Outcomes of Sinus Floor Elevation using a New Approach before Extraction of Periodontally Hopeless Maxillary Molars: A Case Report with 3-year Follow-Up

Zhaoguo Yue,[1] Qi Liu,[2] Haidong Zhang,[1] Jingwen Yang,[3] Lili Miao,[1] and Jianxia Hou[1]

[1]*Department of Periodontology, Peking University School and Hospital of Stomatology, National Engineering Laboratory for Digital and Material Technology of Stomatology, Research Center of Engineering and Technology for Digital Dentistry of Ministry of Health, Beijing Key Laboratory of Digital Stomatology, Beijing, China*
[2]*BYBO Dental Hospital, Beijing, China*
[3]*Department of Prosthodontics, Peking University School and Hospital of Stomatology & National Clinical Research Center for Oral Diseases & National Engineering Laboratory for Digital and Material Technology of Stomatology & Beijing Key Laboratory of Digital Stomatology, Beijing, China*

Correspondence should be addressed to Jianxia Hou; jxhou@163.com

Academic Editor: Konstantinos Michalakis

Introduction. This report is the first to present a case with 3-year follow-up, in which sinus floor elevation was performed before extraction of periodontally hopeless teeth, in order to shorten the edentulous interval between extraction and loading of implants and improve the patient's quality of life. *Case Presentation.* After a series of initial and supportive periodontal therapies, the lateral window was created at the apices of the hopeless teeth, followed by grafting of bone substitute and membrane material at the sinus floor. The tooth was preserved for 13 months prior to extraction followed by immediate implant placement. The patient is satisfied with the oral function partially retained during the treatment period. Predominance of new bone was detected by histologic analysis. The available bone height was augmented from 1–2 to 12–14 mm with little resorption (less than 2 mm of height) after 3 years of follow-up. The dental implant is in good condition without obvious signs of peri-implantitis or mobility after 3 years of loading. *Discussion.* The feasibility of modified sinus floor elevation (MSFE) could be seen in the current case. The potential benefit of MSFE may include shortening the edentulous interval, facilitating bone regeneration, and providing a chance for immediate implant placement. However, further clinical case evaluations and controlled studies are required to determine indications, effectiveness, and safety of such augmentation procedures.

1. Introduction

Severe alveolar bone loss has regularly been found around periodontally hopeless teeth, resulting in inadequate bone volume for implant placement after extraction [1–3]. For the posterior maxilla, when the residual bone height is less than 5 mm, it is typically necessary to perform lateral sinus floor elevation (LSFE) after extraction of compromised teeth [4–6]. A traditional two-stage LSFE may need 6–9 months for socket healing and osteogenesis at the sinus floor before placement of implants becomes possible [7, 8]. Concerning patients with advanced periodontitis whose molars are rated as hopeless, possibly so even bilaterally, long edentulous intervals between extraction and loading of implants may make them unwilling to accept dental implants. Especially when the compromised teeth are free of pain or abscess after

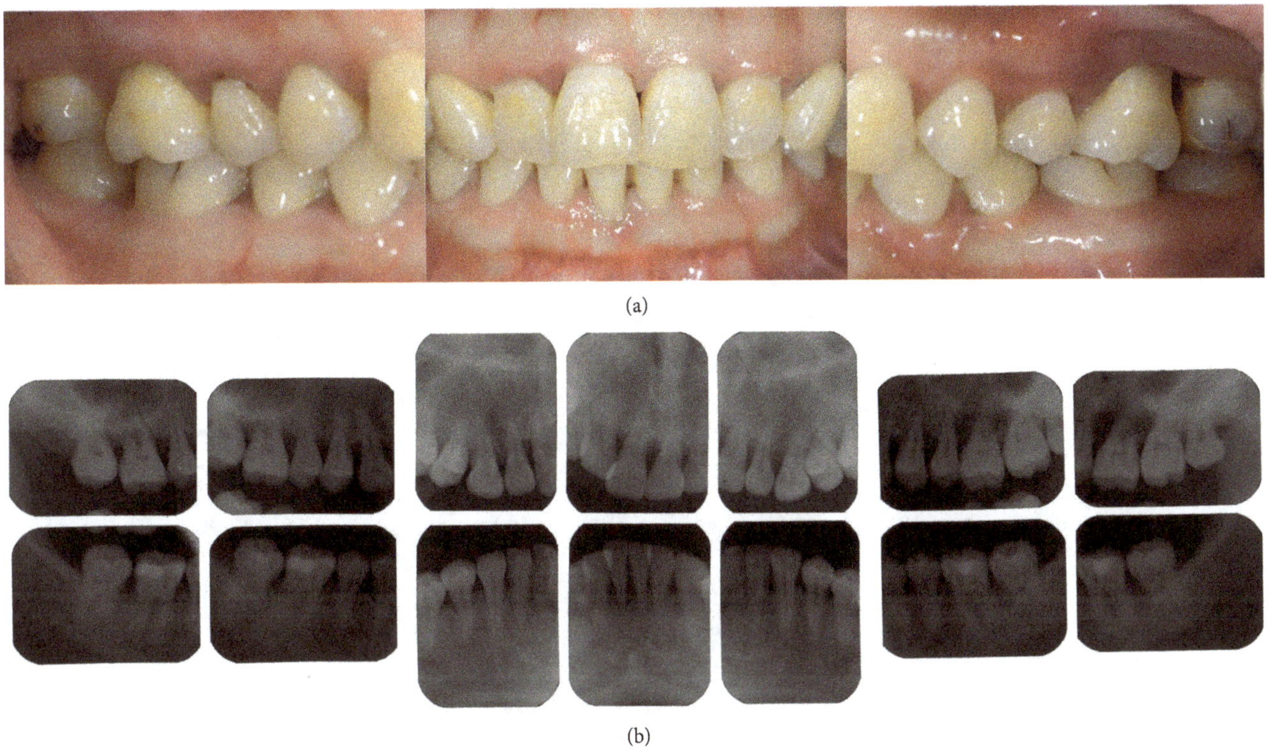

FIGURE 1: The patient had been diagnosed with aggressive periodontitis 4 years ago. Teeth #16 and #26 were severely compromised with bone loss to the apical third of root. (a) Intraoral photographs. (b) Periapical radiographs.

initial periodontal therapy (IPT), residual function is critical, though limited, for the patient's quality of life [9, 10]. As a result, patients, as well as dentists, may hesitate regarding the timing of extraction.

This report presents a new modified technique of LSFE (modified sinus floor elevation [MSFE]), which is performed before the extraction of compromised teeth. This allows clinicians to delay the extraction and shorten the edentulous interval, making LSFE more acceptable for patient.

2. Clinical Presentation

A 33-year-old female presented to the Department of Periodontics of Peking University School of Stomatology, Beijing, China, on June 15, 2017, complaining chiefly about loose molars. Her teeth #16 and #26 had class II–III mobility, and probing depth around the teeth reached 6–10 mm. The alveolar bone of teeth #16 and #26 was resorbed to the apical third of root so that both teeth were rated as hopeless (Figure 1) [11]. Although the periodontal status was compromised, pulp testing revealed a normal response to thermal stimulation. Since teeth #16 and #26 were free from other discomfort and the chewing function was partially preserved, the patient was unwilling to have the molars extracted bilaterally. She was systemically healthy and a nonsmoker with no history of rhinitis or sinusitis. Her treatment consisted of IPT and frequent supportive periodontal therapy (SPT). We preserved tooth #16 until the restorative treatment period. Thorough descaling and root planing were performed on tooth #16. Follow-up visits between short intervals to control biofilm accumulation were scheduled every month. After the gingiva turned pink and firm without bleeding upon probing or deepening pocket (Figure 2), the periodontal status was improved to a remittent level [12], and MSFE was performed on tooth #16. Tooth #26 was extracted and restored by means of a conventional arrangement for LSFE and implant placement.

2.1. Modified LSFE. Preoperative cone beam computed tomography (CBCT) images were obtained for initial screening and evaluation of the residual bone height between sinus floor and alveolar crest near tooth #16, as well as the morphology of the sinus floor. The right maxillary sinus was found clear and healthy with intact sinus floors. Only 1–2 mm of available bone height was observed, indicating LSFE before implant placement (Figure 3(a)).

The MSFE procedure on tooth #16 was performed based on Tatum's method [13]. Under local anesthesia, a crevicular incision was performed, which was designed to be extended to at least one adjacent tooth both mesially and distally. A full-thickness access flap was prepared, debridement of tooth #16 was performed, and an access window (5 mm × 8 mm) was created on the lateral wall of the maxillary sinus using a round diamond bur under irrigation with sterile saline. The lower edge of the window was formed at least 3–5 mm above the floor so as to keep it away from the teeth. The sinus membrane was elevated by at least 10 mm with curettes (Urban Sinus Lift Instrument, Hu-Friedy Mfg. Co., Chicago, IL, USA) from various angles. The elevation range exceeded the apex of the tooth (both buccolingually and mesiodistally). Then, the sinus membrane

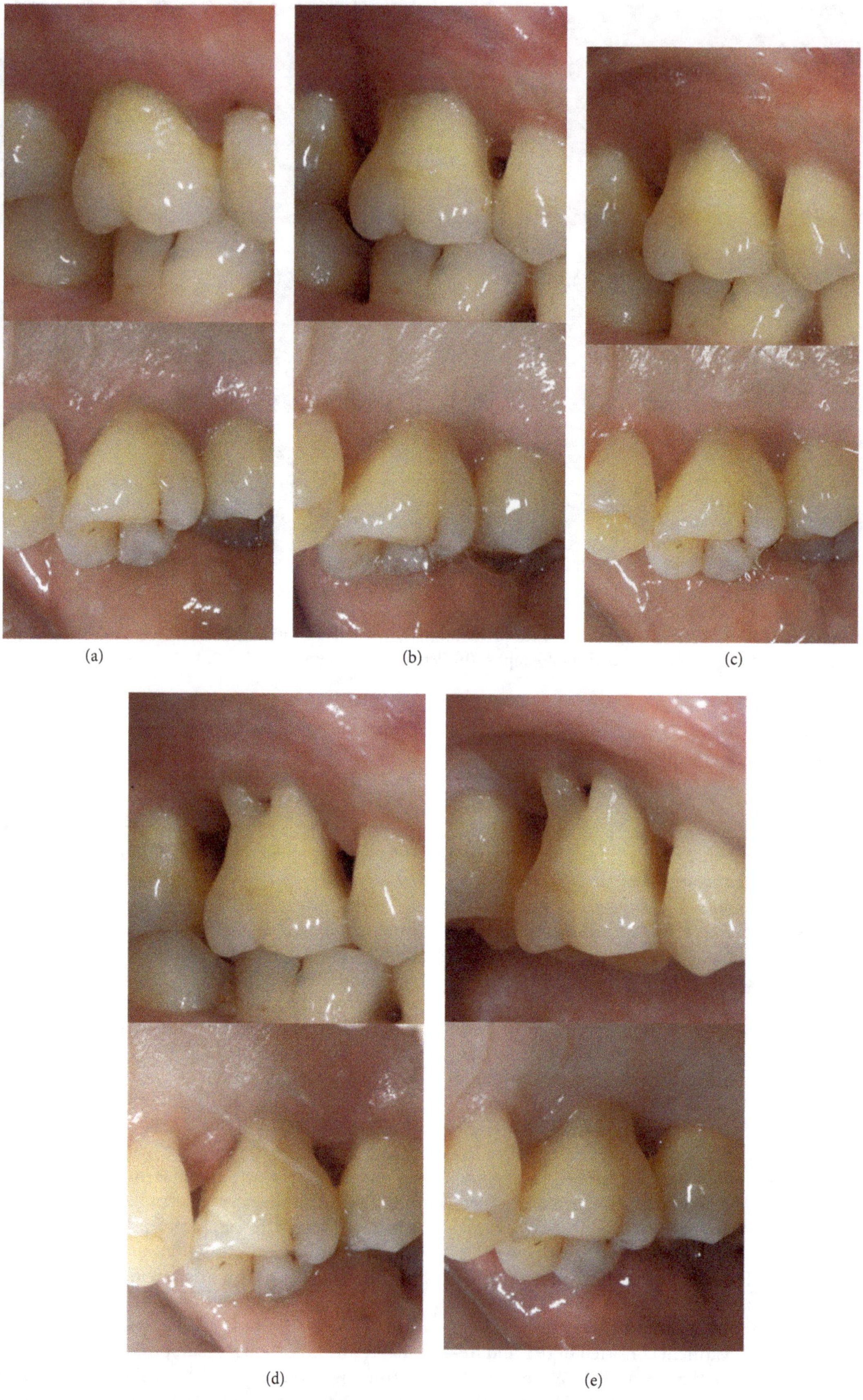

FIGURE 2: Tooth #16 acquired periodontally healthy status after active periodontal treatment. (a) Before periodontal treatment. (b) After 3 months of initial periodontal treatment (IPT) and supportive periodontal treatment (SPT). (c) After 5 months of IPT and SPT. (d) After 7 months of IPT and SPT. (e) After 10 months of IPT and SPT, a remittent status was acquired before the surgery.

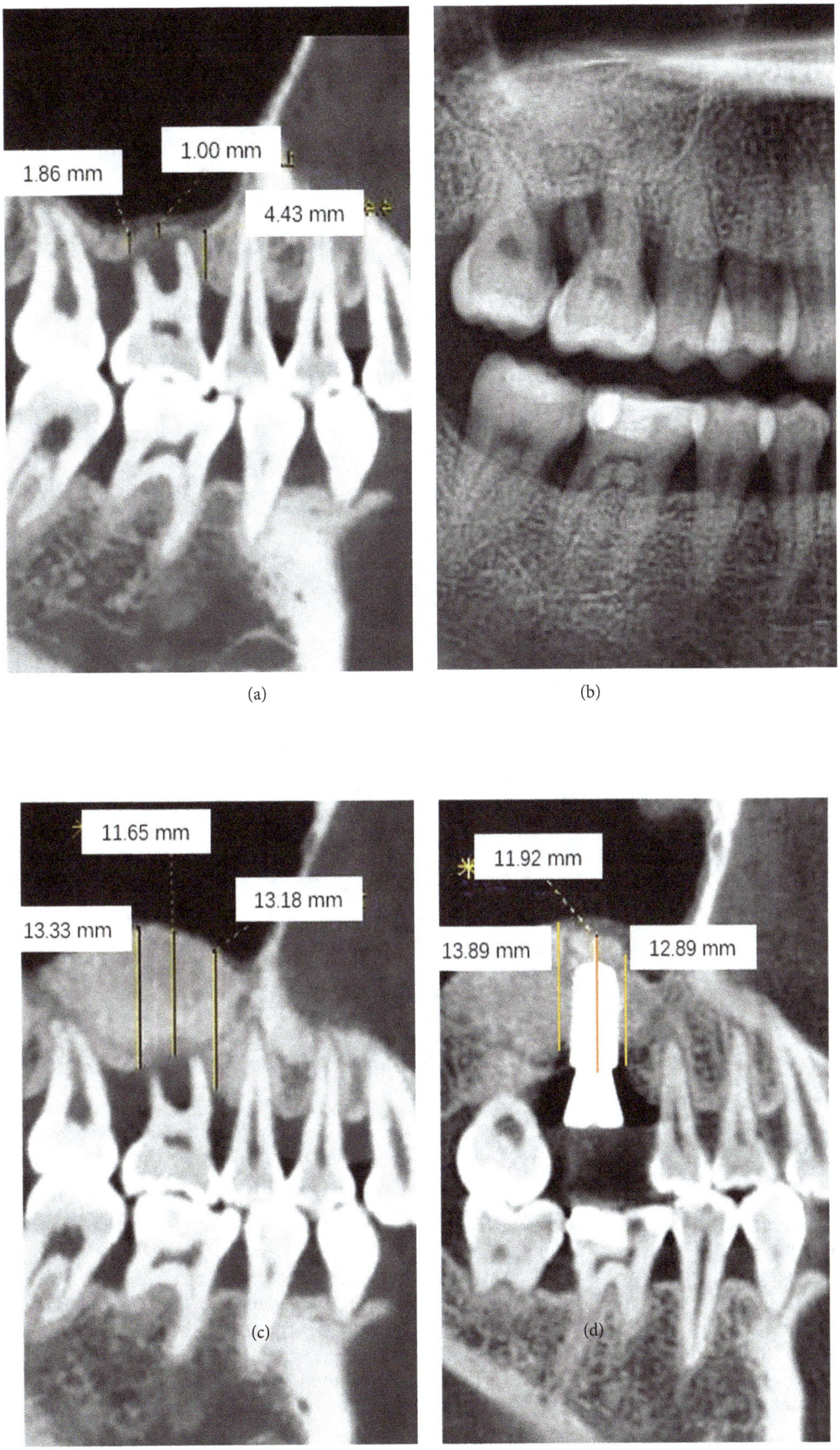

FIGURE 3: Continued.

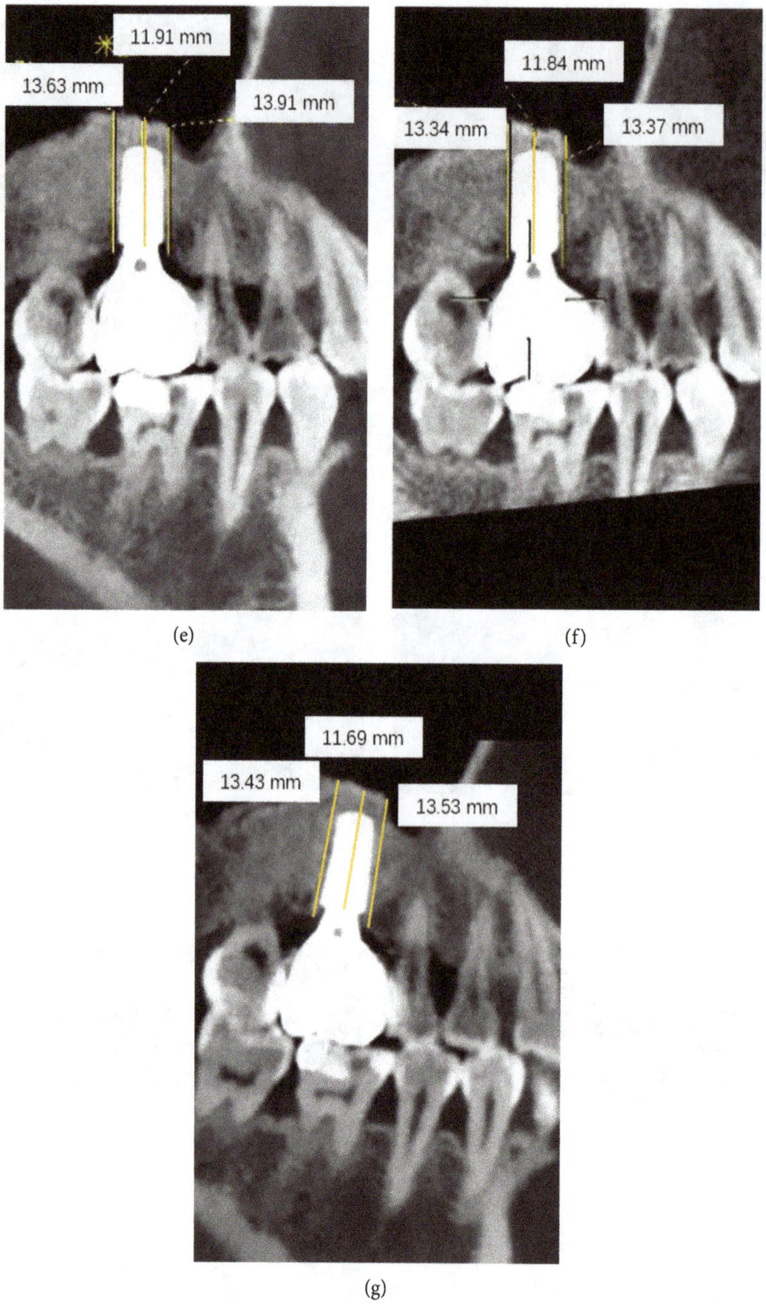

FIGURE 3: CBCT and pantomograph follow-up for tooth #16. (a) Before MSFE. (b) Immediately after MSFE (pantomograph). (c) 3 months after MSFE. (d) 10 months after MSFE. (e) 15 months after MSFE. (f) 26 months after MSFE. (g) 35 months after MSFE.

was lined with a layer of resorbable collagen membrane (Bio-Gide; Geistlich Pharma AG, Wolhusen, Switzerland) 13 mm wide and 25 mm long, and the generated cavity within the maxillary sinus was filled with 1.25 g of small particles of deproteinized bovine bone mineral (Bio-Oss; Geistlich Pharma AG). After grafting, another piece of collagen membrane 12 mm wide and 20 mm long was placed to cover the antrostomy defect. Interrupted sutures were created using non-absorbable suture material (PROLENE 4-0, Ethicon, Somerville, NJ, USA; Figure 4). The patient received antibiotic prophylaxis consisting of 500 mg amoxicillin (Amoxil Capsules, The United Laboratories Co., Hong Kong, China) 30 minutes before the surgery and 3 times daily for the following 7 days postoperatively.

After surgery, the status of tooth #16 was closely monitored. The patient was told to report any adverse event immediately upon occurrence and scheduled to receive SPT every 3 months. At each appointment, periodontal status including PD, BI, and PLI was recorded, and pulp vitality was examined. Thorough descaling and root planing were performed to suppress biofilm formation, and hygiene instructions were given in order to enhance the patient's own plaque control. Although the patient missed the second appointment due to COVID-19, she still had her teeth

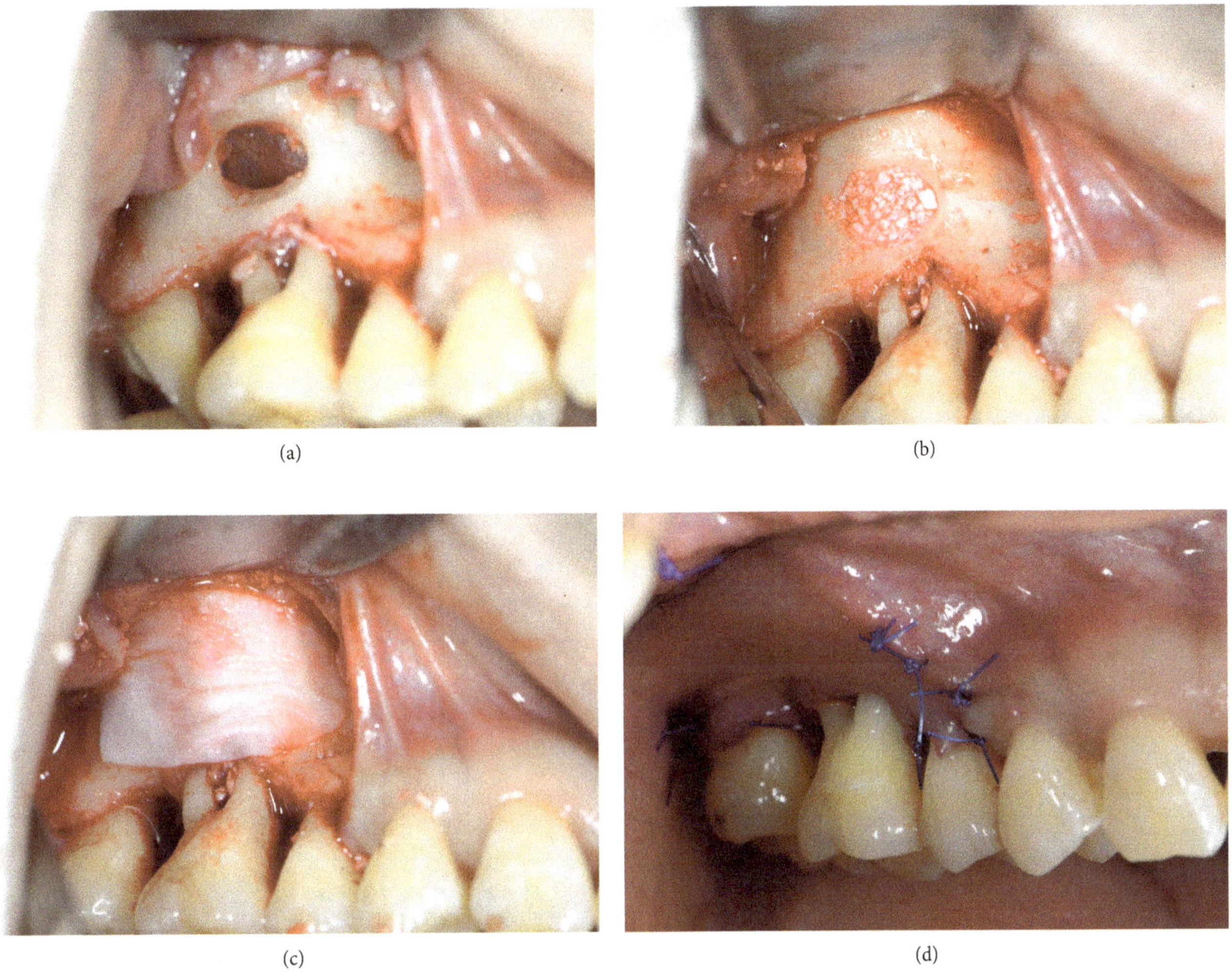

FIGURE 4: The process of the modified lateral sinus floor elevation. (a) Access window on the lateral wall. (b) Grafting materials at the sinus floor. (c) Collagen membrane covering access window. (d) Suturing.

descaled regularly at another clinic. After 10 months, the patient was summoned for the last evaluation of tooth #16 before implant placement. The disease remission status remained stable without sign of active progression, and the vitality was kept normal. The patient described neither discomfort nor complications during the interval, and reported partial chewing function remaining on the right side. A CBCT scan was taken, and an increased bone height of 12–14 mm could be observed at tooth #16. Thus, the site was rated ready for a dental implant (Table 1 and Figure 5(a)).

2.2. Implant Placement and Biopsy Sample Collection. First, tooth #16 was atraumatically extracted with solely vertical force to prevent pressure on the socket walls. After thorough scraping off of all the granulation tissue, the socket walls were confirmed to be intact. Then, a biopsy was taken with a hollow trephine with an internal diameter of 2 mm and a length of 6 mm, and the sample was liberally irrigated with sterile saline before it was fixated in phosphate-buffered formaldehyde. An implant hole was prepared simultaneously. A dental implant with a diameter of 4.8 mm, a length of 10 mm, and a coarsely sand-blasted, acid-etched surface was inserted in the planned site, with a depth where the platform reaches 1 mm below the buccal plate. The implant was inserted with a torque of 35 N·cm. Considering that the gap that remained between walls and implant was less than 2 mm, no bone substitute was filled into it [14]. Finally, the implant was covered with a healing abutment and sutured with non-absorbable sutures (PROLENE 4-0, Ethicon; Figure 5). To double-check the implant position, post-operation periapical radiographs using the paralleling technique were taken (Figure 6(a)).

After 4 months of implant healing without loading, the impressions and bite registration were taken with vinyl-polysiloxane material (Silagum & O-bite, DMG, Beijing, China). A cementable abutment (RC Cementable Abutment, Straumann Holding AG, Basel, Switzerland) with a height of 5.5 mm was selected for building the superstructure. Then, a working cast was scanned, and an anatomic zirconia crown

Table 1: Clinical evaluation of tooth #16 at each follow-up visit.

Treatment Time	PD (mm)	BI	PLI	Pulp Vitality	Peri-implant Marginal Bone Level	Adverse Effect or Complications
Immediately after MSFE	N.A.					Post-operational swelling and pain
3 months after MSFE	2 2 2 3 2 2	1 3	1	Normal (cold test)	N.A.	None
10 months after MSFE (before implant placement)	2–3	1	1	Normal (cold test)	N.A.	None
Implant placement						
Immediately after implant placement	N.A.				1 mm over the platform	None
5 months after implant placement	4 1 2 4 2 3	0 0 0 0 0 0	0 0 0 0 0 0	N.A.	At platform level	None
17 months after implant placement	4 3 3 4 3 3	1 0 1 2 1 0	0 0 1 0 0 0	N.A.	At platform level	None
26 months after implant placement	4 3 3 4 2 2	2 2 3 2 2 2	0 0 1 0 0 0	N.A.	At platform level	None

The data was documented on 6 sites in format as

Mesial-Buccal	Middle-Buccal	Distal-Buccal
Mesial-Palatal	Middle-Palatal	Distal-Palatal

The data was documented on 2 sites in format as

Buccal
Palatal

N.A: Not Available.

was designed and fabricated using computer-aided design (DentalCAD, exocad GmbH, Darmstadt, Germany) and manufacturing system (Linggong, Fujian, China). A screw access was designed on the occlusal surface of the crown. After that, universal single-component priming agent (Monobond Plus, Ivoclar Vivadent, Schaan, Liechtenstein) was applied to the zirconia crown and titanium abutment accordingly. Resin luting cement (Relyx U200, 3M ESPE, St. Paul, MN, USA) was used to lute the two components extraorally according to the manufacturer's recommendations. The superstructure was fixed on the implant with torque of 35 N·cm one month after the impression-taking, and postoperative instructions including oral hygiene care were given to the patient (Figure 7).

2.2.1. Conventional LSFE and Implant Placement. Conventional LSFE was carried out on tooth #26. The tooth was extracted in the initial therapy phase. Seven months after extraction, pre-surgical CBCT was taken. It revealed that the residual bone height remained about 1–2 mm (Figure 8(a)). Then, LSFE was performed, and the procedure was conducted by the same surgeon using the same technique and grafting materials as tooth #16. A layer of resorbable collagen membrane (Bio-Gide; Geistlich Pharma AG)

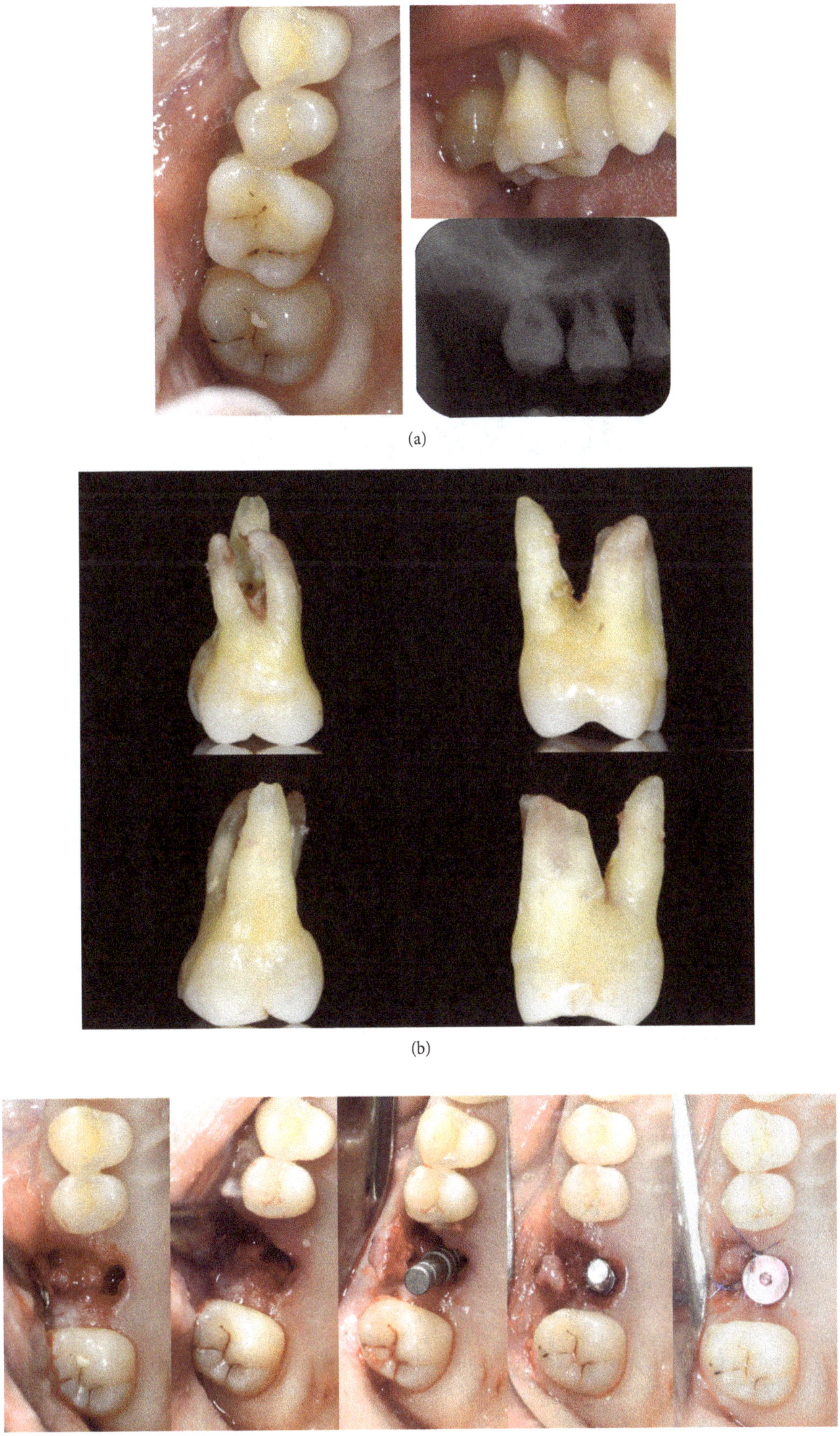

(a)

(b)

(c)

Figure 5: The process of implant placement. (a) Before the extraction. (b) The extracted teeth. (c) Immediate placement of implant.

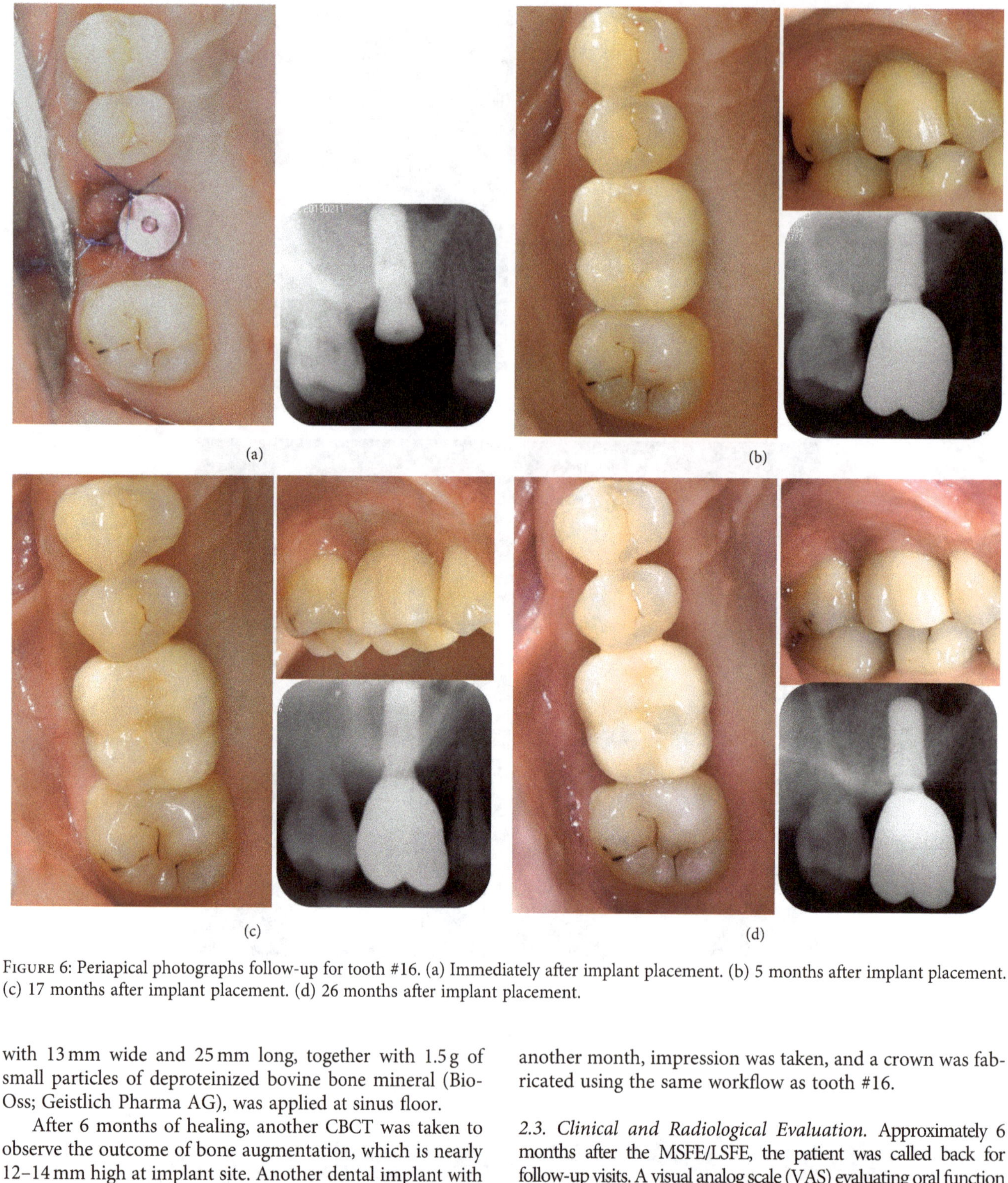

FIGURE 6: Periapical photographs follow-up for tooth #16. (a) Immediately after implant placement. (b) 5 months after implant placement. (c) 17 months after implant placement. (d) 26 months after implant placement.

with 13 mm wide and 25 mm long, together with 1.5 g of small particles of deproteinized bovine bone mineral (Bio-Oss; Geistlich Pharma AG), was applied at sinus floor.

After 6 months of healing, another CBCT was taken to observe the outcome of bone augmentation, which is nearly 12–14 mm high at implant site. Another dental implant with a diameter of 4.8 mm, a length of 10 mm, and a sand-blasted, large-grit, acid-etched surface (SLActive®, Straumann Holding AG) was placed at site with a depth where the platform was aligned with marginal bone. Meanwhile, a bone biopsy was taken as well. The implant was inserted with a torque of 35 N cm and submerged.

After 4 months of the unloaded implant healing, stage-two surgery was performed under local anesthesia to replace the implant cover screws with the healing abutments. After another month, impression was taken, and a crown was fabricated using the same workflow as tooth #16.

2.3. Clinical and Radiological Evaluation. Approximately 6 months after the MSFE/LSFE, the patient was called back for follow-up visits. A visual analog scale (VAS) evaluating oral function over the whole treatment period was handed over to the patient. The patient was asked to rate her oral function level using a 10-grade scale from "0—satisfying" to "10—discomfortable." Clinical evaluation including mucosa conditions and complications, and radiological evaluation including periapical radiographs and CBCT (or pantomograph) were obtained at each follow-up visit.

2.4. Histological Evaluation. The bone biopsy samples were collected during dental implant surgery with the use of a

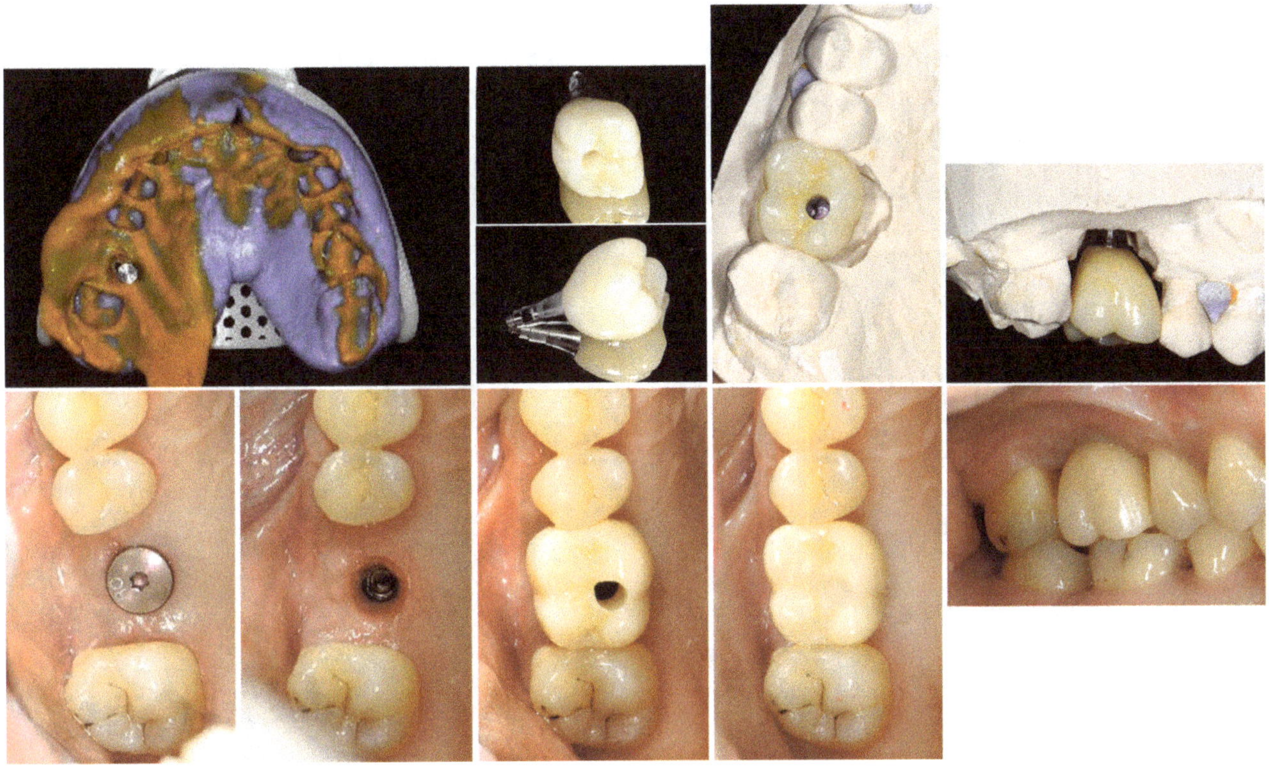

Figure 7: The process of delivering the superstructure.

hollow trephine, fixated in 10% formaldehyde (pH 7.4; +4°C), transferred to 70% ethanol, and stored until used for histomorphometric analysis. The samples were subsequently decalcified in 7% ethylenediaminetetraacetic acid, embedded in low-temperature-polymerizing methyl methacrylate, cut into sections (thickness 4 μm), and stained with both hematoxylin–eosin and modified Mallory aniline blue. The histologic parameters were recorded as described in da Rosa et al. [15].

3. Outcomes

The patient is very satisfied with the whole treatment arrangement. No adverse event or complication was reported. At each re-visit before extraction of tooth #16, vitality of tooth #16 was detected as normal. The probing depth was limited within 3 mm with rare bleeding on probing, indicating a stable periodontal status without sign of progression (Table 1). The VAS was recorded as 2 at 6 months after MSFE, while the score was recorded as 10 on the opposite side (Figure 9). After nearly 3 years of loading, both implants are in good condition without obvious sign of peri-implantitis or mobility (Tables 1 and 2; Figures 6 and 10). The probing depth around teeth #16 and #26 ranged from 2 to 4 mm. The bleeding index occasionally reached 2–3 as plaque accumulating over time.

As for the radiological evaluation, adequate bone height was obtained at the sinus floor on both sides. Comparing with tooth #26, the same level of augmentation could be detected on tooth #16. The available bone height on both sides was augmented from 1–2 to 12–14 mm. Bone volume and marginal bone level after MSFE/LSFE remain stable during 3 years of follow-up. Little resorption (less than 2 mm of height) of bone substitute was observed (Figures 3 and 8).

Both sides shared a similarity in terms of histological analysis. The cylindrical biopsy sample collected from teeth #16 and #26 was found well-consolidated in macroscopic analysis. Newly formed bone as well as lines of osteoblast-forming osteoids could be observed on both sides at the apical side of the biopsy core. Lacunas and osteocytes could be seen in the area of immature bone, whereas limited nonvital bone with empty lacunae also remained in the view. On the MSFE side, scores were 3 for vital bone, 3 for mature newly formed bone, 2 for osteoblasts, 1 for osteoclasts, and 4 for bone marrow (Figure 11). On the LSFE side, scores were 4 for vital bone, 3 for mature newly formed bone, 1 for osteoblasts, 1 for osteoclasts, and 3 for bone marrow.

4. Discussion

Resorption of alveolar bone is a common consequence of periodontitis, which may leave behind inadequate bone volume for implant placement [16]. Especially for maxillary molars, poor periodontal status could even be regarded as a potential predictor for LSFE [16]. In this clinical case, residual bone height at tooth #16 remained only 1–2 mm before extraction, indicating LSFE was inevitable to place

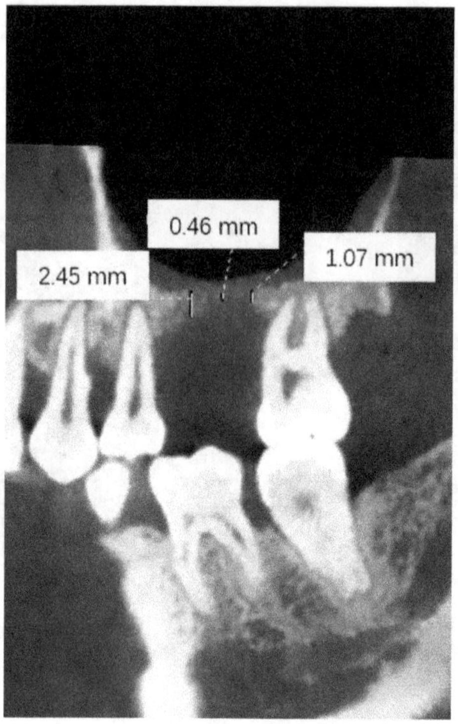

(a)

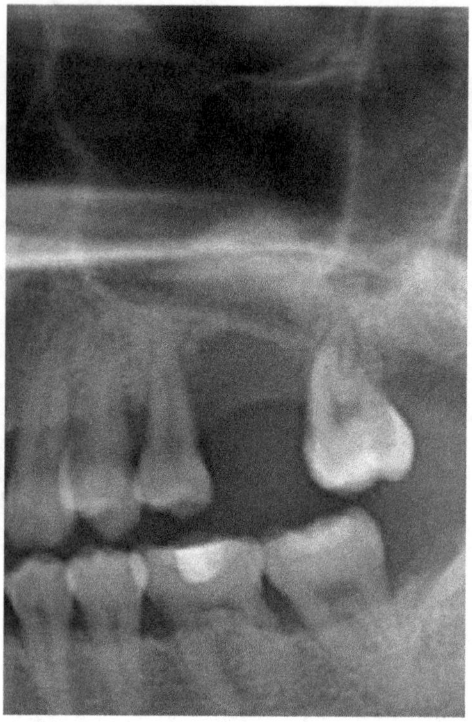

(b)

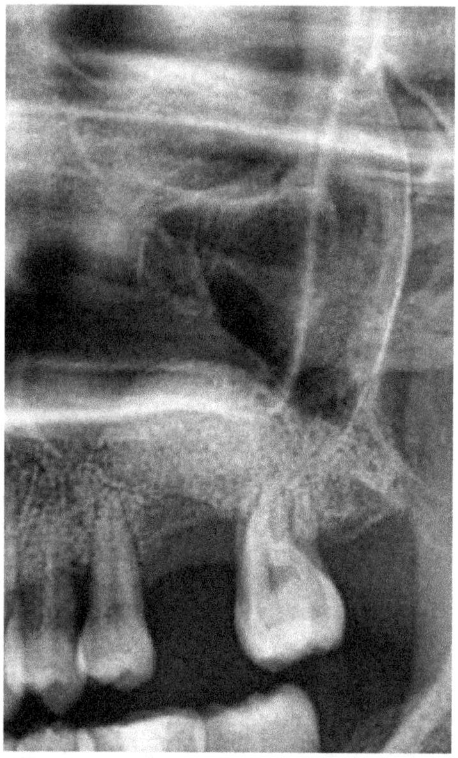

(c)

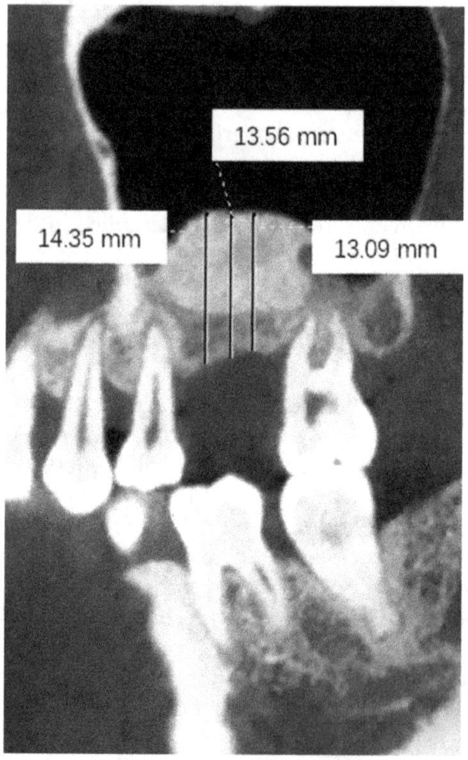

(d)

FIGURE 8: Continued.

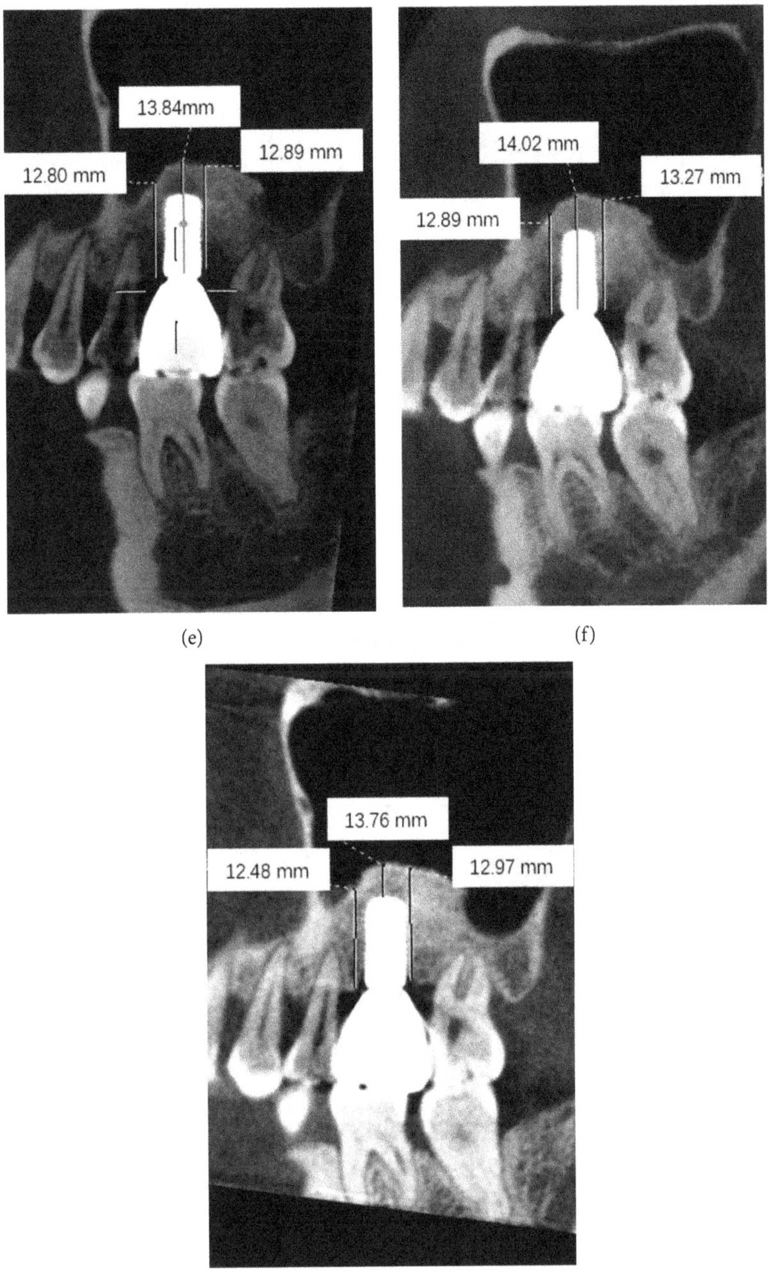

(e) (f)

(g)

FIGURE 8: CBCT and pantomograph follow-up for tooth #26. (a) Before MSFE. (b) Immediately after MSFE (pantomograph). (c) 3 months after MSFE (pantomograph). (d) 7 months after MSFE. (e) 14 months after MSFE. (f) 20 months after MSFE. (g) 32 months after MSFE.

an implant. Thus, a new modified LSFE before the extraction was performed in advance. The possibility of MSFE was foreseen by Beitlitum et al., who demonstrated effectiveness and safety of extending sinus floor augmentation to adjacent teeth beyond the edentulous area [17]. The 3-year follow-up of our case confirmed the feasibility and effectiveness of MSFE. The implant at tooth #16 functioned well with no adverse event or complication ever reported. CBCT revealed adequate increasement on bone volume at the side of MSFE. Furthermore, bone substitute augmented at the sinus floor remained stable with little resorption (less than 2 mm of height).

According to the traditional method of LSFE, compromised teeth are supposed to be extracted 3–4 months before any access to the sinus floor. When it comes to bone heights of only 4 mm or less (≤4 mm), two-stage surgery with bone grafting was required, which means at least another 6 months should elapse before implant placement [7, 8]. This edentulous period in the posterior maxilla leads to obvious reduction of masticatory efficiency. More specifically, the absence of a second molar may cause 5–7% decrease of chewing efficiency [18], whereas a premolar–first molar region bears 90% of the masticatory function of the dentition [19]. This is vital for patients with advanced periodontitis,

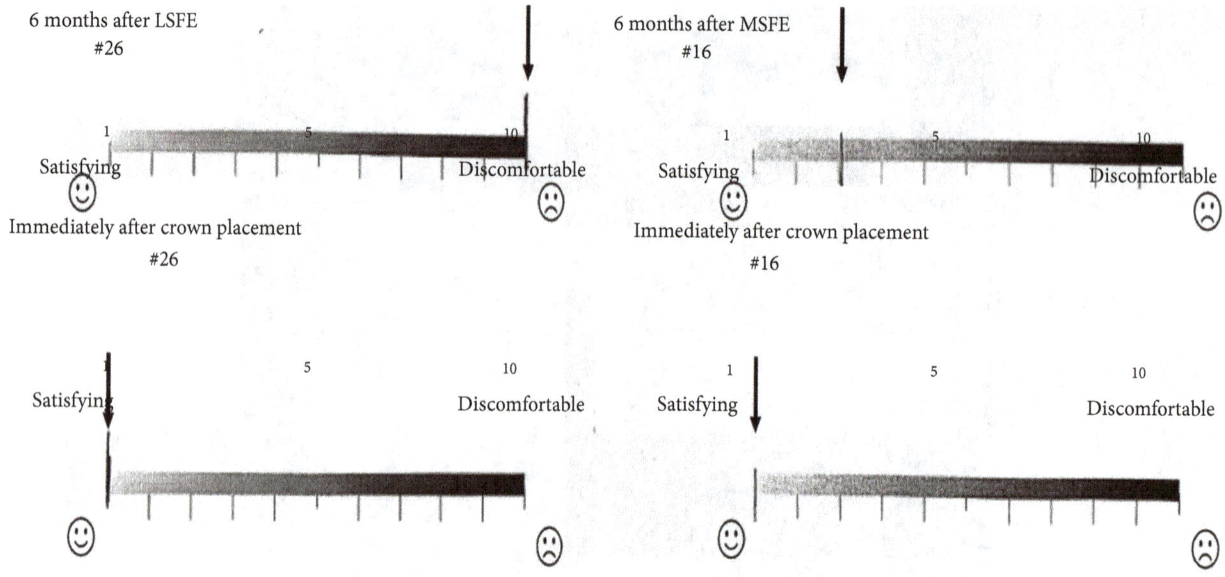

Figure 9: Visual analog scales (VAS) for discomfort were distributed to patient at 6 months after MSFE and immediately after crown placement.

Table 2: Clinical evaluation of tooth #26 at each re-visit.

Treatment Time	PD (mm)			BI			PLI			Peri-implant Marginal Bone Level	Adverse Effect or Complications
Immediately after implant placement	N.A.									At platform Level	None
5 months after implant placement	2	1	2	0	0	0	0	0	0	At platform level	None
	2	3	3	0	0	0	0	0	0		
8 months after implant placement	3	1	2	0	0	0	0	0	0	At platform level	None
	2	3	3	0	0	0	0	0	0		
19 months after implant placement	3	2	2	0	0	0	1	0	0	At platform level	None
	3	3	4	0	0	2	0	0	0		
28 months after implant placement	3	3	4	0	0	2	0	0	1	At platform level	None
	3	4	4	3	2	1	2	0	1		
34 months after implant placement	3	3	4	0	0	2	0	1	1	At platform level	None
	4	3	4	3	1	1	2	0	1		

The data was documented on 6 sites in format as

Mesial-Buccal	Middle-Buccal	Distal-Buccal
Mesial-Palatal	Middle-Palatal	Distal-Palatal

N.A: Not Available.

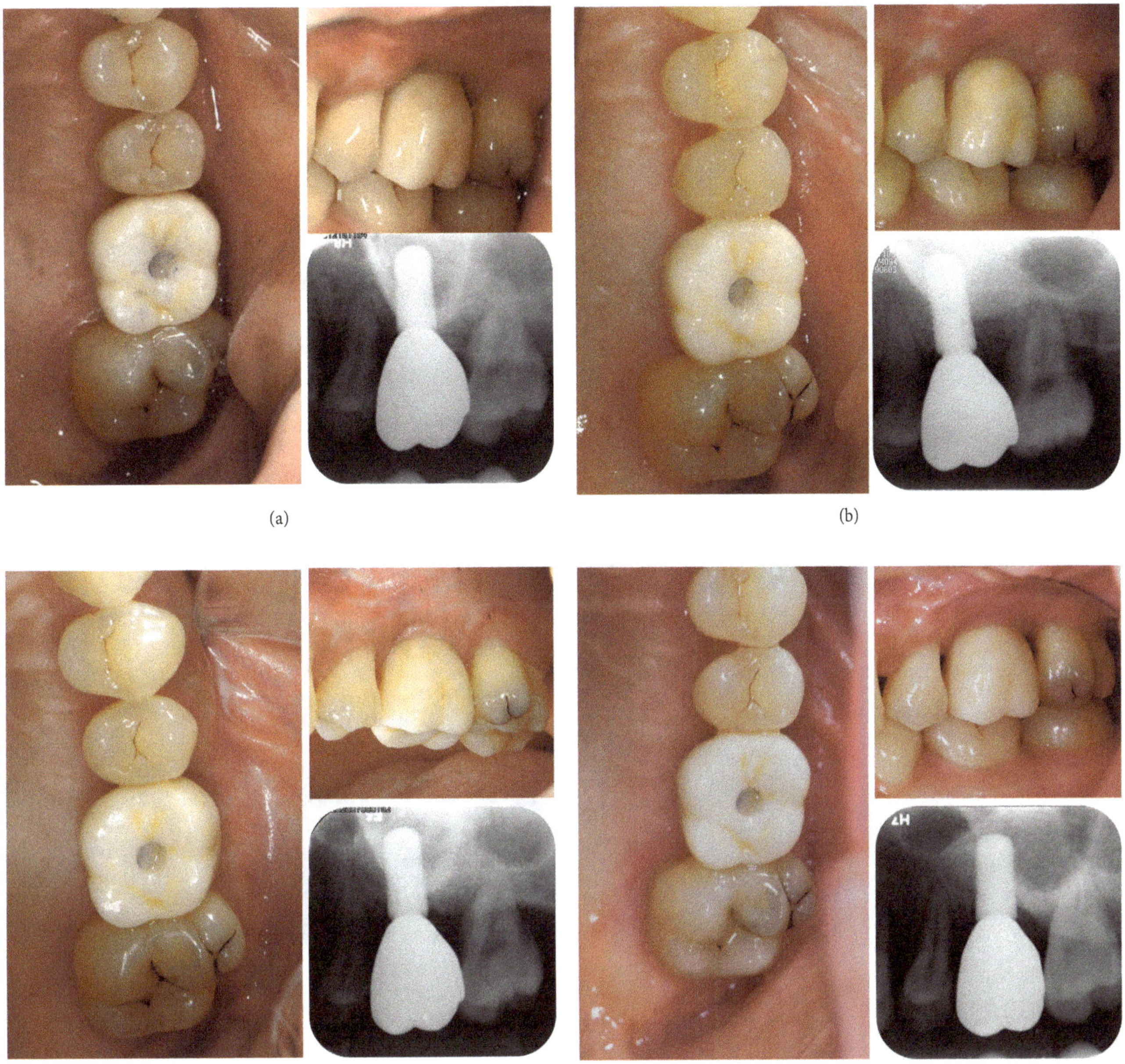

Figure 10: Periapical photographs follow-up for tooth #26. (a) Immediately after crown placement (5 months after implant placement). (b) 19 months after implant placement. (c) 28 months after implant placement. (d) 34 months after implant placement.

since bilateral molars are more likely to be affected than other teeth [1]. For the current case, the VAS score for oral function satisfaction was 2 on the right side as a result of the MSFE on tooth #16. The edentulous period was reduced to 5 months, versus 16 months on the left side which got a VAS score of 10. By arranging LSFE before extraction, limited but vital function of the molar tooth #16 was fully utilized, and oral function during the treatment intervals was improved.

MSFE may also offer the option of immediate implant placement. The bone volume augmented beforehand may be used to achieve initial implant stability, which is essential for successful immediate placement [20]. Fresh sockets after extraction could be practically suitable for inserting implants if the MSFE sites meet with basic conceptions for immediate placement: (a) adequate bone volume after MSFE for selection of proper implant length and width, as well as its initial stability; (b) absence of endodontic disease or progression of periodontal disease; (c) intact socket walls; and (d) thick biotype with more than 2 mm width of keratinized mucosa. In such case, advantages of immediate placement generally recognized by previous studies [21–24] could be exploited on the site, such as earlier loading of the implant or preservation of alveolar bone contour. In current case, another 3–4 months are saved compared with delayed placement.

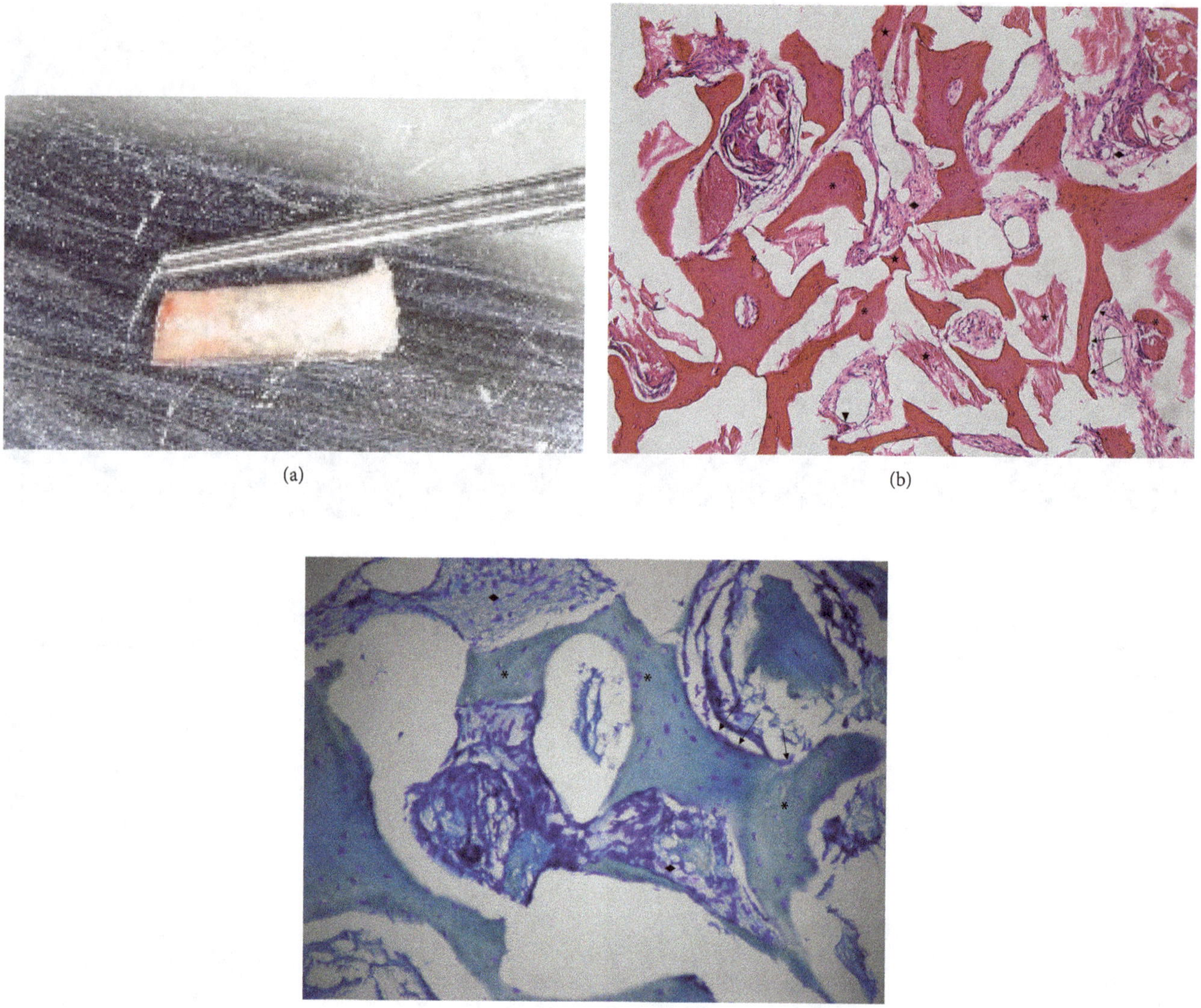

(a) (b) (c)

Figure 11: Histological evaluation of tooth #16. (a) The biopsy sample. (b) Representative section stained with hematoxylin-eosin (H&E) (×10). (c) Representative section stained with modified Mallory aniline blue (×20). Newly formed bone (asterisk), nonvital bone (star), blood marrow (diamond), bone lining cells (arrowhead), and an osteoclast (arrow) are visible.

Bone remodeling is supposed to start upon tooth extraction [25]. Without functional stimulus, the alveolar process continues to retrude towards the basal bone [2, 3]. MSFE minimizes the period of function deficiency and, therefore, has the potential to halt the remodeling at early stage. Moreover, the tooth extraction was shown to abet the pneumatization process of the maxillary sinus due to the absence of stimuli from biting forces [26, 27]. With the tooth kept on site after modified LSFE, biting forces continue to act, providing a chance for preventing resorption of regenerated bone or preventing "re-pneumatization." Thus, quality and quantity of the bone augmented on sinus floor with a modified LSFE technique may be more promising than traditional methods are. In the current case, predominance of new bone was detected via histologic analysis on both sides, with lacunas, osteocytes, and lines of osteoblast-forming osteoids present. Similar histological findings and a comparable level of osteogenesis could be observed on MSFE side and LSFE side. Furthermore, controlled data and studies are necessary to prove or deny superiority of the histological manifestation over traditional approaches.

A potential adverse effect of MSFE may be pulp necrosis. It was reported that elevation of sinus membrane under the teeth would possibly disrupt the innervation and blood supply of individual branches of root apices [28]. However, a retrospect study revealed that most of the pulp devitalization occurred due to severe carious or periodontal lesions. Only 0.7% of probability of tooth devitalization was rated due to sinus floor augmentation [29]. The periapical tissue will not be damaged as long as the integrity of alveolar bone

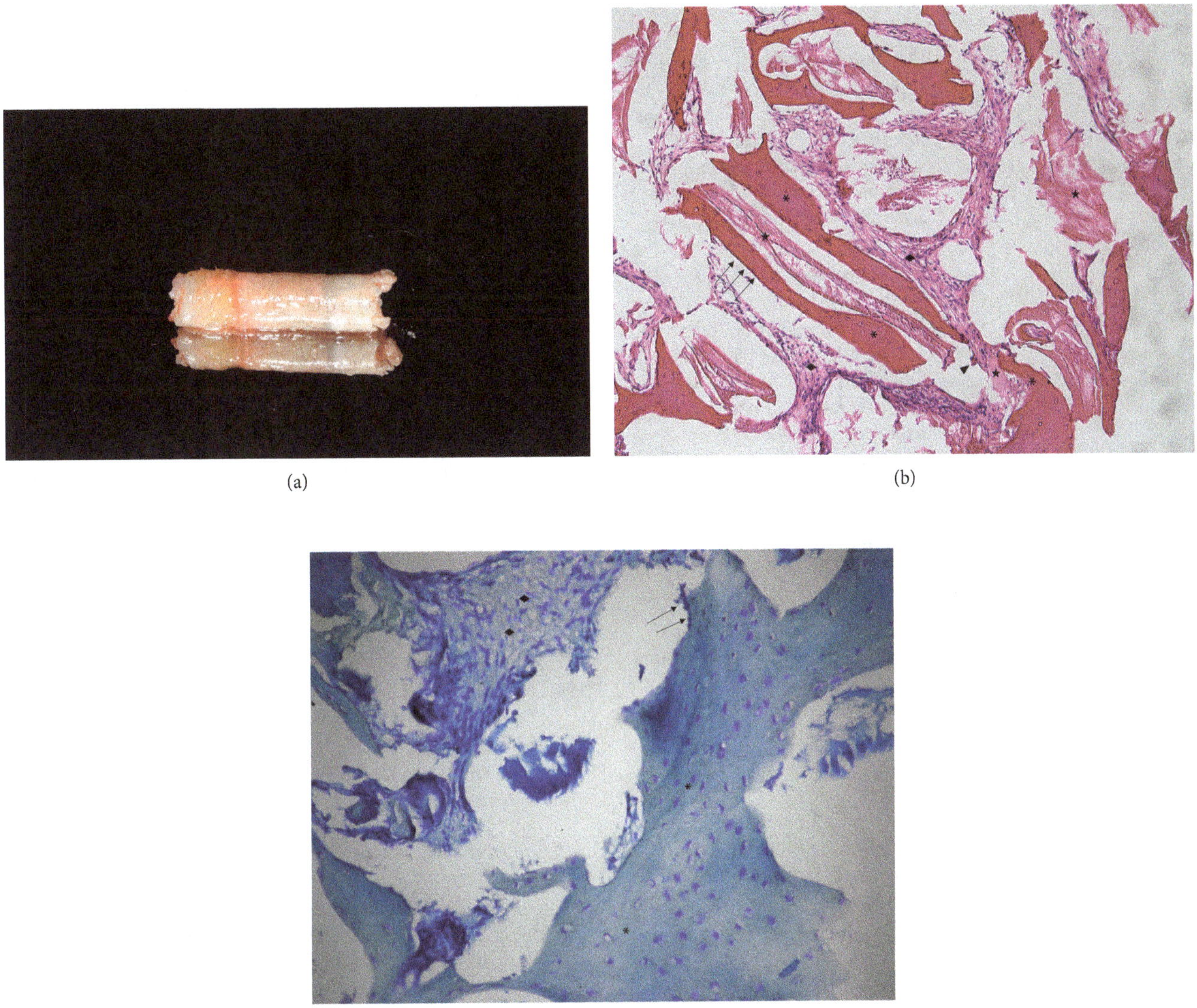

(a) (b) (c)

FIGURE 12: Histological evaluation of tooth #26. (a) The biopsy sample. (b) Representative section stained with hematoxylin-eosin (H&E) (×10). (c) Representative section stained with modified Mallory aniline blue (×20). Newly formed bone (asterisk), nonvital bone (star), blood marrow (diamond), bone lining cells (arrowhead), and an osteoclast (arrow) are visible.

around the apexes of roots remains intact [17]. In the current case, the surgical invasions were carefully confined to the sinus floor without interfering the apex of tooth #16. As a result, the vitality of tooth #16 was detected as normal during the whole period. More clinical data are needed to prove the safety of MSFE.

According to Carranza et al., teeth whose attachment is inadequate to maintain health, comfort, and function are regarded as "hopeless" and should be extracted sooner or later [11]. Once the biofilm was optimally controlled by IPT and frequent SPT, some of the "hopeless" teeth could be freed of acute symptoms and regain part of chewing function [29]. This status refers to reduction of inflammation, such as improvement of PD and control of bleeding on probing, although optimal control of local contributing factors is not achieved. At this time, periodontal disease remission sets in [11], and it is the situation that we consider to be the indication for modified LSFE, which could be summarized as teeth with: (a) more than 50% attachment loss; (b) poor crown-to-root ratio; (c) poor root form; (d) class II or III furcation involvements; (e) more than class II mobility; and (f) difficulty to clean by the patient himself or herself, but are stably manageable under frequent periodontal supportive treatment. Other indications for MSFE refer to the traditional perspective of lateral approach [4–6, 16, 17], such as: (g) inadequate interfurcal bone height for future implant replacement (≤6 mm) together with probing depth exceeding 6 mm; (h) endodontically healthy/treated; (i) absence of sinus disease (e.g., active sinus infection, recurrent chronic sinusitis, or neoplasms of the sinus); and (j) systemically healthy. More cases and long-term follow-up are necessary to prove the validity of the preliminary indication.

5. Summary

Why is this case new information?	The modified sinus floor elevation approach offers an effective method to shorten the edentulous interval between extraction and loading of implants and improve the patient's quality of life, especially for patients with hopeless molars on both sides.
What are the keys to successful management of this case?	The periodontal status of the compromised teeth needs to be managed to a remittent level by means of IPT and SPT preoperatively. Specifically, a significant decrease in inflammation, stabilization of disease progression, and partial restoration of the chewing function should be achieved before surgery.
What are the primary limitations to success in this case?	The difficulty of flap elevation may increase since the hopeless or loose teeth still remain on site. In some cases, the sinus membrane may be thickened or exhibit morbid changes due to chronic inflammation among molars.

Acknowledgments

The authors would like to thank Geistlich Pharma AG, Wolhusen, Switzerland, for providing their materials under the Material Transfer Agreement between Jianxia Hou and Geistlich Pharma AG.

References

[1] O. Helal, G. Göstemeyer, J. Krois, K. Fawzy El Sayed, C. Graetz, and F. Schwendicke, "Predictors for tooth loss in periodontitis patients: systematic review and meta-analysis," *Journal of Clinical Periodontology*, vol. 46, no. 7, pp. 699–712, 2019.

[2] M. G. Araujo and J. Lindhe, "Dimensional ridge alterations following tooth extraction. An experimental study in the dog," *Journal of Clinical Periodontology*, vol. 32, no. 2, pp. 212–218, 2005.

[3] J. Pietrokovski, R. Starinsky, B. Arensburg, and I. Kaffe, "Morphologic characteristics of bony edentulous jaws," *Journal of Prosthodontics*, vol. 16, no. 2, pp. 141–147, 2007.

[4] N. Mohan, J. Wolf, and H. Dym, "Maxillary sinus augmentation," *Dental Clinics of North America*, vol. 59, no. 2, pp. 375–388, 2015.

[5] B. E. Pjetursson and N. P. Lang, "Sinus floor elevation utilizing the transalveolar approach," *Periodontology*, vol. 66, no. 1, pp. 59–71, 2000.

[6] S. Lundgren, G. Cricchio, M. Hallman, M. Jungner, L. Rasmusson, and L. Sennerby, "Sinus floor elevation procedures to enable implant placement and integration: techniques, biological aspects and clinical outcomes," *Periodontology*, vol. 73, no. 1, pp. 103–120, 2017.

[7] N. U. Zitzmann and P. Schärer, "Sinus elevation procedures in the resorbed posterior maxilla. Comparison of the crestal and lateral approaches," *Oral Surgery, Oral Medicine, Oral Pathology, Oral Radiology, and Endodontics*, vol. 85, no. 1, pp. 8–17, 1998.

[8] A. Stern and J. Green, "Sinus lift procedures: an overview of current techniques," *Dental Clinics of North America*, vol. 56, no. 1, pp. 219–233, 2012.

[9] C. Graetz, C. E. Dorfer, M. Kahl et al., "Retention of questionable and hopeless teeth in compliant patients treated for aggressive periodontitis," *Journal of Clinical Periodontology*, vol. 38, no. 8, pp. 707–714, 2011.

[10] R. T. Kao, "Strategic extraction: a paradigm shift that is changing our profession," *Journal of Periodontology*, vol. 79, no. 6, pp. 971–977, 2008.

[11] K. F. Novak, H. H. Takei, and J. H. Do, "Determination of prognosis," in *Carranza's Clinical Periodontology*, M. G. Newman, H. H. Takei, P. R. Klokkevold, and F. A. Carranza, Eds., pp. 394–395, Elsevier, St. Louis, 12th edition, 2015.

[12] I. L. C. Chapple, B. L. Mealey, T. E. Van Dyke et al., "Periodontal health and gingival diseases and conditions on an intact and a reduced periodontium: consensus report of workgroup 1 of the 2017 world workshop on the classification of periodontal and peri-implant diseases and conditions," *Journal of Periodontology*, vol. 89, Suppl 1, pp. S74–S84, 2018.

[13] H. Tatum, "Maxillary and sinus implant reconstructions," *Dental Clinics of North America*, vol. 30, no. 2, pp. 207–229, 1986.

[14] R. B. Smith and D. P. Tarnow, "Classification of molar extraction sites for immediate dental implant placement: technical note," *The International Journal of Oral & Maxillofacial Implants*, vol. 28, no. 3, pp. 911–916, 2013.

[15] J. C. M. da Rosa, B. S. Sotto-Maior, P. de Oliveira, A. C. Rosa, and L. A. Violin Dias Pereira, "Clinical, tomographic, and histologic evaluation of an autogenous bone graft harvested from the maxillary tuberosity for guided bone regeneration: case report with a 4-year follow-up," *The International Journal of Periodontics & Restorative Dentistry*, vol. 41, no. 4, pp. e183–e190, 2021.

[16] C. Walter, D. C. Dagassan-Berndt, S. Kühl, R. Weiger, N. P. Lang, and N. U. Zitzmann, "Is furcation involvement in maxillary molars a predictor for subsequent bone augmentation prior to implant placement? A pilot study," *Clinical Oral Implants Research*, vol. 25, no. 12, pp. 1352–1358, 2014.

[17] I. Beitlitum, W. Habashi, I. Tsesis, E. Rosen, C. E. Nemcovsky, and Y. Manor, "Extended maxillary sinus augmentation to the apical area of the neighboring teeth: advantages and limitations," *The International Journal of Periodontics & Restorative Dentistry*, vol. 38, no. 3, pp. 451–456, 2018.

[18] C. E. Misch, "Single-tooth replacement: treatment options," in *in Contemporary Implant Dentistry*, C. E. Misch, Ed., pp. 327–366, Mosby, St. Louis, 3rd edition, 2008.

[19] J. M. Broadbent, "Chewing and occlusal function," *The Functional Orthodontist*, vol. 17, no. 4, pp. 34–39, 2000.

[20] D. Schwartz-Arad and G. Chaushu, "The ways and wherefores of immediate placement of implants into fresh extraction sites: a literature review," *Journal of Periodontology*, vol. 68, no. 10, pp. 915–923, 1997.

[21] R. J. Lazzara, "Immediate implant placement into extraction sites: surgical and restorative advantages," *The International Journal of Periodontics & Restorative Dentistry*, vol. 9, pp. 333–343, 1989.

[22] M. J. Werbitt and P. V. Goldberg, "The immediate implant: bone preservation and bone regeneration," *The International Journal of Periodontics & Restorative Dentistry*, vol. 12, no. 3, pp. 206–217, 1992.

[23] G. Watzek, R. Haider, N. Mensdorff-Pouilly, and R. Haas, "Immediate and delayed implantation for complete restoration of the jaw following extraction of all residual teeth: a retrospective study comparing different types of serial immediate implantation," *The International Journal of Oral & Maxillofacial Implants*, vol. 10, no. 5, pp. 561–567, 1995.

[24] B. Rosenquist and G. Björn, "Immediate placement of implants into extraction sockets: implant survival," *The International Journal of Oral & Maxillofacial Implants*, vol. 11, no. 2, pp. 205–209, 1996.

[25] L. Schropp, A. Wenzel, L. Kostopoulos, and T. Karring, "Bone healing and soft tissue contour changes following single-tooth extraction: a clinical and radiographic 12-month prospective study," *The International Journal of Periodontics & Restorative Dentistry*, vol. 23, no. 4, pp. 313–323, 2003.

[26] A. Sharan and D. Madjar, "Maxillary sinus pneumatization following extractions: a radiographic study," *The International Journal of Oral & Maxillofacial Implants*, vol. 23, no. 1, pp. 48–56, 2008.

[27] H. Wehrbein and P. Diedrich, "Progressive pneumatization of the basal maxillary sinus after extraction and space closure," *Fortschritte der Kieferorthopädie*, vol. 53, no. 2, pp. 77–83, 1992.

[28] G. E. Romanos, D. E. Papadimitriou, M. J. Hoyo, and J. G. Caton, "Loss of pulp vitality after maxillary sinus augmentation: a surgical and endodontic approach," *Journal of Periodontology*, vol. 85, no. 1, pp. 43–49, 2014.

[29] D. Lundgren, H. Rylander, and L. Laurell, "To save or to extract, that is the question. Natural teeth or dental implants in periodontitis-susceptible patients: clinical decision-making and treatment strategies exemplified with patient case presentations," *Periodontology*, vol. 47, pp. 27–50, 2008.

23

Unicystic Ameloblastoma Mimicking Lateral Periodontal Cyst

Maya Fedhila[1,2] **Raouaa Belkacem Chebil**[1,2] **Sonia Karray**[3] **Badreddine Sriha**[4]
Lamia Oualha[1,2] **and Nabiha Douki**[1,2]

[1]*Department of Oral Medicine and Oral Surgery, SAHLOUL Hospital (Sousse), Dental Faculty of Monastir, University of Monastir, Tunisia*
[2]*Laboratory of Oral Health and Maxillofacial Rehabilitation (LR12ES11), University of Monastir, Tunisia*
[3]*National Center of Medicine in Schools and Universities, Tunisia*
[4]*Faculty of Medicine, University of Sousse, Farhat Hached Hospital of Sousse, Department of Pathology, Sousse, Tunisia*

Correspondence should be addressed to Maya Fedhila; mayafedhila11@gmail.com

Academic Editor: Junichi Asaumi

Intraosseous unicystic ameloblastoma (UA) is a rare subtype of a true neoplasm of odontogenic epithelial origin: ameloblastoma. Despite its rareness, dealing with UA is problematic. It is usually mistaken for an odontogenic cyst, and biopsy is rarely relevant because of its multiple growth patterns. The biggest challenge remains the treatment choice. When we are faced with a mural UA presenting strong similarities with a lateral periodontal cyst and having high rates of recurrence, how is the balance found between the young age, psychological fragility, postoperative process, and need for diagnostic biopsy? That was our dilemma. Our patient is a 23-year-old man with a mural unicystic ameloblastoma, diagnosed with general anxiety disorder. The final decision was to turn to a simple enucleation because of the small size of the lesion, and its radiological features strongly evoked a lateral periodontal cyst. Besides, his young age, psychological condition, and UA's proximity to the surrounding soft tissues guided us toward simple enucleation. Two years later, no sign of radiological recurrence was noted. However, we are aware of a later possibility of resection in case of recurrence.

1. Introduction

Odontogenic lesions are usually discovered through a routine radiography exam, although swelling may appear in the oral cavity. In the setting of this presentation, cysts (e.g., dentigerous cyst, radicular cyst, and keratocyst) are the primary suspected lesion. However, ameloblastoma remains a distinct possibility.

The latter lesion is a slow-growing though locally aggressive tumor representing 9% to 10% of odontogenic tumors. Its frequently reported location is the mandible (angle and ramus region), often associated with an unerupted third molar. It occurs generally during the 3rd to 4th decade of life and has an equal sex distribution [1, 2].

Ameloblastoma is a neoplasm of odontogenic epithelium, arising from epithelial cellular elements and dental tissues in their various phases of development [2]. In pathology, the lesion is characterized by its recapitulation of embryologic ameloblasts and stellate reticulum. It may grow to a great size, causing facial asymmetry, displacement of teeth, malocclusion, and even pathologic fracture [3].

According to the 4th Edition of the World Health Organization update, ameloblastoma is classified into four categories: conventional/multicystic, extraosseous/peripheral, metastasizing, and unicystic [4]. Conventional ameloblastoma is the most common variant (86%), also characterized by the highest recurrence rates [3]. On the contrary, unicystic ameloblastoma (UA) is less recurrent and not due to a secondary cystic change. It is a unique de novo neoplasm representing 15% of ameloblastoma cases [5].

Histologically, we can identify three subtypes of growth patterns [5]:

(i) Luminal showing a flat ameloblastic cyst lining

(ii) Intraluminal characterized by a tumor growth into the cyst lumen, usually with soft luminal projections

(iii) Mural exhibiting infiltrating growth into the wall of the cyst and even beyond into the surrounding bone

UA is particularly known for multiple growth patterns in the same lesion. Hence, a biopsy might give the wrong diagnosis when the specimen shows only one of lesion's multiple growth patterns. It is a dilemma since the treatment of one can promote the recurrence of the other [1].

Currently, conservative and radical treatments exist for UA. The conservative approach consists of a simple enucleation (i.e., surgical removal of the whole lesion including the capsular/pseudocapsular surface), or an enucleation followed by Carnoy's solution [6], or a marsupialization followed by enucleation [1, 7].

On the other hand, radical treatment consists of surgical resection (with or without continuity defect) of the lesion and surrounding bone [1]. The invasive approach is generally indicated for the mural subtype, whereas the conservative one usually suits the luminal or intraluminal pattern growth groups [8].

Therefore, we will introduce a case of a mural UA in the right mandible sector of a 23-year-old man presenting a general anxiety disorder.

2. Case Description

A 23-year-old male presented to the dental unit of Sahloul Hospital in July 2019 due to the reappearance of an old swelling in his right mandible two months prior. He reported a self-resolving swelling episode that occurred one year before that. The patient was also followed in the psychiatry department for generalized anxiety disorder. No history of drug allergy was known. Extraoral physical examination revealed a swelling in the middle of the right mandible body with no associated lymphadenopathy or mouth-opening restriction.

On intraoral examination, the crown of tooth 35 was distally tipped, and a swelling was located in the low vestibule between teeth 35 and 36 (Figure 1). It extended to the jugal mucosa, measuring 0.7 cm by 0.5 cm. It was a nontender mass, hard in consistency, painful to palpation, and covered by normal oral mucosa. The cold test was positive for both 35 and 36, proving their vitality, and axial percussion test was negative for 35 and unsure concerning the first molar.

An orthopantomogram ordered in 2016 (Figure 2) revealed a well-circumscribed, unilocular radiolucent lesion with a sclerotic border between the second premolar and first molar roots, deforming and curving 35 root to the mesial side. The lesion seemed to arise from the lamina dura of 35, extending from the amelocemental junction to the apical third of the teeth along the periodontal space.

On the day of the consultation, radiovisiography (Figure 3) was performed to determine the intraosseous progression of the lesion. A bigger image presenting the same features as that found in the panoramic radiography was depicted The lesion was then approximately 0.2 cm beyond the 35 root and 0.6 cm beyond the 36 distal root. The tooth sides in contact with the lesion (mesial side of the 35 root and mesial side of the 36 mesial root) were lacking periodontal space.

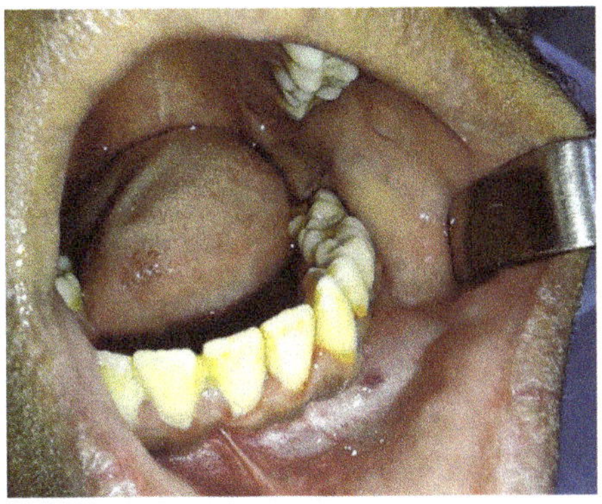

Figure 1: Aspect of the intraoral swelling.

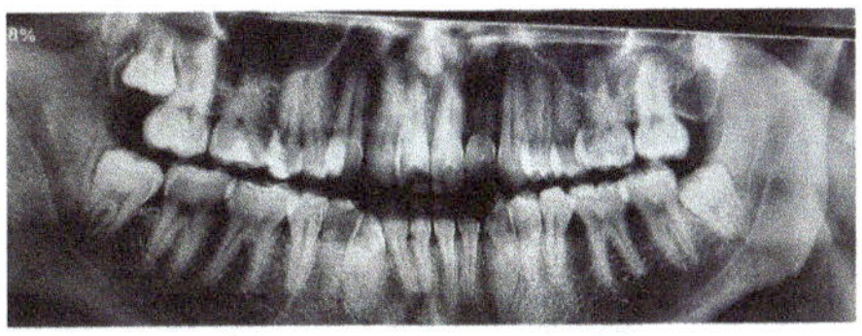

Figure 2: Panoramic radiograph from 2016 demonstrating a well-defined unilocular radiolucent lesion in the left mandible.

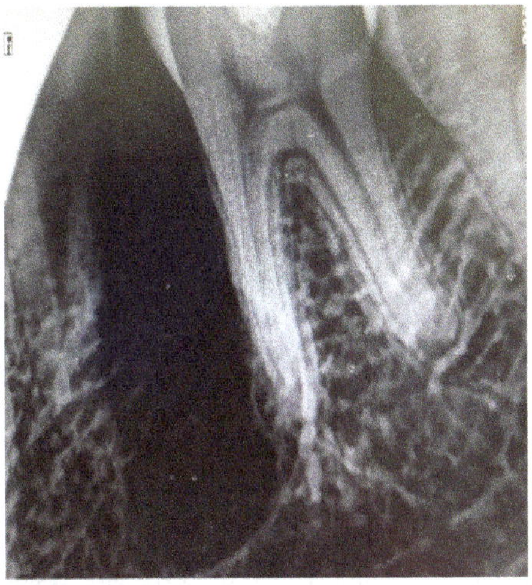

Figure 3: Radiovisiography taken the day of the consultation (2019).

Computed tomography (CT) Dentascan was prescribed and showed a cystic lesion with a radiological tissue density confined in the mandible body (Figure 4). The buccal cortical bone was partially destroyed in its middle segment and thinned out in its upper portion. Deformation of the lingual cortical plate was observed due to the lesion expansion. The cortical bone of the mandibular canal was intact. No sign of root resorption was noted, and only signs of local aggressive behavior were observed.

Considering clinical and radiological findings, a lateral periodontal cyst was strongly suspected because of the

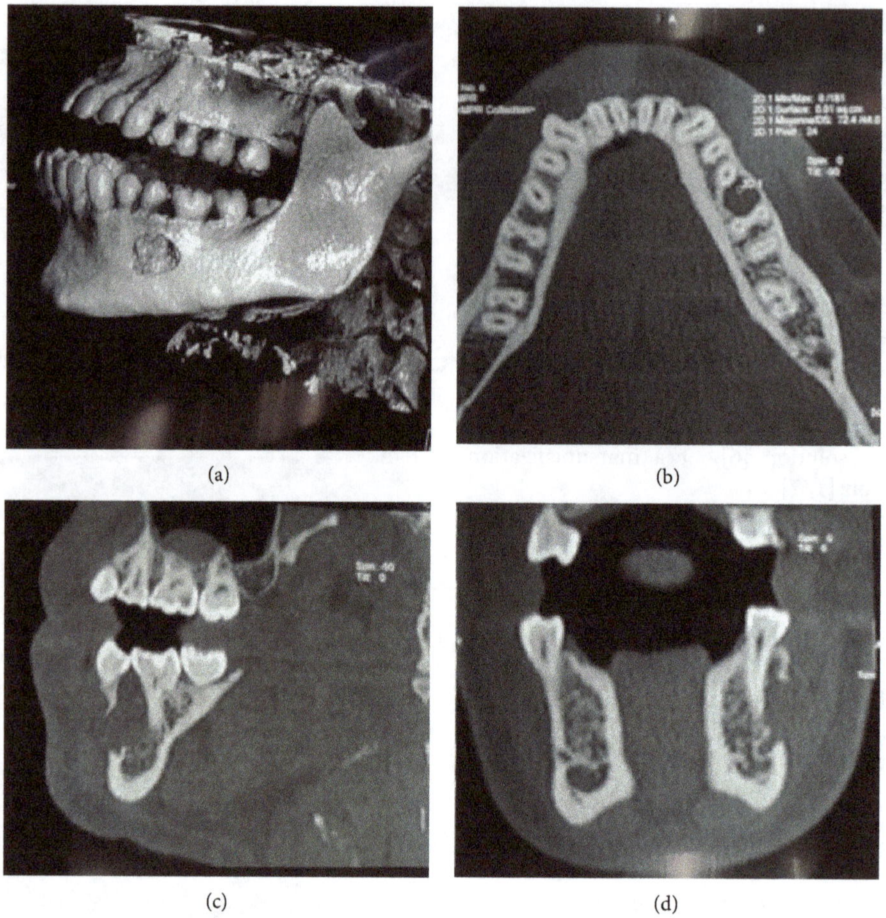

FIGURE 4: Dentascan radiography presenting the lesion on the left mandible on (a): a 3D reconstruction; (b): an axial view; (c): a sagittal view; and (d): a coronal view.

lesion's location, its small size, the vitality of 35 and 36, the lesion's radiological continuity with the 35 lamina dura, and its slow evolution since the first radiograph. Giant cell granuloma and ameloblastoma were also thought of as possible differential diagnoses because of the local aggressive features noted in the CT Dentascan.

Because of the strong suspicion of the lateral periodontal cyst, the small size of the lesion, patient's young age, and his fragile psychological health, we opted for the enucleation of the lesion. We decided not to perform a biopsy since the lesion was too small. Besides, the entire specimen will be needed later to determine all the lesion's histological aspects especially in the case of ameloblastoma.

The patient was informed about the therapeutic options available and the risks of each one. The patient himself asked for the less-traumatic treatment since he was very agitated and could not handle substantial postoperative recovery. Therefore, under local anesthesia, the enucleation of the lesion was performed. The specimen (Figure 5) had a smooth surface. A cystic fluid was present on and around the lesion, appearing more clearly on aspiration. It was removed intact and sent for an anatomical pathology exam (Figure 6). Attention was paid not to make a vigorous curettage that might facilitate recurrence in the case of ameloblastoma. Both teeth around the lesion were left intact.

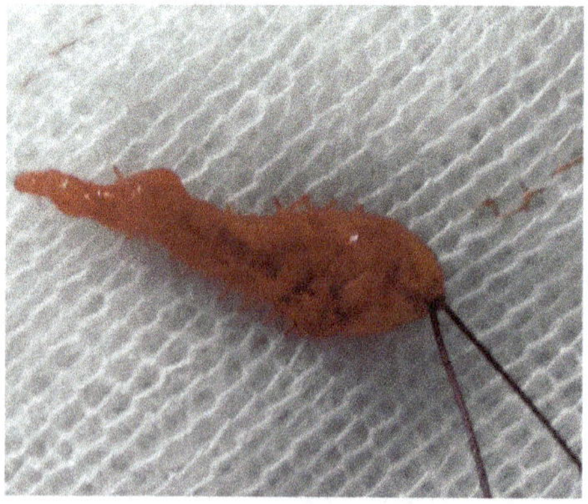

FIGURE 5: Resected specimen.

The histopathologic evaluation reported a single cystic sac with a fibrous wall and the presence of a lining epithelium showing varying thickness without cytonuclear atypia or mitosis (Figure 7). Inside the wall and the nodule associated with the cyst, ameloblastic epithelial clusters with a follicular architecture were observed without mineral deposit (Figure 8). Foci of ameloblastoma cells were noted in and outside the wall, witnessing extraluminal infiltration (Figure 9). Thus, the diagnosis of mural ameloblastoma subtype was made, contrary to the provisional diagnosis of lateral periodontal cyst.

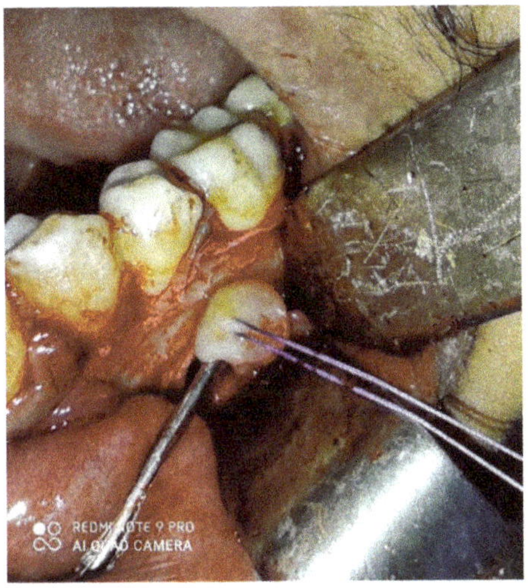

FIGURE 6: Enucleation of the lesion.

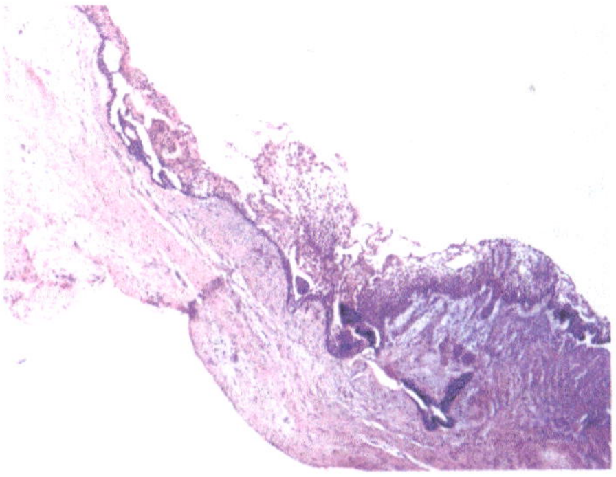

FIGURE 7: Optical microscopic picture presenting ameloblastomatous epithelium lining the cyst cavity. The specimen was stained with hematoxylin and eosin, magnified 40 times.

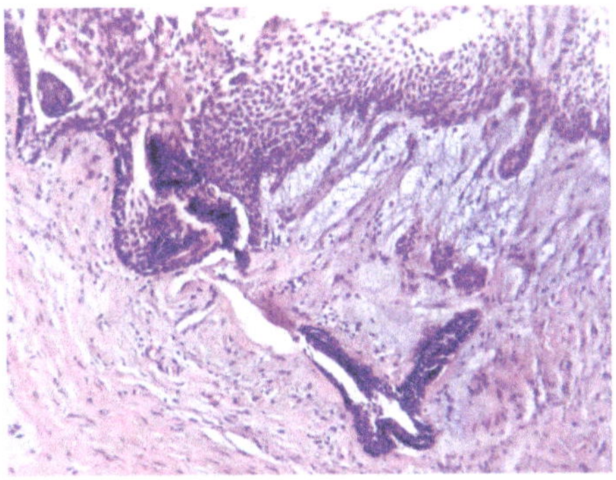

FIGURE 8: Optical microscopic picture showing the invagination of the ameloblastomatous epithelium inside the fibrous wall with the presence of clusters of ameloblast inside the wall. Stained with hematoxylin and eosin, magnified 60 times.

Two years after the enucleation procedure, the patient is still followed up in the outpatient dental clinic. Bone restoration in the affected area was radiologically observed (Figure 10), and no sign of relapse has been noted to this day.

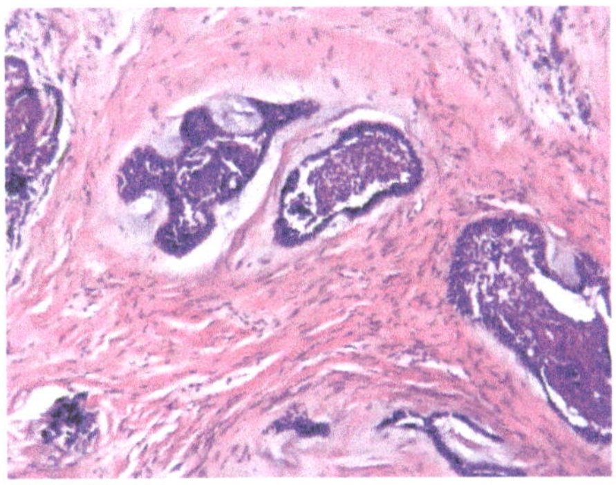

FIGURE 9: Optical microscopic picture showing infiltrating islands of ameloblast cells presenting a follicular architecture, extending into the connective tissue wall suggestive of the mural variant. Stained with hematoxylin and eosin, magnified 100 times.

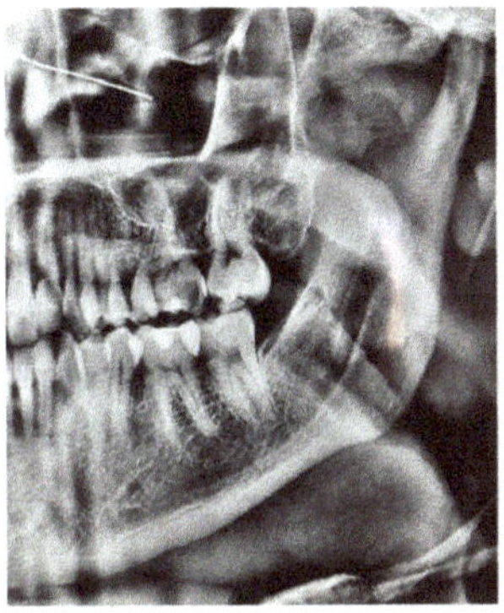

FIGURE 10: Portion of a 2021 control panoramic radiography focused on the old lesion emplacement.

3. Discussion

Unicystic ameloblastoma was first described by Robinson and Martinez in 1977 as one of the three ameloblastoma subtypes: a unique and rare de novo neoplasm. It is reported in 15% of intraosseous ameloblastoma [9]. UA is mostly observed among young patients as noted in our case report. Currently, no gender preference is reported [1, 10]. Eighty percent of the time, UA is reported to be surrounding the crown of impacted teeth [1, 11]. Because of this frequent location, its demarcated unicystic radiolucency, and its low aggressive behavior (compared to conventional ameloblastoma), UA may be mistaken with an odontogenic cyst [12].

Nevertheless, our lesion did not have the usual frequent location reported in the literature (ramus and mandible angle) [13] since it appeared between the 35 and 36 roots. None of these teeth was impacted, and the lesion had no contact with any of their crowns. On the contrary, it was lengthening in continuity with the mesial side of the 35 root and the distal side of the mesial 36 root. Concerning the two remaining root walls (distal side of the 35 root and mesial side of the distal 36 root), periodontal space was no longer radiologically noticeable since the lesion extended a few cm beyond roots' length.

In fact, the location of the lesion, its small radiologically sized aspect, and its intimate contact with the lamina dura made us primarily consider the diagnosis of a lateral periodontal cyst. Some authors reported this same UA differential diagnosis [14, 15], though none of the lesions presented were that small despite years of evolution and had that location. Actually, the intraradicular location is quite rare. Only one article reported a multilocular lesion between the 2nd and 3rd molars, although signs of radicular resorption were observed [13]. Therefore, a biopsy is paramount to elucidate the difference since the culprit lesion has a higher rate of recurrence [16]. In fact, it is only when the pathologist examines the entire specimen that the diagnosis of UA and specifically its subtype can be revealed. In this case presented, considering the small size of the lesion and the differential diagnosis considered, we did not perform a biopsy so the specimen could be removed intact (during the enucleation) and analyzed entirely.

To confirm a UA diagnosis, the minimum criterion is the presence of a single cystic sac lined by variable epithelium ranging from that with typical ameloblastic characteristics to a metaplastic epithelium consisting of nonkeratinizing squamous cell layers [17]. However, it is very important to be aware of the UA histological subtype as it determines, with the procedure, the recurrence rate of the lesion [10, 14].

Ackerman et al. assessed three UA subtypes after a clinicopathologic study of 53 cases [5]:

(i) The first one is a luminal UA: when the tumor is confined to the luminal surface of the cyst. Its recurrence rate is the lowest, ranging from 10% to 25% since the ameloblastic cells are contained and do not invade adjacent tissue

(ii) The second one is the intraluminal UA: a nodular proliferation into the lumen. No infiltration of the tumor cell into the connective tissue is observed as well. It is usually microscopically similar to conventional ameloblastoma

(iii) The third one is the mural UA with the higher recurrence rate, 50% to 80% risk. Invasive islands of ameloblastomatous epithelium in the connective tissue wall are observed, though they do not involve the entire epithelium. The infiltration can even extend beyond into the surrounding bone, hence its high recurrence rate

Later in 2003, Philipsen and Reichart described another UA grouping as follows [18]:

(i) Subgroup 1: luminal

(ii) Subgroup 1.2: luminal and intraluminal

(iii) Subgroup 1.2.3: luminal, intraluminal, and intramural

(iv) Subgroup 1.3: luminal and intramural

Treatment—whether conservative or radical—is usually controversial, as it depends on pathology results which may reveal only one of the multiple growth patterns of the lesion [1]. However, the invasive approach is mostly the chosen therapy for the highest recurrence rate groups such as the 1.2.3 and 1.3 subgroups that show intramural growths [8, 10]. Treatment consists of a segmental or marginal resection of the lesion followed by reconstructive plate adjustment or grafting (from the fibula or iliac crest) [19]. It is expected to have the lowest recurrence rate among all treatments: 3.6% if adequate bone margins are removed.

However, opting for this procedure must be well thought out and requires a balanced judgment, so its success does not lead to overtreatment [6, 20]. This option is associated with severe postoperative complications: deformity, oral dysfunctions, etc. [1, 21]. In fact, despite a successful reconstruction; removal of teeth, masticatory dysfunction, and abnormal jaw movement are common and stand against full patient recovery, especially for the fragile [6]. For instance, regarding children, Tanaka et al. demonstrated that minimal surgical treatment must be the first choice [21]. In fact, lack of mandible growth during the developmental period can cause severe facial deformation encroaching deeply on their quality of life [6, 21].

Furthermore, psychological fragility either in children or in adults is put to the test through this severe procedure [22]. Actually, regarding patients with psychological conditions, no specific recommendations were found. It is only reported that in particular cases, positive and negative outcomes must be predicted to find a balanced solution [6, 20].

In our case, our patient had a fragile psychological state as he was suffering from general anxiety disorder (GAD), a chronic disabling psychological disease, for now 10 years [23]. In fact, his condition, including his young age, the small size of the lesion, and the high possibility of a lateral periodontal cyst, was the key point to our decision. Besides, resection procedures and surgery are in general very traumatic, especially for patients with psychological conditions, requiring long and difficult convalescent periods [6]. A study tried to explore the evolution of anxiety of patients who had previous orofacial deformity after an orthognathic surgery [22]. They noticed that even when surgery improved their quality of life and their social connections, it did not change patients' personality, especially regarding anxiety traits. Furthermore, patients might experience significant depression after surgery [22]. In our case, the patient was very disturbed and anxious about his lesion and swelling.

Hence, after comparing the radiological and clinical features of the lesion (its small size, its location between premolar roots, and its continuity with the lamina dura) to the young age and psychological condition of our patient, we opted for a simple enucleation. This procedure would involve less patient morbidity, and the effect on his quality of life is minimal. In fact, literature reported as in our case that some surgeons advocate a conservative approach, especially for young patients to prevent future problems with oral functions and esthetics [1, 24].

Nevertheless, keeping in mind the possibility of an ameloblastoma, we paid attention not to realize a vigorous curettage of the bone as it might implant foci of ameloblastoma more deeply in the bone [25]. A regular follow-up was set with frequent checking appointments. Aside from enucleation, two other conservative procedures exist: marsupialization followed by enucleation and enucleation followed by the application of Carnoy's solution. Enucleation alone has, according to Lau and Sammann, the higher recurrence rate among treatments, 30.5% [20], while the use of Carnoy's solution (suggested by Stoelinga and Bronkhorst in 1988) [26] decreases the risk of recurrence after a conservative surgical treatment. In the present case, we did not use the solution after the enucleation because the lesion destroyed the cortical plate in some portions, becoming in contact with soft tissues and the alveolar vascular nervous plexus. So in this case, the use of Carnoy's solution would have mummified all the anatomical elements surrounding the lesion [27].

Concerning marsupialization, it was not an option either, because of the small size of our lesion, contrary to a 2007 case report presenting a wide lesion in the left region of the mandible managed with a marsupialization [6]. According to a systematic review of Lau and Samman, this procedure has 18% risk of recurrence [20].

Most of the time, conservative treatment is reserved for UA 1 and 1.2 subgroups since no infiltration of ameloblastoma exists beyond the lesion lumen [8]. However, to this day, no real consensus was set concerning UA treatment. No adequate evidence proves which treatment modality is the most effective. Because of the relative rarity of the tumor, a definitive conclusion to this debate is controversial and difficult to reach [6, 20].

In the end, we wanted to give our patient every chance to keep a normal life without encroaching on his already fragile psychology with a difficult procedure and postoperative convalescence. After all, considering the circumstances, the patient is out of danger and satisfied, and we still have 20% to 50% chance of total success [5]. Nevertheless, the patient was informed about the possibility of recurrence considering the true diagnosis of the lesion. After two years, no sign of relapse was observed, although, if recurrence would happen later, a radical procedure should be considered.

Acknowledgments

The authors thank the Department of Pathology of the Farhad Hached Hospital for their collaboration and support, Dr Ahmed Sami Hammami (Medical University of Monastir, Tunisia) for his support during this process, Mr. Elliott Pearl (AuthorAID in the Eastern Mediterranean) for English language proofreading, Mrs. Karen Shashok (AuthorAID in the Eastern Mediterranean) for her assistance, and the 30th American Dental Congress.

References

[1] C. C. Black, R. R. Addante, and C. A. Mohila, "Intraosseous ameloblastoma," *Oral Surgery, Oral Medicine, Oral Pathology, Oral Radiology, and Endodontics*, vol. 110, no. 5, pp. 585–592, 2010.

[2] R. S. Ramesh, S. Manjunath, T. H. Ustad, S. Pais, and K. Shivakumar, "Unicystic ameloblastoma of the mandible–an unusual case report and review of literature," *Head & Neck Oncology*, vol. 2, no. 1, p. 1, 2010.

[3] K. M. Masthan, N. Anitha, J. Krupaa, and S. Manikkam, "Ameloblastoma," *Journal of Pharmacy & Bioallied Sciences*, vol. 7, Suppl 1, pp. S167–S170, 2015.

[4] J. M. Wright and M. Vered, "Update from the 4th edition of the World Health Organization classification of head and neck tumours: odontogenic and maxillofacial bone tumors," *Head and Neck Pathology*, vol. 11, no. 1, pp. 68–77, 2017.

[5] G. L. Ackermann, M. Altini, and M. Shear, "The unicystic ameloblastoma: a clinicopathological study of 57 cases," *Journal of Oral Pathology*, vol. 17, no. 9-10, pp. 541–546, 1988.

[6] J. Kim, E. Nam, and S. Yoon, "Conservative management (marsupialization) of unicystic ameloblastoma: literature review and a case report," *Maxillofacial Plastic and Reconstructive Surgery*, vol. 39, no. 1, pp. 1–6, 2017.

[7] S. Briki, W. Elleuch, F. Karray, M. Abdelmoula, and I. Tanoubi, "Cysts and tumors of the jaws treated by marsupialization: a description of 4 clinical cases," *Journal of Clinical and Experimental Dentistry*, vol. 11, no. 6, pp. e565–e569, 2019.

[8] P. A. Reichart and H. P. Philipsen, *Odontogenic Tumors and Allied Lesions*, London: Quintessence, London, 2004.

[9] D. G. Gardner and R. L. Corio, "Plexiform unicystic ameloblastoma: a variant of ameloblastoma with a low-recurrence rate after enucleation," *Cancer*, vol. 53, no. 8, pp. 1730–1735, 1984.

[10] M.-H. Hsu, M.-L. Chiang, and J.-K. Chen, "Unicystic ameloblastoma," *Journal of Dental Sciences*, vol. 9, no. 4, pp. 407–411, 2014.

[11] Z. Agani, V. Hamiti-Krasniqi, J. Recica, M. P. Loxha, F. Kurshumliu, and A. Rexhepi, "Maxillary unicystic ameloblastoma: a case report," *BMC Research Notes*, vol. 9, no. 1, pp. 1–4, 2016.

[12] S. Ueno, S. Nakamura, K. Mushimoto, and R. Shirasu, "A clinicopathologic study of ameloblastoma," *Journal of Oral and Maxillofacial Surgery: Official Journal of the American Association of Oral and Maxillofacial Surgeons*, vol. 44, no. 5, pp. 361–365, 1986.

[13] G. Isacsson, L. Andersson, H. Forsslund, I. Bodin, and M. Thomsson, "Diagnosis and treatment of the unicystic ameloblastoma," *International Journal of Oral and Maxillofacial Surgery*, vol. 15, no. 6, pp. 759–764, 1986.

[14] Z. Chaudhary, V. Sangwan, U. S. Pal, and P. Sharma, "Unicystic ameloblastoma: a diagnostic dilemma," *National Journal of Maxillofacial Surgery*, vol. 2, no. 1, pp. 89–92, 2011.

[15] V. Savithri, M. Janardhanan, and S. Rakesh, "Unicystic ameloblastoma as a differential diagnosis for odontogenic cysts," *Oral and Maxillofacial Pathology Journal*, vol. 5, no. 1, 2014.

[16] H. Konouchi, J. Asaumi, Y. Yanagi et al., "Usefulness of contrast enhanced-MRI in the diagnosis of unicystic ameloblastoma," *Oral Oncology*, vol. 42, no. 5, pp. 481–486, 2006.

[17] A. Dunsche, O. Babendererde, J. Lüttges, and I. N. Springer, "Dentigerous cyst versus unicystic ameloblastoma–differential diagnosis in routine histology," *Journal of Oral Pathology & Medicine*, vol. 32, no. 8, pp. 486–491, 2003.

[18] J. S. Chana, Y. M. Chang, F. C. Wei et al., "Segmental mandibulectomy and immediate free fibula osteoseptocutaneous flap reconstruction with endosteal implants: an ideal treatment method for mandibular ameloblastoma," *Plastic and Reconstructive Surgery*, vol. 113, no. 1, pp. 80–87, 2004.

[19] B. Saravanakumar, J. Parthiban, V. Aarthi Nisha, T. Sarumathi, and C. A. Prakash, "Unicystic ameloblastoma of the mandible- report of two cases with review of literature," *Journal of Clinical and Diagnostic Research*, vol. 8, no. 5, pp. -Zd07–Zd09, 2014.

[20] S. L. Lau and N. Samman, "Recurrence related to treatment modalities of unicystic ameloblastoma: a systematic review," *International Journal of Oral and Maxillofacial Surgery*, vol. 35, no. 8, pp. 681–690, 2006.

[21] N. Tanaka, A. Murata, A. Yamaguchi, and G. Kohama, "Clinical features and management of oral and maxillofacial tumors in children," *Oral Surgery, Oral Medicine, Oral Pathology, Oral Radiology, and Endodontic*, vol. 88, no. 1, pp. 11–15, 1999.

[22] P. Brunault, J. Battini, C. Potard et al., "Orthognathic surgery improves quality of life and depression, but not anxiety, and patients with higher preoperative depression scores improve less," *International Journal of Oral and Maxillofacial Surgery*, vol. 45, no. 1, pp. 26–34, 2016.

[23] J. R. T. Davidson, D. E. Feltner, and A. Dugar, "Management of generalized anxiety disorder in primary care: identifying the challenges and unmet needs," *The Primary Care Companion for CNS Disorders*, vol. 12, no. 2, article 27451, 2010.

[24] S. Ueno, K. Mushimoto, and R. Shirasu, "Prognostic evaluation of ameloblastoma based on histologic and radiographic typing," *Journal of Oral and Maxillofacial Surgery: Official Journal of the American Association of Oral and Maxillofacial Surgeons*, vol. 47, no. 1, pp. 11–15, 1989.

[25] T. J. Li, M. Kitano, K. Arimura, and K. Sugihara, "Recurrence of unicystic ameloblastoma: a case report and review of the literature," *Archives of Pathology & Laboratory Medicine*, vol. 122, no. 4, pp. 371–374, 1998.

[26] P. J. Stoelinga and F. B. Bronkhorst, "The incidence, multiple presentation and recurrence of aggressive cysts of the jaws," *Journal of Cranio-Maxillofacial Surgery*, vol. 16, no. 4, pp. 184–195, 1988.

[27] S. Sivanmalai, K. Kandhasamy, N. Prabu, C. N. Prince, and C. S. Prabu, "Carnoy's solution in the mangement of odontogenic keratocyst," *Journal of Pharmacy & Bioallied Sciences*, vol. 4, no. 6, pp. 183–185, 2012.

24

Biomechanics for Orthodontic Intrusion of Severely Extruded Maxillary Molars for Functional Prosthetic Rehabilitation

Ivan Pedro Taffarel,[1,2] Thiago Martins Meira,[1,3] Lara Karolina Guimarães,[1] Oscar Mario Antelo,[1,4] and Orlando Motohiro Tanaka[1,2,5]

[1]*School of Life Sciences, Pontifícia Universidade Católica do Paraná, Curitiba, Brazil*
[2]*Brazilian Board of Orthodontics and Dentofacial Orthopedics, Brazil*
[3]*Bahia State University (UNEB), Guanambi, Bahia, Brazil*
[4]*Universidad Intercontinental, Cidade de Mexico, Mexico*
[5]*The Center for Advanced Dental Education, Saint Louis University, USA*

Correspondence should be addressed to Orlando Motohiro Tanaka; tanakaom@gmail.com

Academic Editor: Wasiu L. Adeyemo

The objective of this clinical case is thus to present a Class II, division 1, subdivision malocclusion with a severely extruded maxillary left hemiarch, which, due to the loss of mandibular teeth, makes prosthetic rehabilitation of the edentulous spaces impossible. A significant intrusion was performed with mini-implants followed by miniplates associated with fixed appliance and elastomeric chains. The results of this process showed that the biological responses of the teeth and the surrounding bony structure to the intrusion were demonstrated to be normal and acceptable. A clinically significant intrusion of the left maxillary molars, along with the recovery of the interocclusal space and the prosthetic rehabilitation, was obtained with a fixed orthodontic appliance that was associated to the biomechanics with TADs. It also allowed the obtaining of Class I canine relationship, demonstrated periodontal health and favored the prosthetic rehabilitation with good occlusion, aesthetics, and satisfactory function.

1. Introduction

Posterior teeth that are supraerupted due to the early loss of their antagonists are commonly seen in adults that have limited or no access to dentistry during childhood and adolescence [1]. An early loss of any molar is bound to cause supraeruption of the opposing molar into the available space. Overeruption of such a molar can lead to occlusal interference and functional disturbances and cause great difficulty during prosthetic reconstruction [2].

Orthodontic treatment of overerupted molars has always been considered challenging for most orthodontists, as it is one of the most difficult movements to achieve during orthodontic treatment [3]. This is primarily due to the greater root volume of these teeth [4]. Pure intrusion can only be achieved when an adequate anchorage system is available to support the light and continuous forces that are directed through the tooth's center of resistance [5].

Various approaches have been proposed to intrude overerupted molars, including the use of removable appliances with elastics [6], modified palatal arches [7], elastomeric chains [8], magnets [9], and skeletal anchorage systems [10].

Currently, temporary anchorage devices (TADs), such as mini-implants and miniplates, are the treatment of choice for enhancing orthodontic tooth movement. These devices promote absolute anchorage, and the teeth can be moved immediately after the placement, with no need for patient collaboration. TADs reduce the orthodontic treatment period, minimize the discomfort during treatment, favor aesthetics, and increase the predictability of the final result.

The purpose of this clinical report is to describe a case of Class II, division 1, subdivision malocclusion that had severe maxillary left molar extrusion, and the direct use of mini-implants and miniplate for maxillary molar intrusion was chosen to create the necessary space for prosthetic rehabilitation.

2. Case Report

2.1. Diagnosis and Etiology. The patient was a 26.2-year-old female, who had presented for an initial consultation at the orthodontic office with the chief complaint that "the top teeth have gone down."

In the extraoral examination, she presented a concave profile and an asymmetric smile. Clinically presented, she had a Class II, division 1, subdivision malocclusion (4.0 mm), overjet, moderate overbite, and an absence of the first and second mandibular molars and maxillary right first molar. With severe extrusion of the maxillary molars, more severe on the left side, the maxillary midline deviated 2.0 mm to the right, and the mandibular deviated 1.0 mm to the left. (Figures 1 and 2).

In the radiographic examination, it was verified that there was an impacted maxillary left third molar and endodontic treatment and intra-radicular metal pins in maxillary right first premolar, left maxillary first, and second molars. Both mandibular third molars were mesially tilted, and the maxillary incisor had big restorations. (Figure 3). Cephalometric radiograph presented a skeletal Class I (ANB = 2°), upright maxillary incisors and slightly proclined mandibular incisors (Table 1).

2.2. Treatment Objectives. The treatment objective of this patient was thus to correct Class II on the left side, attain an ideal overjet and overbite, correct the midline deviation, intrude maxillary posterior teeth, and recover space for prosthetic rehabilitation. This was in addition to maintaining the optimal facial balance and aesthetics.

2.3. Treatment Alternatives. Alternative treatments are as follows:

(1) Reduction of the crown height of the second right maxillary molar or an extraction of the maxillary left first, second, and third molars to create space surgically for prosthesis rehabilitation

(2) An intrusion of the maxillary molars with the fixed appliance of the maxillary molars in both sides, using TADs

(3) Intruding maxillary molars with the fixed appliance of the maxillary molars in both sides with corticotomy, removing some piece of the alveolar bone to make adequate space for prosthesis rehabilitation on the left side

(4) Surgically leveling both intruding maxillary posterior teeth

(5) Surgically leveling the intruding maxillary left posterior teeth and intruding the right maxillary molar with TADs

In the mandibular arch, the third molars were rectified by making them upright, along with prosthesis rehabilitation in both sides.

2.4. Treatment Progress. Initially, Roth .022-in × .028-in prescription brackets were bonded only to the maxillary arch (Figure 3(a)), and after starting the alignment and leveling stages with a .018-in SS archwire, four mini-implants were installed, one buccal and one palatal (Figures 4(a), 4(c), and 4(d)), with the objective of absolute anchorage for posterior tooth intrusion and Class II correction on the left side and a correction of the maxillary midline deviation.

The mini-implants on the left side as adjunctive for the intrusion also facilitated the distalization and thus corrected Class II on this side. After a year of treatment, brackets were bonded into the mandibular arch. In spite of the good evolution, there was a reduction in the vertical distance of the maxillary left posterior teeth in relation to the mini-implant, thus making it necessary to replace the buccal mini-implant with a miniplate (Figures 5(a)–5(c)).

The intrusion of both molars was achieved by using a combination of a mini-implant, TMA spring, and elastic chains. NiTi springs were also used for the anterior retraction and thus facilitated the correction of the Class II dental relation and the maxillary midline deviation (Figures 5(d)–5(f)).

The mandibular third molars were not considered as their extractions were programmed. Prior to the removal of the maxillary and mandibular fixed appliances, temporary acrylic crowns were affixed over the lower implants, to maintain the recovered vertical dimension (Figure 6).

2.5. Treatment Results. Facially, her smile became symmetrical, balanced, and harmonious (Figure 7, facial). After the correction of the Class II relationship, the maxillary midline deviation, maintenance of the overjet and overbite, and after the recovery of the prosthetic space, a new alignment and leveling, along with subsequent intercuspation and finalization phases, were performed. After the removal of the appliance, a fixed canine-to-canine retention (0.6 mm), was bonded, and a wraparound-type removable appliance were used for the full duration of a year, after which it was used for another year, but only at night during sleeping hours (Figures 7 and 8).

The panoramic radiograph shows that the maxillary left molars' alveolar bone level is in good shape, reasonable root parallelism, and implant-prosthetic rehabilitation in the mandibular arch (Figure 9). The cephalometric measurements and superimposition revealed a proclination of the maxillary incisors and the maintenance of a good profile line (Figure 9, Table 1).

The occlusal line was leveled with the isolated intrusion of maxillary right second molar and the intrusion of both left molars, combined with alveolar bone upward movement (Figure 10).

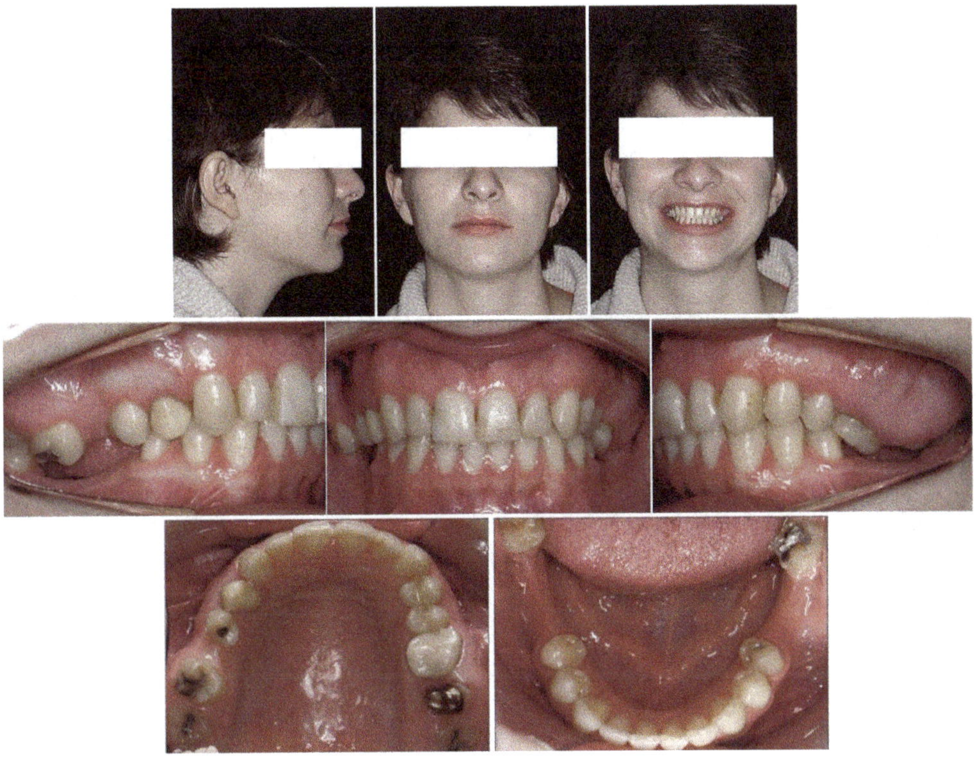

FIGURE 1: Pretreatment facial and intraoral photographs.

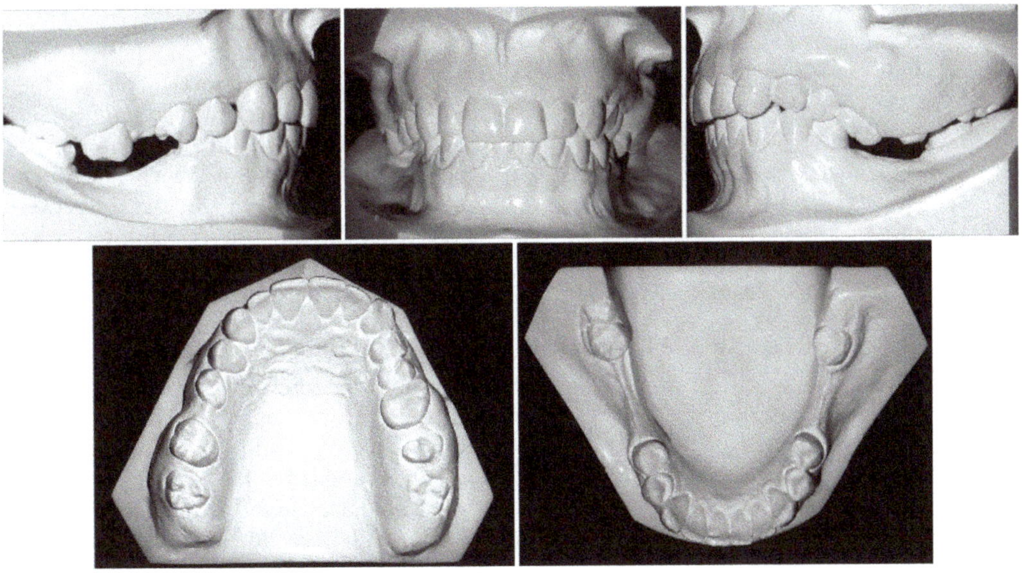

FIGURE 2: Pretreatment dental casts.

3. Discussion

This patient's treatment demonstrated the efficacy of the direct use of orthodontic mini-implants for the correction of extruded, maxillary first molars.

It is common for adult patients with dental loss, particularly of molars and premolars, to have an extrusion of the antagonist, thus rendering prosthetic rehabilitation difficult [11]. In these cases, the use of TADs along with orthodontic biomechanics is used to obtain better case control while minimizing unwanted side effects [9, 11, 12], as described in the present case report in an interdisciplinary approach.

When prosthodontic treatment of a missing molar has been delayed, the traditional treatment has been used to

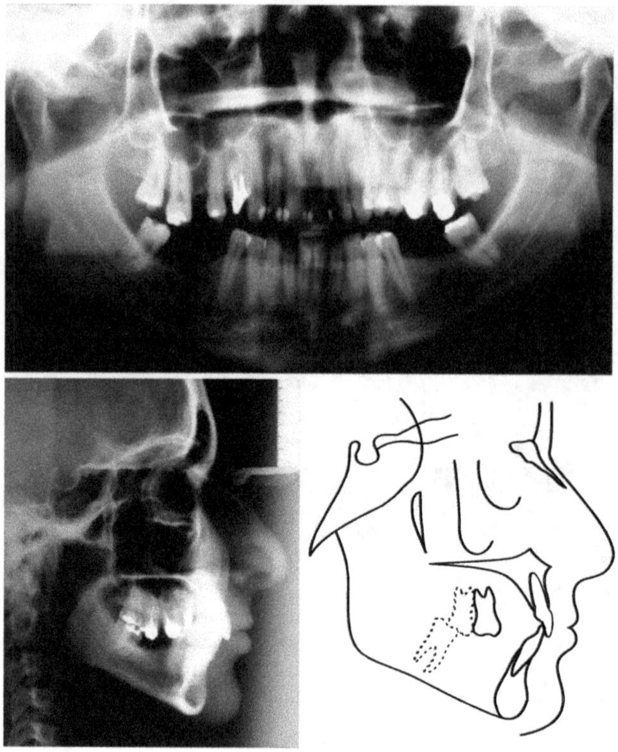

FIGURE 3: Pretreatment panoramic radiograph, lateral cephalometric radiograph, and tracing.

TABLE 1: Cephalometric measurements.

Measurements	Norms	Pretreatment	Posttreatment
SNA angle (°)	82	89	88
SNB angle (°)	80	84	85
ANB angle (°)	2	5	3
Ao-Bo (mm)	♀ 0 ± 2 ♂ 1 ± 2	-3	0
Facial angle (°)	87	87	88
Convexity (°)	0	13	88
FMA (°)	25	21	20
GoGn-SN (°)	32	27	23
Y-axis (°)	59	61	59
1-NA (mm)	4	3	7
1-NA (°)	22	13	28
1-NB (mm)	4	7	6
1-NB (°)	25	30	29
IMPA (°)	90	97	101
Interincisal angle (°)	132	134	121
Z angle (°)	75	78	77

Follow up.

reduce the crown length of the tooth opposite the extruded tooth [13], or to adjust the path of intrusion. Intrusion by subapical osteotomy [14] and extraction of the extruded molar are more aggressive alternatives, but most patients today refuse to sacrifice a healthy tooth.

Many patients often decline the latter option and would prefer a restoration of the mandibular occlusion. Depending on the patient's cooperation, the treatment would include either a shortening of the arch length or the selection of a treatment plan with extensive reduction of the supererupted maxillary molar, thus requiring endodontic treatment, periodontal surgery, and crown restoration, or even surgical impaction of the extruded teeth [4] as presented in the present clinical case.

In this reported clinical case, the first step was the use of mini-implants. Two mini-implants were installed on each side, one buccally and another palatally, to have more controlled movement and to make it less complex for the professional, with more predictable results [15]. For pure intrusion, a total of three mini-implants could be used in a tooth, in agreement with Paccini et al. [16]. Alternatively, a combination of selective alveolar corticotomies with a full-coverage splint which is modified to incorporate superelastic NiTi coil springs [1] can be viable in efficiently intruding the overerupted maxillary molars and reduce surgical risks, treatment time, and costs for both orthodontists.

To avoid root resorption, intrusive force levels should be kept optimal. While optimal force has not yet been suggested for intrusion with miniscrews, forces greater than what is generally accepted for intrusion in conventional treatments are reported to be applied with miniscrews and miniplates [17]. In the present clinical case, light forces of approximately 50 g were used in each molar, as reported by Melsen et al. [5], although some authors suggest intrusive forces of 150 g [11] and 100 g [18].

Although our clinical case has presented a good evolution with TADs, it was necessary to replace the mini-implant more cervical. However, it would imply positioning it in the alveolar mucosa, which would be contraindicated. Therefore, a miniplate was chosen for the left side, where the extrusion was larger and due to the little space between the roots of the posterior for the mini-implant, to further continue the movement of intrusion and to increase the vertical distance with the tooth antagonists.

In a finite element study, a unilateral force promoted higher stress in the root apex and higher dental tipping, and the bilateral forces promoted better distribution without evidence of dental tipping. However, the bilateral intrusion technique suggested a lower probability of root apex resorption [19], as applied in the present case.

There was no clockwise rotation of the mandible, which is a commonly seen side effect in the correction of anterior open bite. This is different from the present case report as there was an absence of teeth in the opposite arch. The periapical radiographs showed improvement in the crown-to-root ratios, no adjacent tooth extrusion, and no root resorption, which was in agreement with the results obtained by Oliveira et al. [1].

The increasing demands by adult patients for interdisciplinary dental treatment, in general, often lead to a need for methods with minimal complications, as well as rapid and comfortable solutions that require no tooth support, no aesthetic compromise, and minimal patient compliance. As such, mini-implants and miniplates have been found to be

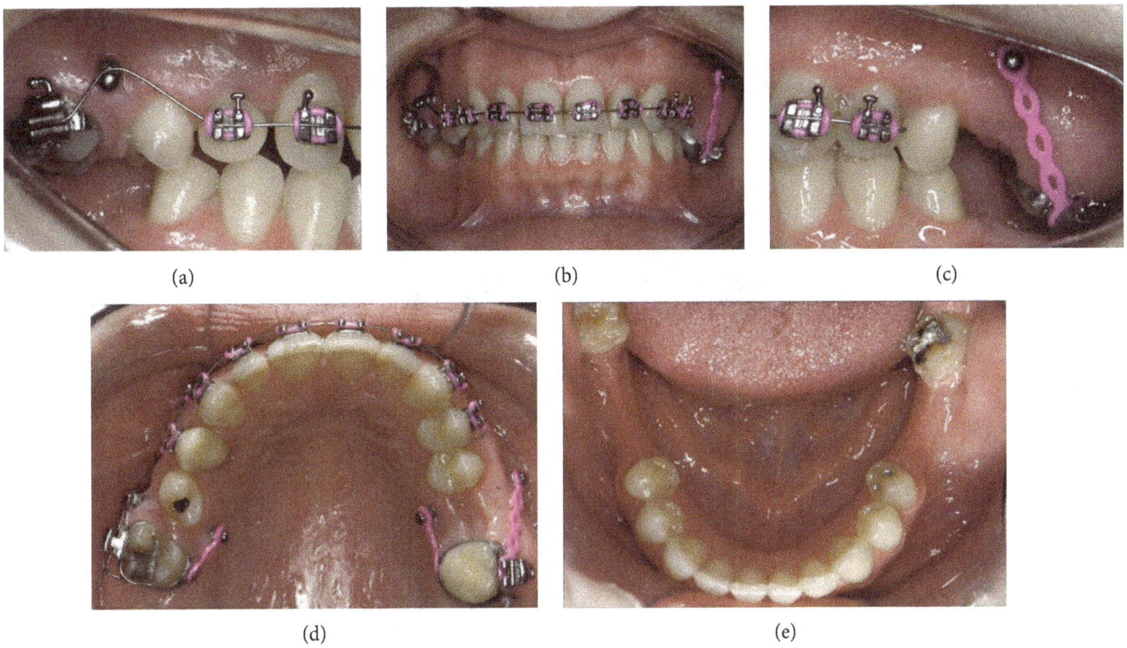

FIGURE 4: Progress starting the intrusion of maxillary left molars.

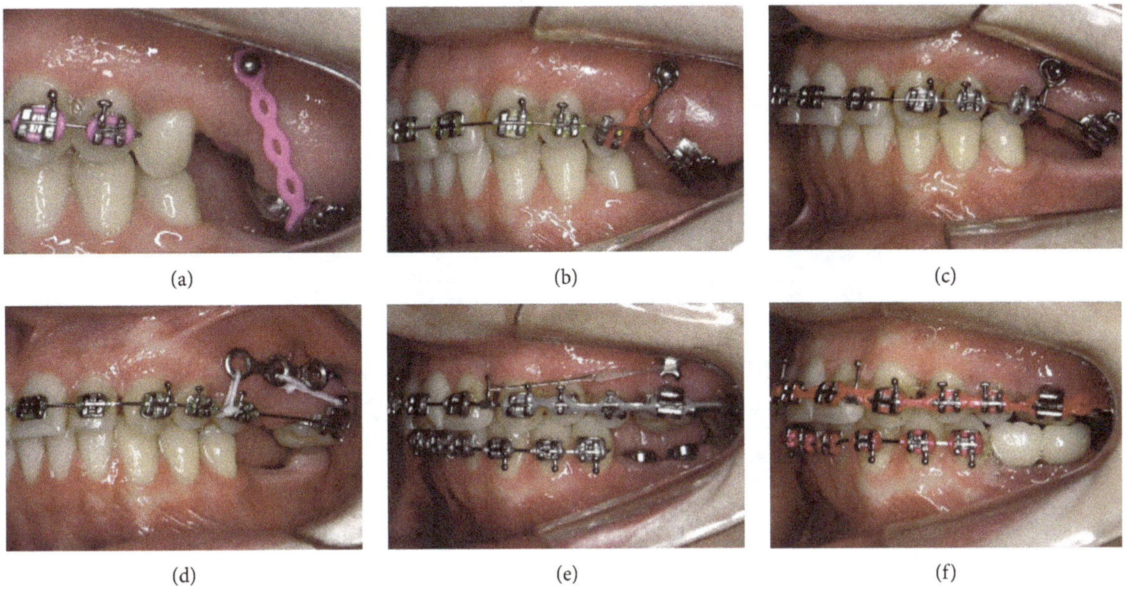

FIGURE 5: Progress sequence of the intrusion of maxillary left molars from first to finishing stages.

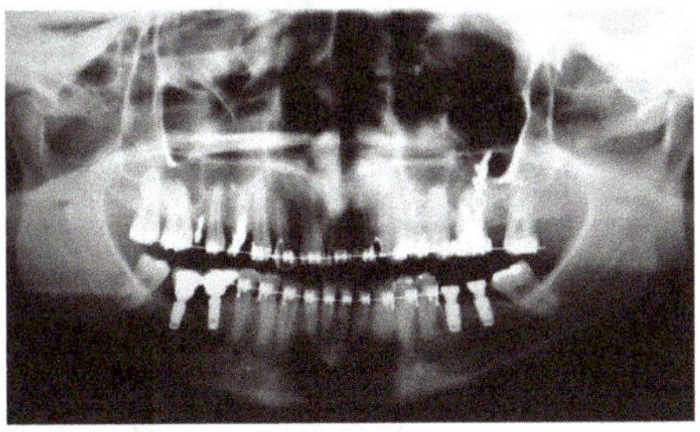

FIGURE 6: Progress panoramic radiograph.

an effective method of treatment for molar intrusion, with relatively simple installation and removal.

These devices have been used in the orthodontic office with increasing frequency, particularly in cases where an inadequate number of dental units stand in the way of an effective anchorage, or even when only used to simplify orthodontic mechanics and make it more predictable. Hence, in the present clinical case, TADs were used to make molar intrusion possible in this case, which involved extremely overerupted maxillary left molars.

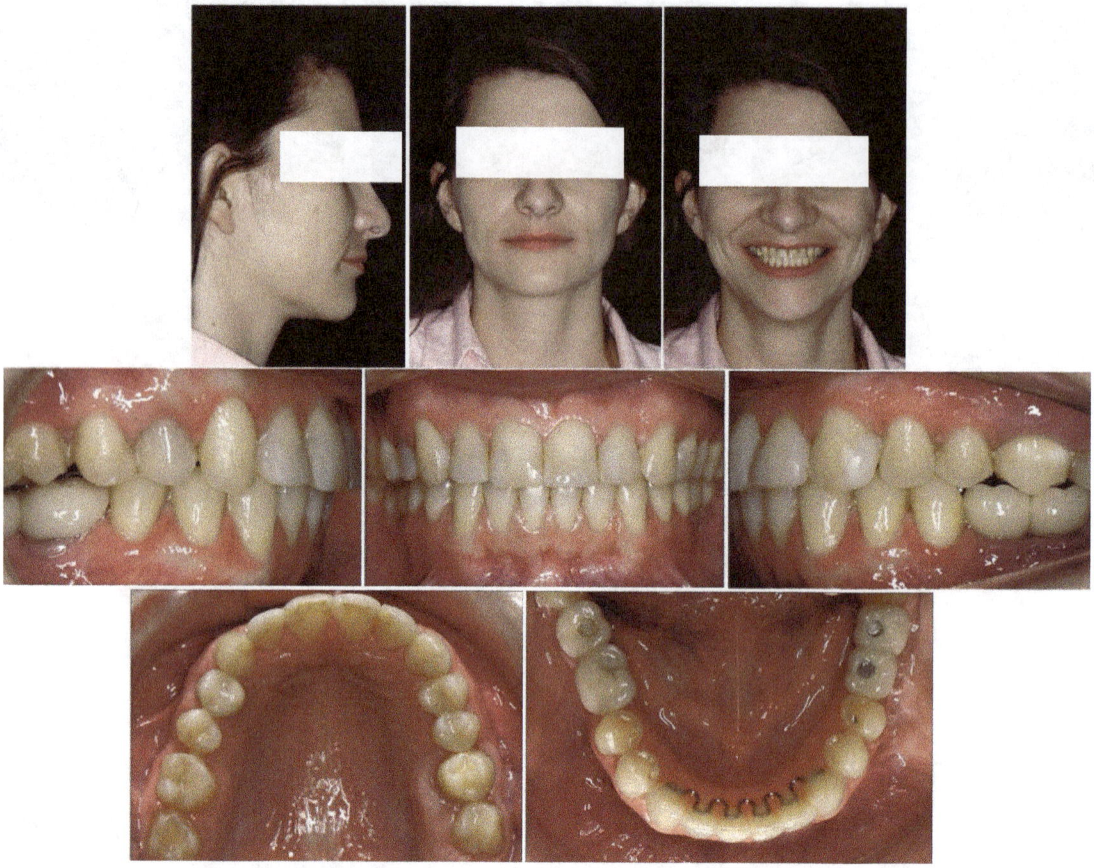

FIGURE 7: Posttreatment facial and intraoral photograph.

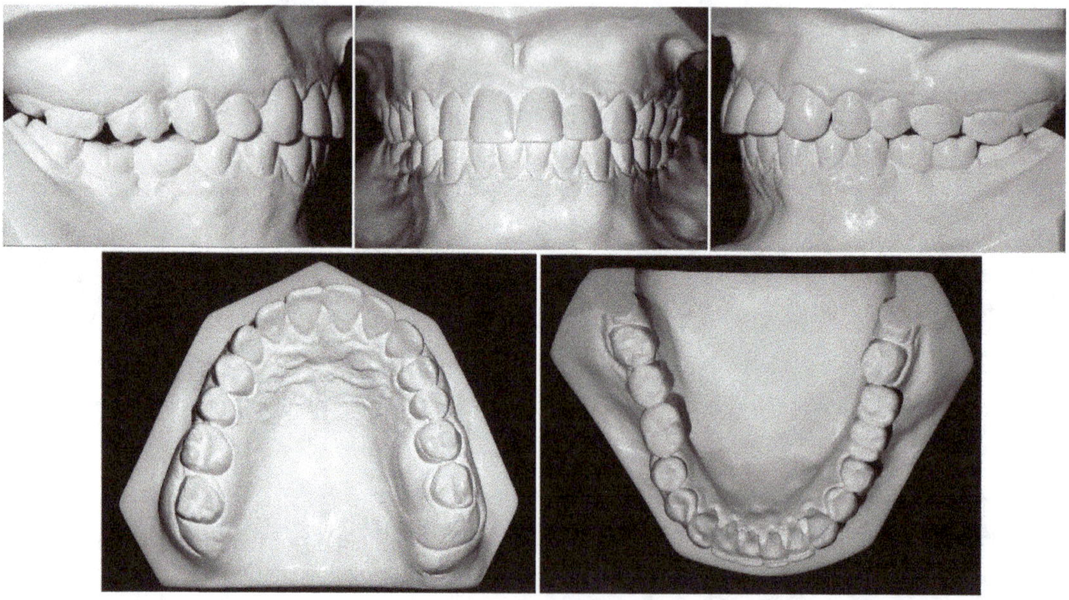

FIGURE 8: Posttreatment dental casts.

4. Conclusion

A clinically significant intrusion of the left maxillary molars, with the recovery of the interocclusal space and prosthetic rehabilitation, was obtained with the fixed orthodontic appliance associated with the biomechanics with TADs. A Class I canine relationship was also obtained, with a correction of midline deviation and a restoration of occlusion with implants, along with good occlusion, aesthetics, and satisfactory function.

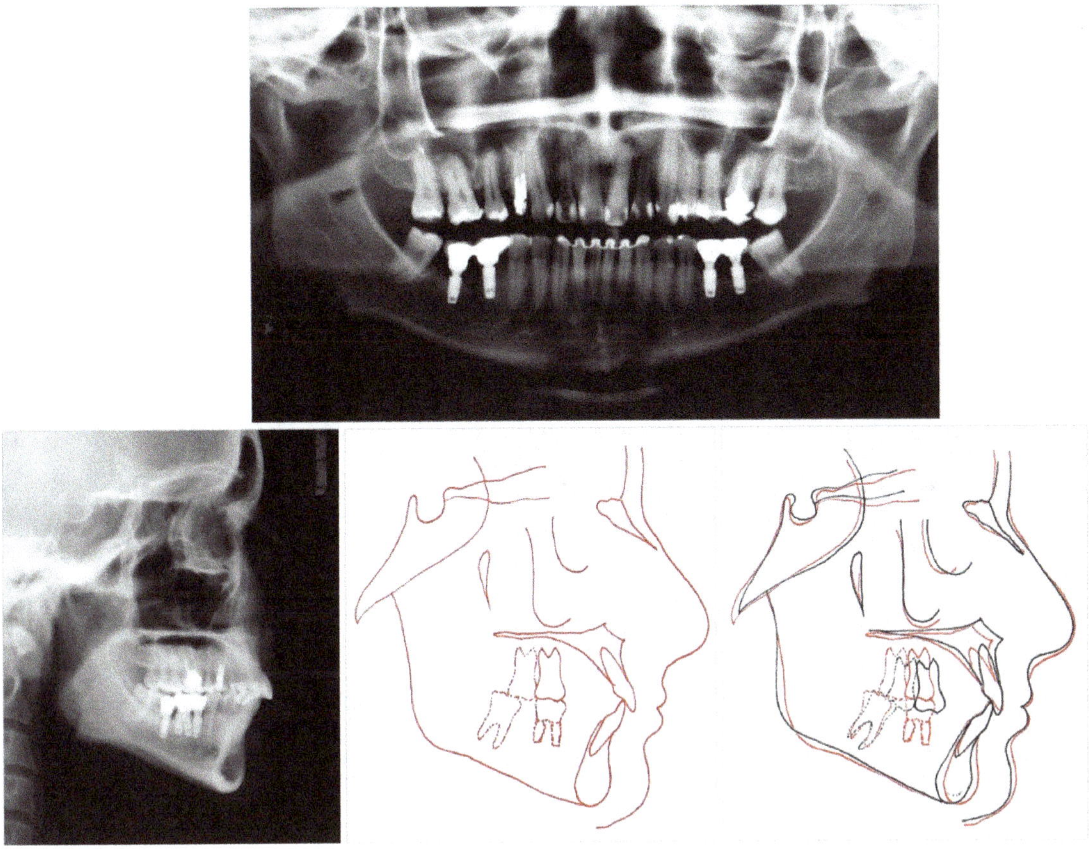

FIGURE 9: Posttreatment panoramic radiograph, lateral radiograph, lateral cephalometric radiograph tracing, and superimposition: before treatment (black) and after treatment (red).

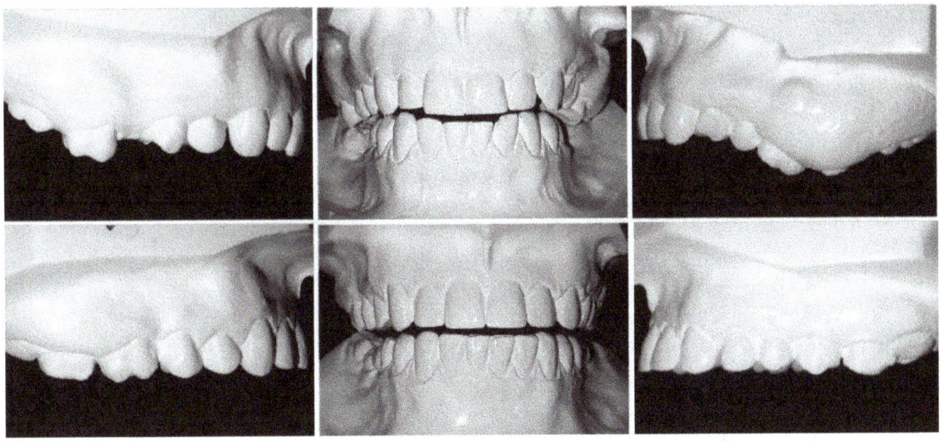

FIGURE 10: Pretreatment and posttreatment dental casts. Uneven occlusal plane.

References

[1] D. D. Oliveira, B. F. de Oliveira, H. H. de Araujo Brito, M. M. de Souza, and P. J. Medeiros, "Selective alveolar corticotomy to intrude overerupted molars," *American Journal of Orthodontics and Dentofacial Orthopedics*, vol. 133, no. 6, pp. 902–908, 2008.

[2] F. Heravi, S. Bayani, A. S. Madani, M. Radvar, and N. Anbiaee, "Intrusion of supra-erupted molars using miniscrews: clinical success and root resorption," *American Journal of Orthodontics and Dentofacial Orthopedics*, vol. 139, no. 4, article S088954061001005X, pp. S170–S175, 2011.

[3] C. J. Burstone and F. Farzin-Nia, "Production of low-friction and colored TMA by ion implantation," *Journal of Clinical Orthodontics*, vol. 29, no. 7, pp. 453–461, 1995.

[4] C. R. M. Pinzan-Vercelino, F. S. Bramante, J. de Araújo Gurgel, E. C. C. E. Vergani, and R. de Souza Gregórioc, "Intrusion of maxillary molar using mini-implants: a clinical report and follow-up at 5 years," *The Journal of Prosthetic Dentistry*, vol. 118, no. 1, article S0022391316306205, pp. 1–4, 2017.

[5] B. Melsen, N. Agerbaek, and G. Markenstam, "Intrusion of incisors in adult patients with marginal bone loss," *American Journal of Orthodontics and Dentofacial Orthopedics*, vol. 96, no. 3, pp. 232–241, 1989.

[6] G. Alessandri Bonetti and D. Giunta, "Molar intrusion with a removable appliance," *Journal of Clinical Orthodontics*, vol. 30, no. 8, pp. 434–437, 1996.

[7] A. Enacar, M. Pehlivanoglu, and C. A. Akcan, "Molar intrusion with a palatal arch," *Journal of Clinical Orthodontics*, vol. 37, no. 10, pp. 557–559, 2003.

[8] M. G. Woods and R. S. Nanda, "Intrusion of posterior teeth with magnets. An experiment in growing baboons," *The Angle Orthodontist*, vol. 58, no. 2, pp. 136–150, 1988.

[9] K. H. Sherwood, J. Burch, and W. Thompson, "Intrusion of supererupted molars with titanium miniplate anchorage," *The Angle Orthodontist*, vol. 73, no. 5, pp. 597–601, 2003.

[10] Y. C. Park, S. Y. Lee, D. H. Kim, and S. H. Jee, "Intrusion of posterior teeth using mini-screw implants," *American Journal of Orthodontics and Dentofacial Orthopedics*, vol. 123, no. 6, pp. 690–694, 2003.

[11] C. C. Yao, J. J. Lee, H. Y. Chen, Z. C. Chang, H. F. Chang, and Y. J. Chen, "Maxillary molar intrusion with fixed appliances and mini-implant anchorage studied in three dimensions," *The Angle Orthodontist*, vol. 75, no. 5, pp. 754–760, 2005.

[12] H. S. Park, B. K. Jang, and H. M. Kyung, "Maxillary molar intrusion with micro-implant anchorage (MIA)," *Australian Orthodontic Journal*, vol. 21, no. 2, pp. 129–135, 2005.

[13] L. A. Norton and I. Lopes, "Specific mechanics for abutment uprighting," *Australian Dental Journal*, vol. 25, no. 5, pp. 273–278, 1980.

[14] Y. A. Mostafa, K. M. Tawfik, and N. H. El-Mangoury, "Surgical-orthodontic treatment for overerupted maxillary molars," *Journal of Clinical Orthodontics*, vol. 19, no. 5, pp. 350-351, 1985.

[15] T. M. Araújo, R. L. Lima Filho, and A. M. Bolognese, "Skeletal anchorage with miniimplants," *Revista Dental Press Ortodontia e Ortopedia Facial*, vol. 11, pp. 126–156, 2007.

[16] J. V. Paccini, F. A. Cotrim-Ferreira, F. V. Ferreira, K. M. Freitas, R. H. Cancado, and F. P. Valarelli, "Efficiency of two protocols for maxillary molar intrusion with mini-implants," *Dental Press J Orthod*, vol. 21, no. 3, pp. 56–66, 2016.

[17] G. Han, S. Huang, J. W. Von den Hoff, X. Zeng, and A. M. Kuijpers-Jagtman, "Root resorption after orthodontic intrusion and extrusion: an intraindividual study," *The Angle Orthodontist*, vol. 75, pp. 912–918, 2005.

[18] N. D. Kravitz, B. Kusnoto, P. T. Tsay, and W. F. Hohlt, "Intrusion of overerupted upper first molar using two orthodontic miniscrews. A case report," *The Angle Orthodontist*, vol. 77, no. 5, pp. 915–922, 2007.

[19] M. M. Sugii, B. C. F. Barreto, W. Francisco Vieira-Junior, K. R. I. Simone, A. Bacchi, and R. A. Caldas, "Extruded upper first molar intrusion: comparison between unilateral and bilateral miniscrew anchorage," *Dental Press J Orthod*, vol. 23, no. 1, pp. 63–70, 2018.

25

Treatment of an Adult Skeletal Class III Patient with Surgically Assisted Rapid Palatal Expansion and Facemask

Hossein Behnia,[1] Hossein Mohammad-Rahimi,[2] and Mohammad Behnaz[3]

[1]*Department of Oral and Maxillofacial Surgery, Dental School, Shahid Beheshti University of Medical Sciences, Tehran, Iran*
[2]*Dental Research Center, Dental Research Institute, Dental School, Shahid Beheshti University of Medical Sciences, Tehran, Iran*
[3]*Department of Orthodontics, Dental School, Shahid Beheshti University of Medical Sciences, Tehran, Iran*

Correspondence should be addressed to Mohammad Behnaz; m.behnaz@sbmu.ac.ir

Academic Editor: Luis M. J. Gutierrez

This case report presents the treatment of a 21-year-old male patient with class III skeletal malocclusion, an open bite, and vertical growth pattern. He was managed with surgically assisted rapid palatal expansion (SARPE) along with an orthopedic facemask. The duration of treatment was 16 months. Significant improvement and favourable outcome were observed concerning both facial appearance and paraclinical parameters after completion of treatment.

1. Introduction

Excessive length of the mandibular body, maxillary hypoplasia, or a combination of both can lead to skeletal class III malocclusion [1, 2]. It has a reported incidence of 5% to 14% in different populations [3]. The treatment of skeletal class III malocclusion in adults is challenging for orthodontists [4]. Maxillary transverse deficiency is common in these patients, which makes their management even more difficult [5].

Various treatment options have been suggested for class III patients including dentofacial orthopedics (e.g., facemask), camouflage treatment, and orthognathic surgery [6]. However, the three-step surgical-orthodontic approach has been mentioned as the gold standard for most cases of skeletal class III malocclusion, particularly adults. This technique includes a presurgical-orthodontic phase for levelling and alignment of teeth followed by an orthognathic surgery and a postsurgical-orthodontic phase to adjust the occlusion [7, 8]. Although orthodontists conventionally and widely use this approach, it has some disadvantages: it prolongs the treatment time, orthodontic decompensation may worsen the facial profile, and it is associated with patient discomfort during the presurgical-orthodontic phase due to unideal changes in occlusion [9].

Due to the reasons above, researchers have suggested alternative treatment modalities such as the surgery-first approach [9] and application of orthopedic facemask with rapid palatal expansion (RPE) [10, 11]. In recent years, the combined use of facemask and RPE has shown favourable outcomes in class III patients especially in those with a maxillary constriction [12]. However, such studies often used nonsurgical approaches for RPE. Therefore, the outcome of this technique may not be satisfactory for adult patients [13].

We hypothesized that surgically assisted rapid palatal expansion (SARPE) along with an orthopedic facemask might lead to desirable outcomes in adult patients with skeletal class III malocclusion and maxillary constriction. This case report describes the management of an adult patient with class III skeletal malocclusion, an open bite, and vertical growth pattern.

2. Case Presentation

2.1. Diagnosis and Etiology. A 21-year-old male was referred to the Orthodontics Department of the School of Dentistry, Shahid Beheshti University of Medical Sciences, in 2016. His chief complaint was dental crowding in the maxilla and

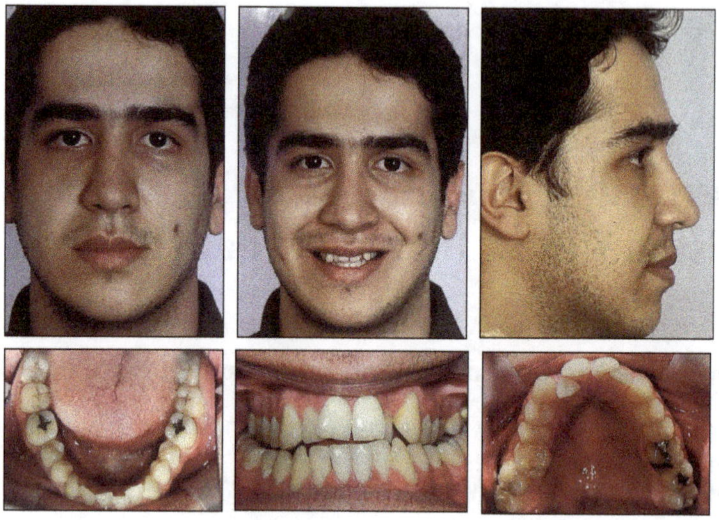

FIGURE 1: Pre-treatment facial and intraoral photographs.

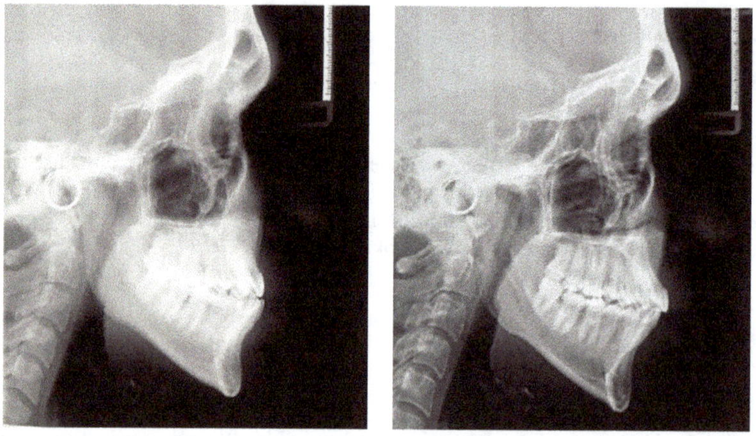

(a) (b)

FIGURE 2: Lateral cephalometry: (a) pretreatment; (b) posttreatment.

unfavourable profile view. The patient mentioned that he preferred a nonsurgical treatment approach.

Clinical examination was carried out, and a lateral cephalogram was obtained for a definite diagnosis. Moreover, a diagnostic cast was fabricated. Preoperative photography is presented in Figure 1.

The lateral cephalometric measurements indicated skeletal class III malocclusion pattern (ANB: -5.0°, Wits appraisal: 7.2 mm, SNA: 77.7°, SNB: 78.3°) with a vertical growth pattern (SN-MP: 42.4° and S-Go/N-Me: 57.7%). The inclination of the maxillary incisors was close to normal range (U1-SN: 99.3°); however, the mandibular incisors were retroclined because of dentoalveolar compensation (IMPA: 85.9°). The patient had a slightly obtuse nasolabial angle (103.2°), and his lower lip was protrusive relative to the E line (0.4 mm) (Figure 2(a)).

Based on clinical and radiographic examinations, the patient was diagnosed with class III skeletal malocclusion with an open bite tendency and edge-to-edge incisor relationship. The patient had maxillary constriction, which led to posterior crossbite. Dental crowding of the maxilla was also observed. Moreover, the patient had a concave profile.

The etiology of his condition was found to be hereditary. Tooth size-arch length discrepancy was also present due to maxillary constriction.

2.2. Treatment Objectives. Based on the diagnosis and etiologies, the treatment objectives were set as follows: (i) skeletal expansion of the maxilla, (ii) forward movement of the maxilla, (iii) correction of posterior crossbite, (iv) protrusion of the maxillary anterior teeth, (v) correction of dental crowding in the maxilla, (vi) establishing Angle's class I occlusion, (vii) correction of overjet and overbite, (viii) achieving a stable occlusal relationship, and (ix) achieving satisfying facial esthetics.

2.3. Treatment Alternatives. Orthognathic surgery (Le Fort I) and anterior repositioning of the maxilla is the conventional treatment for adult patients with skeletal class III malocclusion due to maxillary retrognathism. In patients with skeletal

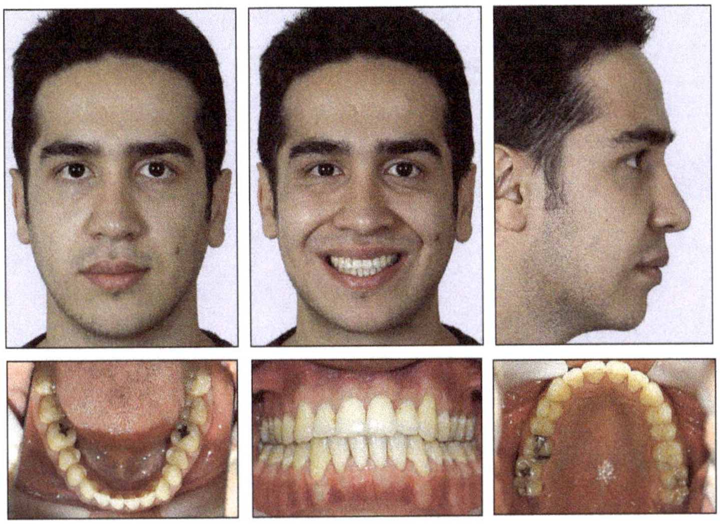

FIGURE 3: Posttreatment facial and intraoral photographs.

maxillary constriction, SARPE is also required in addition to Le Fort I surgery; thus, these patients need a two-step surgical procedure, which is more complex and may be associated with more complications.

Facemask has been suggested as an alternative approach to decrease the number of surgical procedures required. However, application of this approach often fails in achieving the desired outcome.

2.4. Treatment Progress. Due to the patient's preference, a nonsurgical approach for camouflage therapy was first started. We started RPE using a hyrax device. After four months, we decided to stop the treatment following the observation of flaring of the posterior teeth and gingival recession.

Considering the skeletal constriction of the maxilla, SARPE was considered for the patient. Initially, we waited for two months for the previous treatment outcomes to relapse. Next, full banding and bonding of the maxillary teeth were performed to correct the alignment of the maxillary teeth. Also, space was created between the maxillary central incisors, especially in the root area. This space helped to protect and preserve the roots of the incisor teeth during the surgical incision in the midpalatal region for SARPE. To create this space, a spring was placed between the central incisors. This treatment was started nine months before the surgical procedure.

After achieving the desired outcomes by fixed orthodontic treatment, SARPE was performed. Briefly, following the induction of general anesthesia, an osteotomy was done in the midpalatal region. Then, the intermaxillary suture was cut. Downfracture of the maxilla was not performed during the surgery.

Following the surgical procedure, a previously fabricated hyrax device was used for palatal expansion as a tooth-borne appliance. The active expansion continued for 12 days (twice a day). After this period, 6 mm space was achieved between the maxillary central incisors, which was desirable. The device remained in the mouth for the retention period of about four months.

A facemask was used to treat the maxillary deficiency in the sagittal plane. The facemask was connected to the hooks embedded in the hyrax device using elastics. The duration of the active phase of treatment by the facemask was three months.

Finally, occlusal settling and final detailing of dentition were performed by fixed orthodontics and intermaxillary elastics. Orthodontic treatment was accomplished about one year after surgery.

2.5. Treatment Results. The treatment outcome was desirable. Skeletal relationships were appropriate. An ideal occlusal relationship was achieved. Dental crowding and posterior crossbite were corrected. No gingival recession was observed after treatment. Postoperative photography is presented in Figure 3.

Lateral cephalometric analysis showed skeletal improvement (ANB: 2.0°, Wits appraisal: 0.6 mm, SNA: 79.7°, SNB: 77.3°). SN-MP decreased from 42.4° to 39.0°, which led to less hyperdivergent growth pattern when compared to the pretreatment facial status. Moreover, as a result of treatment, the maxillary incisors were proclined (U1-SN: 107.6°) to make room for the posterior teeth. Also, the mandibular incisors were uprighted from IMPA 85.9° to IMPA 90.3° (Figure 2(b)). Detailed information of pre- and posttreatment lateral cephalometric analysis is available in Table 1.

3. Discussion

The management of adult patients with maxillary deficiency in addition to class III skeletal malocclusion is complicated [5]. The aim of this study was to propose a new approach for the treatment of such patients in case of failure of camouflage therapy without performing the two-step surgical procedure. The present case report showed successful management of a 21-year-old patient with class III skeletal malocclusion using a combination of SARPE and facemask, which led to a desirable outcome.

Table 1: Cephalometric measurements.

	Pretreatment	Posttreatment	Norm ± SD
Skeletal (vertical analysis)			
FH-SN (°)	6.4	4.0	6.0 ± 4.0
MP-SN (°)	42.4	39.0	33.0 ± 6.0
Sum of angles (Jarabak) (°)	402.4	399.0	380.0 ± 6.0
S-Go/N-Me (%)	57.7	624	65.0 ± 4.0
Skeletal (sagittal analysis)			
SNA (°)	77.7	79.3	82.0 ± 3.5
SNB (°)	78.3	77.3	80.9 ± 3.4
ANB (°)	-0.6	2.0	1.6 ± 1.5
Wits appraisal (°)	-5.0	0.6	−1.0 ± 1.0
Dental			
U1-SN (°)	99.3	107.6	103.1 ± 5.5
IMPA (°)	85.9	90.3	95.0 ± 7.0
Interincisal angle (U1-L1) (°)	132.4	123.0	130.0 ± 6.0
U1-NA (mm)	5.8	7.4	4.3 ± 2.7
L1-NB (mm)	5.8	7.9	4.0 ± 1.8
Soft tissue			
Upper lip to E-plane (mm)	-4.4	-2.3	−8.0 ± 2.0
Lower lip to E-plane (mm)	0.4	-0.1	−2.0 ± 2.0
Nasolabial angle (Col-Sn-UL) (°)	103.3	91.1	102.0 ± 8.0

FH-SN: angle between Frankfurt horizontal line and sella-nasion plane; MP-SN: angle mandibular plane (MP) and sella-nasion plane; S-Go/N-Me: the ratio of length sella-gonion to nasion-menton; SNA: sella-nasion-A point; SNB: sella-nasion-B point; ANB: A point-nasion-B point; U1-SN: upper incisor to sella-nasion plane angle; IMPA: lower incisor to MP angle; interincisal angle: angle between the mandibular and maxillary incisors; U1-NA: distance from upper incisor to NA line; L1-NA: distance from lower incisor to NA line.

The treatment of choice for management of adult patients with skeletal class III malocclusion may include camouflage orthodontic treatment or orthognathic surgery. Camouflage therapy is the treatment of choice for nongrowing adult patients with mild or moderate class III skeletal malocclusion and favourable facial status. However, if patients have severe class III skeletal malocclusion, orthognathic surgery may be preferred [14, 15]. A favourable outcome can be expected by accurate diagnosis, proper case selection, and efficient treatment planning.

In the present case report, we first initiated the camouflage therapy. However, following the occurrence of flaring of the posterior teeth and gingival recession, we decided to change the treatment plan. According to the literature, in case of deterioration of periodontal status as a result of camouflage orthodontic treatment, the orthognathic surgical approach should be preferably adopted [16]. The occurrence of gingival recession in camouflage therapy is believed to be related to the patient's periodontal biotype. Moreover, the movement of mandibular incisors is limited in patients with thin alveolar bone due to the risk of dehiscence [17].

As mentioned earlier, the conventional orthognathic surgery for skeletal class III malocclusion patients is composed of a three-step surgical-orthodontic approach including preoperative orthodontics, orthognathic surgery, and postoperative orthodontic treatment [7]. Various problems have been reported for this approach. The long duration of orthodontic treatment especially in the presurgical phase may discourage the patients and negatively affect their compliance [18]. Dowling et al. reported that the length of conventional surgical-orthodontic treatment is about 22 months and includes 16 months of presurgical-orthodontic treatment and six months of postsurgical-orthodontic treatment [19]. However, these time periods may vary depending on the operator's skills [20]. Some other disadvantages have also been reported for this approach including the gingival recession, root resorption, and worsened facial esthetics, which may occur during the presurgical-orthodontic phase [18, 21]. To prevent them, researchers have suggested a two-step orthognathic surgical approach that does not require preoperative orthodontics [18, 22–24]. This new approach has a significantly shorter treatment period [22], which in addition to immediate improvement of facial esthetics [25, 26] often results in higher patient satisfaction and their improved cooperation.

Despite these advantages, we did not perform orthognathic surgery. In orthognathic surgery of patients with skeletal class III malocclusion, researchers recommend the bimaxillary osteotomy procedures, which include Le Fort I and bilateral sagittal split osteotomy [27]. The orthognathic surgery itself has various complications such as paresthesia, hematoma, and infection. Furthermore, only a few patients are willing to undergo orthognathic surgery [28].

We selected a three-step approach for our adult patient, which included an initial orthodontic treatment, SARPE, and facemask therapy. This approach yielded favourable results regarding facial esthetics, occlusal relationships, and cephalometric measurements. The maxillary expansion procedures can help in achieving better outcomes in the treatment of patients with skeletal class III malocclusion. Furthermore, they increase the final stability of orthodontic treatment by providing appropriate overjet for the buccal segments [29, 30].

After SARPE, we used a facemask for protraction of the maxillary segment by applying elastic forces to the hyrax. Similar to our study, it has been reported that maxillary expansion besides the application of facemask will lead to favourable outcomes in class III patients. This approach has both skeletal and dental effects on the patient's occlusion [6, 16, 31, 32].

Unlike the aforementioned studies that adopted a nonsurgical approach for maxillary expansion, we used SARPE for our patient. This surgical approach is the recommended procedure for adult patients with maxillary constriction, who have passed their growth spurt [33, 34]. Timms and Vero [35] suggested that the best time for SARPE is between 25 and 30 years of age. However, it should be noted that skeletal maturation is more important than the chronological age of the patient.

The results of the present study showed that in an adult patient with skeletal class III malocclusion and maxillary constriction, successful treatment outcomes can be achieved by a combination of SARPE and application of facemask. However, clinical trials are required to assess the efficacy of this treatment approach further.

References

[1] J. Delaire, "Maxillary development revisited: relevance to the orthopaedic treatment of Class III malocclusions," *European Journal of Orthodontics*, vol. 19, no. 3, pp. 289–311, 1997.

[2] M. Tabuchi, H. Fukuoka, K. Miyazawa, and S. Goto, "Skeletal class III malocclusion with unilateral congenitally missing maxillary incisor treated by maxillary protractor and edgewise appliances," *The Angle Orthodontist*, vol. 80, no. 2, pp. 405–418, 2010.

[3] W. Liu, P. Sun, C. Xin, Y. Du, and B. Ding, "Effects of maxillary protraction therapy on facial soft tissue in patients with skeletal class III malocclusion," *Biomedical Research*, vol. 28, no. 22, 2018.

[4] J.-H. Kim, M. A. G. Viana, T. M. Graber, F. F. Omerza, and E. A. BeGole, "The effectiveness of protraction face mask therapy: a meta-analysis," *American Journal of Orthodontics and Dentofacial Orthopedics*, vol. 115, no. 6, pp. 675–685, 1999.

[5] J. H. Park, J. Yu, and J.-M. Chae, "Lateral open bite and crossbite correction in a class III patient with missing maxillary first premolars," *American Journal of Orthodontics and Dentofacial Orthopedics*, vol. 152, no. 1, pp. 116–125, 2017.

[6] A. Abraham, E. Peter, K. Philip, J. George, and R. Sreevatsan, "Early management of class III malocclusion with bonded maxillary expansion and facemask therapy-a case report," *International Dental Journal of Student Research*, vol. 4, no. 4, pp. 202–206, 2016.

[7] W. Proffit and J. Miguel, "The duration and sequencing of surgical-orthodontic treatment," *The International journal of adult orthodontics and orthognathic surgery*, vol. 10, no. 1, pp. 35–42, 1995.

[8] W. R. Proffit and R. P. White Jr., "Development of surgeon-orthodontist interaction in orthognathic surgery," *Seminars in Orthodontics*, vol. 17, no. 3, pp. 183–185, 2011.

[9] P. Brachvogel, J. Berten, and J. Hausamen, "Surgery before orthodontic treatment: a concept for timing the combined therapy of skeletal dysgnathias," *Deutsche Zahn-, Mund-, und Kieferheilkunde mit Zentralblatt*, vol. 79, no. 7, pp. 557–563, 1991.

[10] T. Baccetti, J. S. McGill, L. Franchi, J. A. McNamara Jr., and I. Tollaro, "Skeletal effects of early treatment of class III malocclusion with maxillary expansion and face-mask therapy," *American Journal of Orthodontics and Dentofacial Orthopedics*, vol. 113, no. 3, pp. 333–343, 1998.

[11] S. W. Smith and J. D. English, "Orthodontic correction of a class III malocclusion in an adolescent patient with a bonded RPE and protraction face mask," *American Journal of Orthodontics and Dentofacial Orthopedics*, vol. 116, no. 2, pp. 177–183, 1999.

[12] K.-S. Cha, "Skeletal changes of maxillary protraction in patients exhibiting skeletal class III malocclusion: a comparison of three skeletal maturation groups," *The Angle Orthodontist*, vol. 73, no. 1, pp. 26–35, 2003.

[13] T. Baccetti, L. Franchi, and J. A. McNamara Jr., "Cephalometric variables predicting the long-term success or failure of combined rapid maxillary expansion and facial mask therapy," *American Journal of Orthodontics and Dentofacial Orthopedics*, vol. 126, no. 1, pp. 16–22, 2004.

[14] J. Lin and Y. Gu, "Preliminary investigation of nonsurgical treatment of severe skeletal class III malocclusion in the permanent dentition," *The Angle Orthodontist*, vol. 73, no. 4, pp. 401–410, 2003.

[15] H.-S. Baik, H.-K. Han, D.-J. Kim, and W. R. Proffit, "Cephalometric characteristics of Korean class III surgical patients and their relationship to plans for surgical treatment," *The International Journal of Adult Orthodontics and Orthognathic Surgery*, vol. 15, no. 2, pp. 119–128, 2000.

[16] P. Liu, H. Chen, X. Shi, and J. Guo, "Conservative treatment of a young adult patient with a moderate skeletal class III malocclusion by applying the temporary anchorage devices and the surgically assisted rapid palatal expansion," *Clinical Case Reports*, vol. 5, no. 12, pp. 2003–2011, 2017.

[17] H.-P. Müller and T. Eger, "Masticatory mucosa and periodontal phenotype: a review," *International Journal of Periodontics & Restorative Dentistry*, vol. 22, no. 2, 2002.

[18] Y. K. Lian, A. M. C. Hsieh, M. S. Tsai et al., "Treatment efficiency and stability of skeletal class III malocclusion with a surgery-first approach," *Orthodontics & Craniofacial Research*, vol. 21, no. 2, pp. 90–95, 2018.

[19] P. Dowling, L. Espeland, O. Krogstad, A. Stenvik, and A. Kelly, "Duration of orthodontic treatment involving orthognathic surgery," *The International Journal of Adult Orthodontics and Orthognathic Surgery*, vol. 14, no. 2, pp. 146–152, 1999.

[20] D. Mavreas and A. E. Athanasiou, "Factors affecting the duration of orthodontic treatment: a systematic review," *European Journal of Orthodontics*, vol. 30, no. 4, pp. 386–395, 2008.

[21] R. Koole and P. Egyedi, "The case for postoperative orthodontics in orthognathic surgery," *Journal of Cranio-Maxillofacial Surgery*, vol. 18, no. 7, pp. 293–296, 1990.

[22] H.-S. Hwang, M.-H. Oh, H.-K. Oh, and H. Oh, "Surgery-first approach in correcting skeletal class III malocclusion with mandibular asymmetry," *American Journal of Orthodontics and Dentofacial Orthopedics*, vol. 152, no. 2, pp. 255–267, 2017.

[23] S.-H. Baek, H.-W. Ahn, Y.-H. Kwon, and J.-Y. Choi, "Surgery-first approach in skeletal class III malocclusion treated with 2-jaw surgery: evaluation of surgical movement and postoperative orthodontic treatment," *Journal of Craniofacial Surgery*, vol. 21, no. 2, pp. 332–338, 2010.

[24] K. J. Hong and J. G. Lee, "2 phase treatment without preoperative orthodontics in skeletal class III malocclusion," *Journal of the Korean Association of Oral and Maxillofacial Surgeons*, vol. 25, no. 1, pp. 48–53, 1999.

[25] E. J. W. Liou, P. H. Chen, Y. C. Wang, C. C. Yu, C. S. Huang, and Y. R. Chen, "Surgery-first accelerated orthognathic surgery: postoperative rapid orthodontic tooth movement," *Journal of Oral and Maxillofacial Surgery*, vol. 69, no. 3, pp. 781–785, 2011.

[26] F. Hernández-Alfaro, R. Guijarro-Martínez, A. Molina-Coral, and C. Badía-Escriche, ""Surgery First" in Bimaxillary Orthognathic Surgery," *Journal of Oral and Maxillofacial Surgery*, vol. 69, no. 6, pp. e201–e207, 2011.

[27] G. Iannetti, M. T. Fadda, T. M. Marianetti, V. Terenzi, and A. Cassoni, "Long-term skeletal stability after surgical correction in class III open-bite patients," *Journal of Craniofacial Surgery*, vol. 18, no. 2, pp. 350–354, 2007.

[28] C. S. Sousa and R. N. T. Turrini, "Complications in orthognathic surgery: a comprehensive review," *Journal of Oral and Maxillofacial Surgery, Medicine, and Pathology*, vol. 24, no. 2, pp. 67–74, 2012.

[29] J. A. McNamara Jr., "An orthopedic approach to the treatment of class III malocclusion in young patients," *Journal of clinical orthodontics: JCO*, vol. 21, no. 9, pp. 598–608, 1987.

[30] M. D. Adkins, R. S. Nanda, and G. F. Currier, "Arch perimeter changes on rapid palatal expansion," *American Journal of Orthodontics and Dentofacial Orthopedics*, vol. 97, no. 3, pp. 194–199, 1990.

[31] M. Saadia and E. Torres, "Sagittal changes after maxillary protraction with expansion in class III patients in the primary, mixed, and late mixed dentitions: a longitudinal retrospective study," *American Journal of Orthodontics and Dentofacial Orthopedics*, vol. 117, no. 6, pp. 669–680, 2000.

[32] R. Lione, L. T. Huanca Ghislanzoni, E. Defraia, L. Franchi, and P. Cozza, "Bonded versus banded rapid palatal expander followed by facial mask therapy: analysis on digital dental casts," *European Journal of Orthodontics*, vol. 38, no. 2, pp. 217–222, 2016.

[33] J. A. Lehman Jr. and A. J. Haas, "Surgical-orthodontic correction of transverse maxillary deficiency," *Clinics in Plastic Surgery*, vol. 16, no. 4, pp. 749–755, 1989.

[34] R. A. Bays and J. M. Greco, "Surgically assisted rapid palatal expansion: an outpatient technique with long-term stability," *Journal of Oral and Maxillofacial Surgery*, vol. 50, no. 2, pp. 110–113, 1992.

[35] D. J. Timms and D. Vero, "The relationship of rapid maxillary expansion to surgery with special reference to midpalatal synostosis," *British Journal of Oral Surgery*, vol. 19, no. 3, pp. 180–196, 1981.

26

Recovering of Dizziness of a Patient with Sinusitis after Root Canal Therapy for Upper Second Molar

Ibrahem Amro,[1] **Lyana Shawar**,[1] **Raed abu Hantash**,[2] **Basem Abuquba**,[2] **and Akram Amro**[2]

[1]*Lebanon Dental Clinic, State of Palestine*
[2]*Al-Quds University, State of Palestine*

Correspondence should be addressed to Lyana Shawar; lyan.shwr@gmail.com

Academic Editor: Jose López-López

This case report illustrates the recovery of dizziness of a young healthy patient after root canal therapy of upper second molar. The patient developed dizziness and unbalanced walking four months ago. After cardiac, ENT, neurological, physiotherapy and medical investigations, his entire checkup showed no abnormalities. The patient visited a dental clinic for a routine checkup; after dental clinical and radiographical examination, a chronic abscess infection in an upper second molar region close to the sinus was diagnosed. Root canal therapy was performed that resulted in a disappearance of the dizziness and full recovery was achieved. *Conclusion.* Infected upper teeth with periapical lesion are associated with dizziness as a complication of odontogenic-related sinusitis. Dental and medical cooperation contributes to a better management diagnosis of the dizziness.

1. Introduction

Dizziness is the sensation of disturbed or impaired spatial orientation without a false or distorted sense of motion [1]; there are many conditions and diseases may cause dizziness. One of the most common diagnoses was sinusitis in addition to labyrinthitis, otitis media, benign positional vertigo, and unspecified presyncope that were among the most common causes of dizziness [2].

Sinusitis is one of the most common respiratory infections as a result of pathogenic bacteria through the oral cavity or nasal ostium [3]. The signs and symptoms of sinusitis may include per orbital edema, headache, facial pain, tooth pain, fever, earache, a sore throat, cough, nasal congestion, dizziness, nasal obstruction, and foul breath [4].

One of the common types of sinusitis is the OS which may occur when the Schneiderian membrane is disrupted by many conditions [5] such as infections which originate from maxillary teeth, maxillary dental trauma odontogenic pathology of maxillary bone, or iatrogenic causes like dental implant, extractions, and maxillary osteotomies in orthognathic surgery [3].

Lee and Lee (2010) investigated the clinical features and treatments of (OS) and found that dental infection was a major predisposing factor of OS.

Brook (2016) reviewed the different management strategies of sinusitis of odontogenic origin; he pointed out that both surgical and dental treatments of the odontogenic pathological conditions combined with medical therapy are indicated.

Root canal therapy is a debridement procedure that is based on the removal of the irritants (bacteria) and inactivation of endotoxins and other toxic products from the canal and periapical areas to get a successful treatment [6], [7]. Root canal treatment depended on chemical and mechanical ways [6]. Mechanical way is based on using manual and rotary files. The rotary system has many benefits; it reduces the intracanal bacteria [8] and increases the quality of root fillings [9].

2. Case Presentation

This case study indicates the effectiveness of root canal therapy to treat OS and disappearance of symptoms. Patient

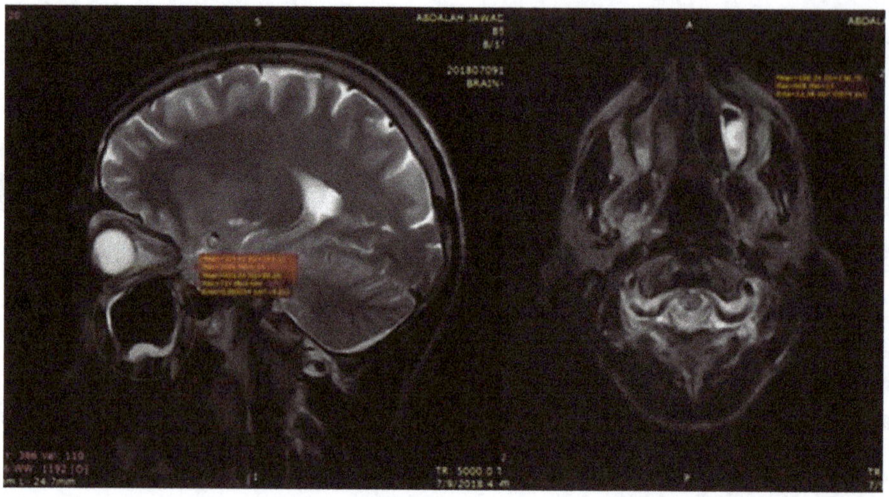

Figure 1: MRI sagittal and axial views show thickness of mucosal layer of maxillary sinus.

consent was obtained, and then history was taken. A 26-year-old male who is medically fit had suffered from dizziness in walking and standing. He had a headache while eating and tilting his head forward.

The patient consulted internal, cardiac, and neurological and ENT specialists to treat the dizziness; all medical investigations were negative and all given conservative management failed to improve his dizziness.

After a further audiologist examination, videonystagmography study showed normal study with no signs of peripheral dizziness cause in origin. The static position test at different head positions with and without eye closure showed no significant spontaneous or any positional nystagmus. Cervical spine MRI was normal and brain MRI showed chronic sinusitis (Figure 1).

According to the MRI findings, the patient was treated with many types of antibiotic which were azithromycin 500 mg three times daily/one course and then amoxicillin with clavulanic acid 500 mg three times daily/one course. The physician changed the antibiotic to ciprofloxacin (500 mg twice daily).

After this history of none responsive conservative medical management, the patient came for the dental examination and baseline assessment and examination was performed; dental examination showed no swelling or inflammation to be detected; pain was reported as 7 out of 10. Intraoral examination showed sinus tract with pus mobility grade 2. Radiograph examination in orthopantomogram and periapical (Figures 2 and 3) showed radiolucency around upper 6 and 7 and arrived at the border of the maxillary sinus using rubber dam for isolation starting with using a cold and percussion test to determine the vitality of pulp, upper 6 positive on cold but there is no pain on percussion and upper 7 pain on percussion but negative on cold. Our initial diagnosis was upper left second molar previously initiated therapy with chronic apical abscess with sinus tract; the upper left first molar was diagnosed with irreversible pulpitis; normal apical tissues used gutta-percha to determine the caused tooth of sinus track (Figures 4 and 5). According to X-ray, signs, and a gutta test, the upper left second molar was the caused

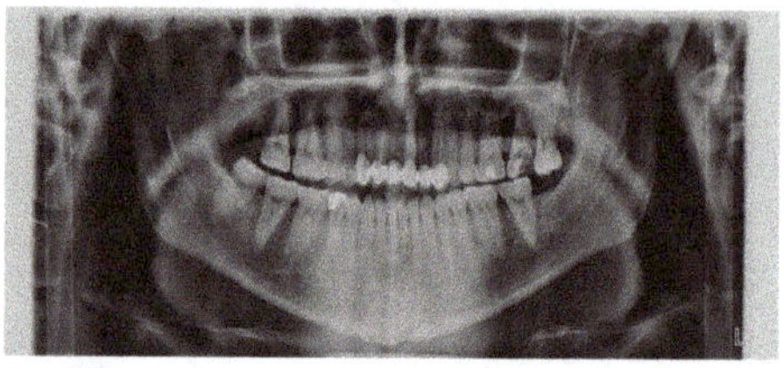

Figure 2: Orthopantomogram before treatment showed the upper left second molar opened with periapical radiolucency.

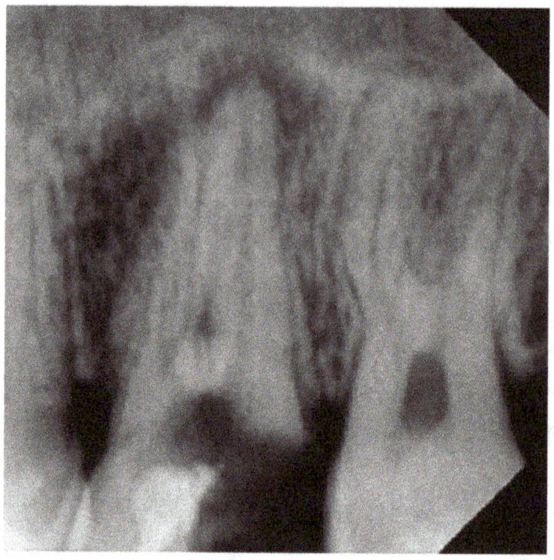

Figure 3: Periapical X-ray before treatment.

tooth; a management plan was based on root canal therapy to preserve tooth and reduce the sign and symptoms of infection. Preoperative periapical X-ray was taken to determine the initial length of canals. There was no need for anesthesia as it is a nonvital tooth; as mentioned before, the tooth was previously initially treated so the canal orifice was opened, using low-speed turbine to remove the soft dentine and get a good vision. K file numbers 10, 15, and 20 were used to open canals, and normal saline was used as an initial irrigation to get rid of pus.

After ensuring that all canals were opened in working length, a rotary system crown-down technique was used

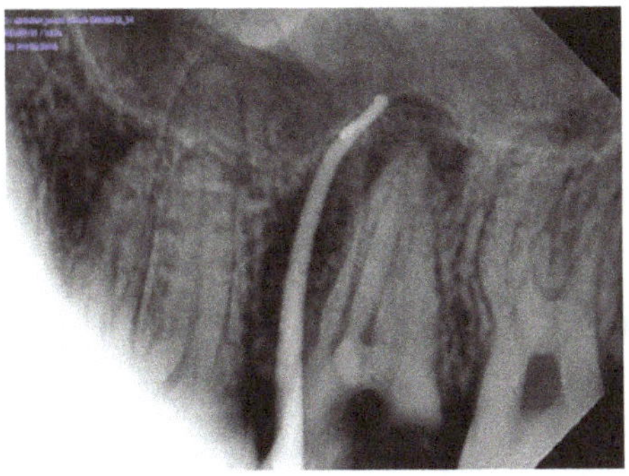

Figure 4: Periapical X-ray shows gutta-percha inserted through sinus.

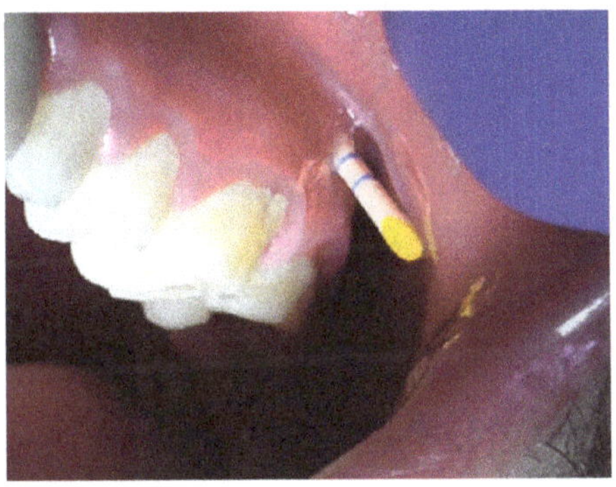

Figure 5: Gutta-percha inserted through sinus.

to shape canals starting with an initial file in 15 mm sodium hypochlorite 5% that was used for irrigation and hydrogen peroxide, saline between them; protaper rotary system finishing file (F1) was used to finish shaping in full working length of 21 mm. Irrigation with sodium hypochlorite was done, and then normal saline was used for final irrigation, canal was dried using F1 paper point, and calcium hydroxide with iodoform as an internal canal medication (Figure 6).

After one week, the patient showed less dizziness on walking, no pain was reported while eating, and periapical X-ray showed reduce radiolucency CBCT after obturation.

After 2 weeks further, the patient came to our clinic with severe pain on cold and hot; the upper left first molar was assessed and diagnosed with deep caries. Symptomatic irreversible pulpitis root canal treatment was completed in one visit. After 2 weeks further, using rubber dam isolation treatment started to speed up round bur to remove temporary filling. F1 rotary file had been used to remove all formed calcium hydroxide canals. The process involved irrigation with normal saline, then soaking the canals for around 10 min with sodium hypochlorite, activation (with water pick) for 30 seconds per canal, irrigation with normal saline, and using paper point (F1) to dry the canals. Complete obturation was performed by using F1 Gutta percha and hot Gutta system with endomethazone and eugenol as a sealer. Glass ionomer was used to close the pulp chamber then completing the tooth filling using composite (Figure 7).

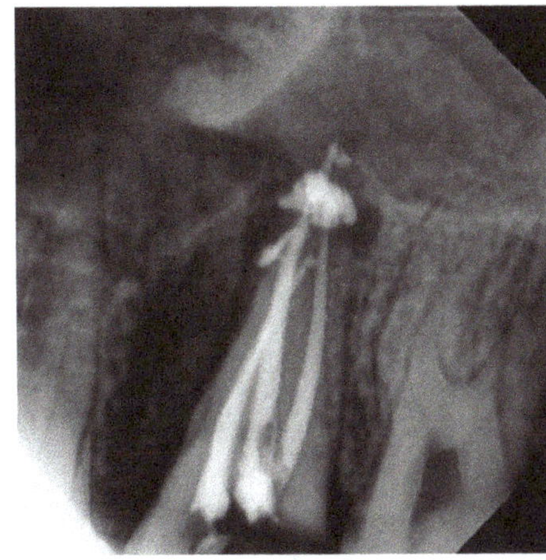

Figure 6: Upper left first molar with calcium hydroxide shows the tooth with direct contact with sinus.

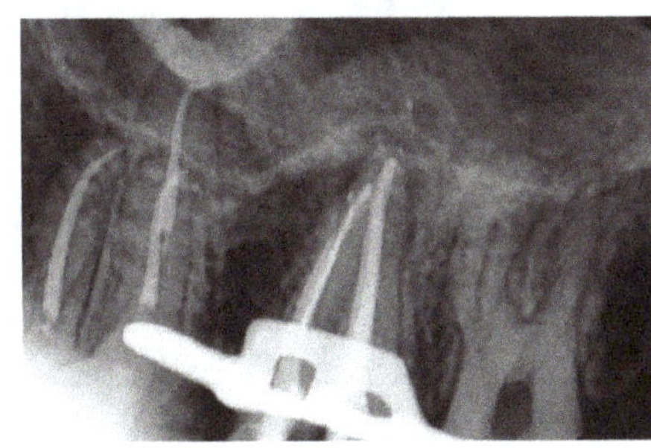

Figure 7: Periapical due to upper 7 obturation.

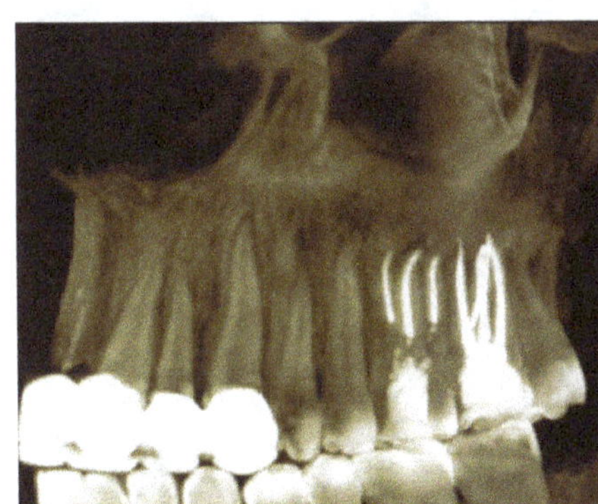

Figure 8: CBCT.

CBCT after obturation (Figures 8 and 9).

2.1. Follow-Up. Two months after the intervention, the patient reported a complete recovery of dizziness and sinusitis; pain was reported as 0 m which reflects a primary recovery of OS; a follow-up after 2 weeks periapical X-ray showed decrease of radiolucency (Figure 10).

CBCT after 10 months shows disappearance of radiolucency around the apex (Figure 11).

3. Discussion

The association between dizziness and sinusitis was not surprising as it was well documented in literature. The auditory

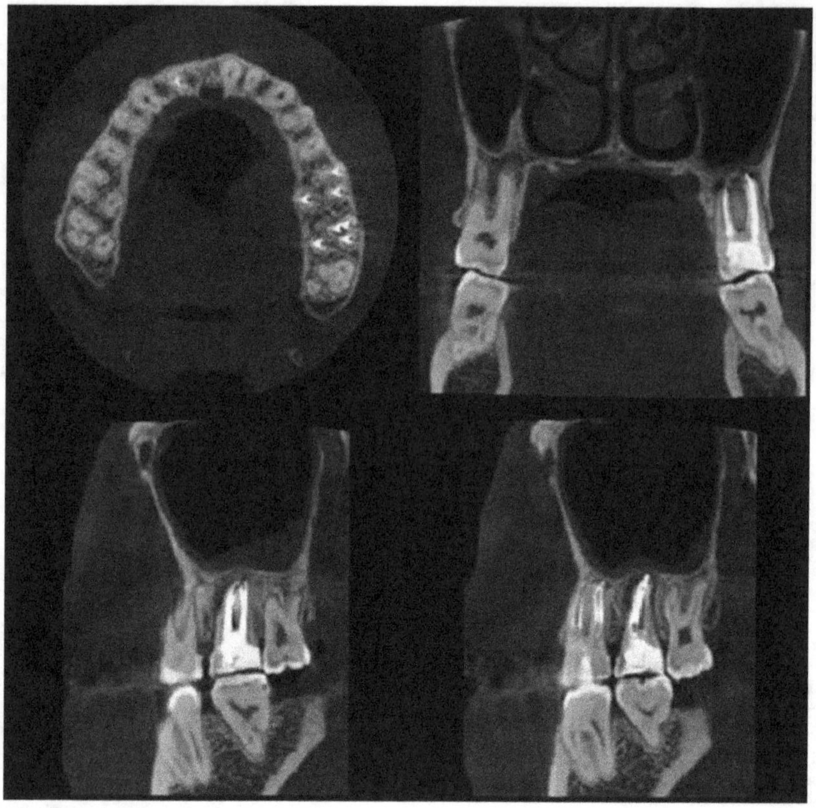

Figure 9: CBCT after obturation. Axial, coronal, and sagittal views.

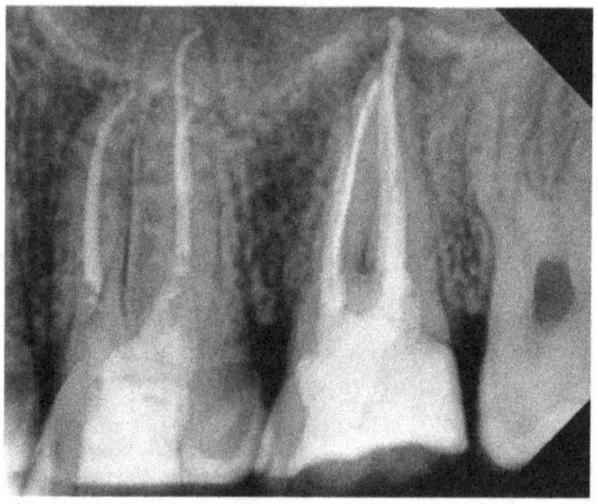

Figure 10: Periapical X-ray after 2 weeks of obturation.

tube is a narrow osteocartilaginous channel connecting the nasal cavity with the tympanic cavity [10]. It is a responsibility for pressure equilibrium and ventilation of the middle ear, so according to the anatomical and functional connections, auditory tubes are affected in upper respiratory trunk infection as sinusitis that lead to middle ear and unbalance disorder [11].

OS infections are considered to be predisposing factors for sinusitis, because of the anatomical relation. The antral mucosa has been weakened and broken down and the Schneiderian membrane is perforated [4] by chronic dental infection/inflammation as a reason to bacterial colonization [12].

In the maxillary teeth, the second molar roots are the closest to the maxillary sinus floor, followed by the roots of the first molar, second premolar, and first premolar. These short distances between roots and maxillary sinus explain the easy extension of an infectious process from these teeth to the maxillary sinus [4].

The OS is a polymicrobial infection, aerobic-anaerobic bacteria, with anaerobes outnumbering the aerobes [3]. There are two types of bacteria which are most commonly found in OS, which are *Staphylococcus Aureus* and *Gram-negative bacilli* [3, 13, 14] As was mentioned in patient's history, treatment was based on eliminating this opportunist bacteria.

This justifies why antibiotic treatment without dental treatment failed to eliminate the causing bacteria which lead to treatment failure.

Sinusitis is a common etiology of dizziness, but sinusitis of odontogenic cause associated with dizziness had not been discussed in literature according to the knowledge of the authors, which is the main finding of this article.

This case report showed that there is a correlation between dental infection and sinusitis, which makes the sinus vulnerable for a major source of infection, especially with bad oral hygiene patient. Many patients with maxillary sinusitis were treated symptomatically without treating the underlying causes.

In this case, dizziness was recovered, after the sinusitis had improved, with no major intervention other than root canal therapy, which shows the importance of the proper

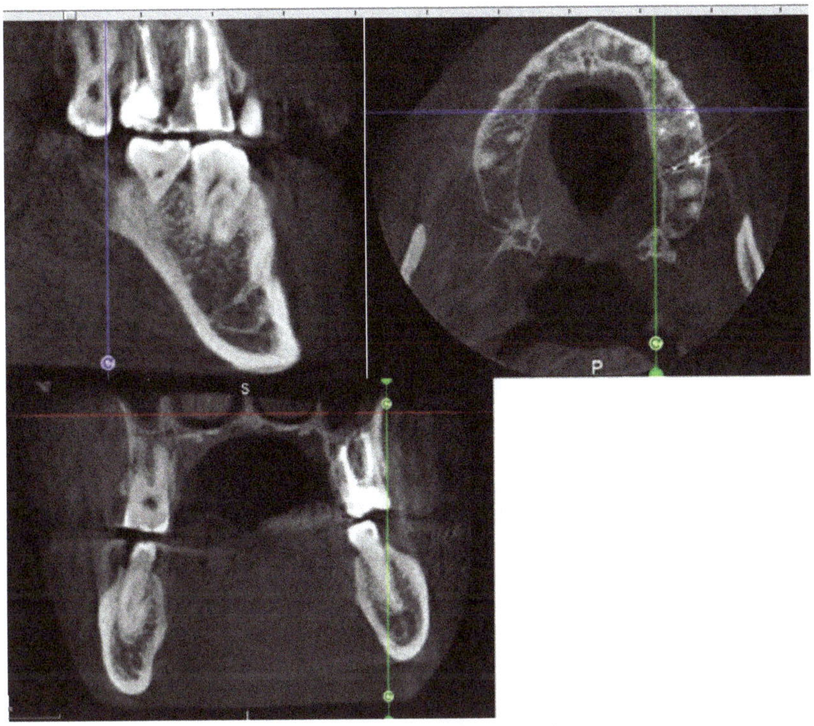

Figure 11: CBCT after 10 months of obturation.

diagnosis and management of the primary cause, rather than treating temporarily the signs of a complication.

The implication of this finding may be that patients that come with dizziness and the evidence of sinusitis, periapical lesions should be investigated. In this case, it was showed that an open source of contamination will lead to the failure of any pharmacological management of local sinusitis on the long run, which makes this finding an essential element in future history taking from patients with sinusitis-related dizziness.

One of the limitations of this study was that it did not take into consideration the types of bacteria that caused OS to find out which types of bacteria could help in the treatment and could also contribute to a better understanding of this medical interaction. The authors of this study recommend further research in this field, trying to investigate this medical complication with related bacteria or normal flora of oral cavity.

The finding in this case underlines the necessity of management of the infected maxillary teeth not just to preserve the tooth health but also to prevent further complication that sinusitis is only one example of them, with all its complication starting from with dizziness and ending up of tumor [15].

4. Conclusion

Failure to diagnose sinusitis of dental origin will lead to further complications including dizziness. Elimination of bacterial sources is essential for preventing recurrence of sinusitis and its chronicity. Referral of sinusitis patient to the dentist may augment treatment and accelerate healing in OS-related dizziness.

Recommendations of this study include the evaluation of any dizzy patient must include dental history and examination, to exclude any causes of dental origin.

Acknowledgments

The authors wish to express their gratitude to Dr. Emad Qirresh at Al Quds University.

References

[1] A. Bisdorff, M. Von Brevern, T. Lempert, and D. E. Newman-Toker, "Classification of vestibular symptoms: towards an international classification of vestibular disorders," *Journal of Vestibular Research*, vol. 19, no. 1-2, pp. 1–13, 2009.

[2] P. D. Sloane, J. Dallara, C. Roach, K. E. Bailey, M. Mitchell, and R. McNutt, "Management of dizziness in primary care," *The Journal of the American Board of Family Practice*, vol. 7, no. 1, pp. 1–8, 1994.

[3] I. Brook, "Sinusitis of odontogenic origin," *Otolaryngology-Head and Neck Surgery*, vol. 135, no. 3, pp. 349–355, 2006.

[4] D. C. Amanda Armington, D. C. Lorraine Ginter, D. C. Shawn Hatch et al., *Sinus Pain and Rhinosinusitis*, University of Western States, 2017.

[5] K. C. Lee and S. J. Lee, "Clinical features and treatments of odontogenic sinusitis," *Yonsei medical journal*, vol. 51, no. 6, pp. 932–937, 2010.

[6] R. Haghgoo and F. Moradi, "Evaluation of antimicrobial efficacy of nanosilver solution, sodium hypochlorite and normal

saline in root canal irrigation of primary teeth," *Contemporary clinical dentistry*, vol. 9, no. 6, pp. 227–232, 2018.

[7] T. A. F. de Melo, G. S. L. Gründling, F. Montagner et al., "LPS levels in root canals after the use of ozone gas and high frequency electrical pulses," *Brazilian oral research*, vol. 30, no. 1, 2016.

[8] G. B. Shuping, D. Ørstavik, A. Sigurdsson, and M. Trope, "Reduction of intracanal bacteria using nickel-titanium rotary instrumentation and various medications," *Journal of endodontics*, vol. 26, no. 12, pp. 751–755, 2000.

[9] A. Molander, D. Caplan, G. Bergenholtz, and C. Reit, "Improved quality of root fillings provided by general dental practitioners educated in nickel–titanium rotary instrumentation," *International endodontic journal*, vol. 40, no. 4, pp. 254–260, 2007.

[10] J. M. Prades, J. M. Dumollard, F. Calloc'h, N. Merzougui, C. Veyret, and C. Martin, "Descriptive anatomy of the human auditory tube," *Surgical and Radiologic Anatomy*, vol. 20, no. 5, pp. 335–340, 1998.

[11] A. G. M. Schilder, M. F. Bhutta, C. C. Butler et al., "Eustachian tube dysfunction: consensus statement on definition, types, clinical presentation and diagnosis," *Clinical Otolaryngology*, vol. 40, no. 5, pp. 407–411, 2015.

[12] K. G. Legert, M. Zimmerman, and P. Stierna, "Sinusitis of odontogenic origin: pathophysiological implications of early treatment," *Acta oto-laryngologica*, vol. 124, no. 6, pp. 655–663, 2004.

[13] I. Brook, "Microbiology of acute and chronic maxillary sinusitis associated with an odontogenic origin," *The Laryngoscope*, vol. 115, no. 5, pp. 823–825, 2005.

[14] I. Brook, "Microbiology of acute sinusitis of odontogenic origin presenting with periorbital cellulitis in children," *Annals of Otology, Rhinology & Laryngology*, vol. 116, no. 5, pp. 386–388, 2007.

[15] M. A. Kiresur, A. Ananthaneni, V. S. Guduru, and R. S. Devi, "Keratocystic odontogenic tumor involving the maxillary sinus: a rare entity," *Clinical Cancer Investigation Journal*, vol. 5, no. 1, p. 92, 2016.

27

The Digital Abutment Check: An Improvement of the Fully Digital Workflow

Sebastian Hinz,[1] Daniel Ellmann,[2] Christian Wegner,[1] Wolfgang Bömicke,[3] and Tobias Bensel[1]

[1]*Department of Prosthodontics, Faculty of Medicine, Martin Luther University Halle-Wittenberg, Magdeburger Straße 16, 06112 Halle (Saale), Germany*
[2]*R+K CAD/CAM Technologie GmbH & Co.KG, Ruwerstieg 43, 12681 Berlin, Germany*
[3]*Department of Oral, Dental and Maxillofacial Diseases, Heidelberg University Hospital, Im Neuenheimer Feld 400, Heidelberg 69120, Germany*

Correspondence should be addressed to Sebastian Hinz; sebastian.hinz@uk-halle.de

Academic Editor: Mine D ndar

By using modern digitalization techniques, an existing denture can be digitized and aid the provision of a new implant-supported denture according to a fully digital workflow. This includes fully navigated implant surgery and results in an immediately provided prosthetic restoration. However, even with the current digital workflow, it is challenging to achieve a definitive prosthetic restoration in a single treatment session. In order to achieve a definitive denture in as few treatment sessions as possible, we have implemented the digital abutment test. This test modified the existing data set and determined the final restoration. In the present case, the preexisting maxillary removable complete denture was converted into a fixed immediate restoration using the fully digital workflow. The workflow is divided into two treatment phases, each with three treatment sessions, where part of the second phase involves an innovative digital abutment check. The illustrated case shows an effective use of current digital possibilities. Special attention was also paid to a minimally invasive course of therapy.

1. Introduction

Once the hard and soft tissues of the oral cavity have been digitally recorded, e.g., by intraoral scanners and modern 3D radiograph technology, these data can serve as the basis for further digital process steps [1]. Before implant surgery, the final position of the implants can be determined virtually using planning software and 3D radiograph images. The position of the inserted implants is of crucial importance for the final design of the anchored prosthesis and the long-term survival of the dentures [2–4]. In this context, template-guided implant surgery allows for the accurate placement of dental implants [2, 3]. A precise surgical template can be fabricated by merging the intraoral-scan data with the 3D radiographic data [5–7]. For the surgeon, the use of a surgical template results in a predictable and safe treatment procedure. Patients additionally benefit from a shorter treatment time, fewer postoperative restrictions, and an overall increase in comfort [8]. As a consequence, template-guided implant placement is becoming increasingly popular. [8–11].

The implants were placed according to the COMFOUR® system (CAMLOG Vertriebs GmbH, Wimsheim, Germany). Four implants are used to immediately rehabilitate the edentulous jaw with a fixed interim restoration. The advantages of the system lie in the maximum expansion of the support polygon through a precisely planned implant position, but especially implant angulation; the distal implants are usually inserted at an angle between 15 and 30 degrees [3, 4, 12–14]. This allows the prosthetic support field to be expanded

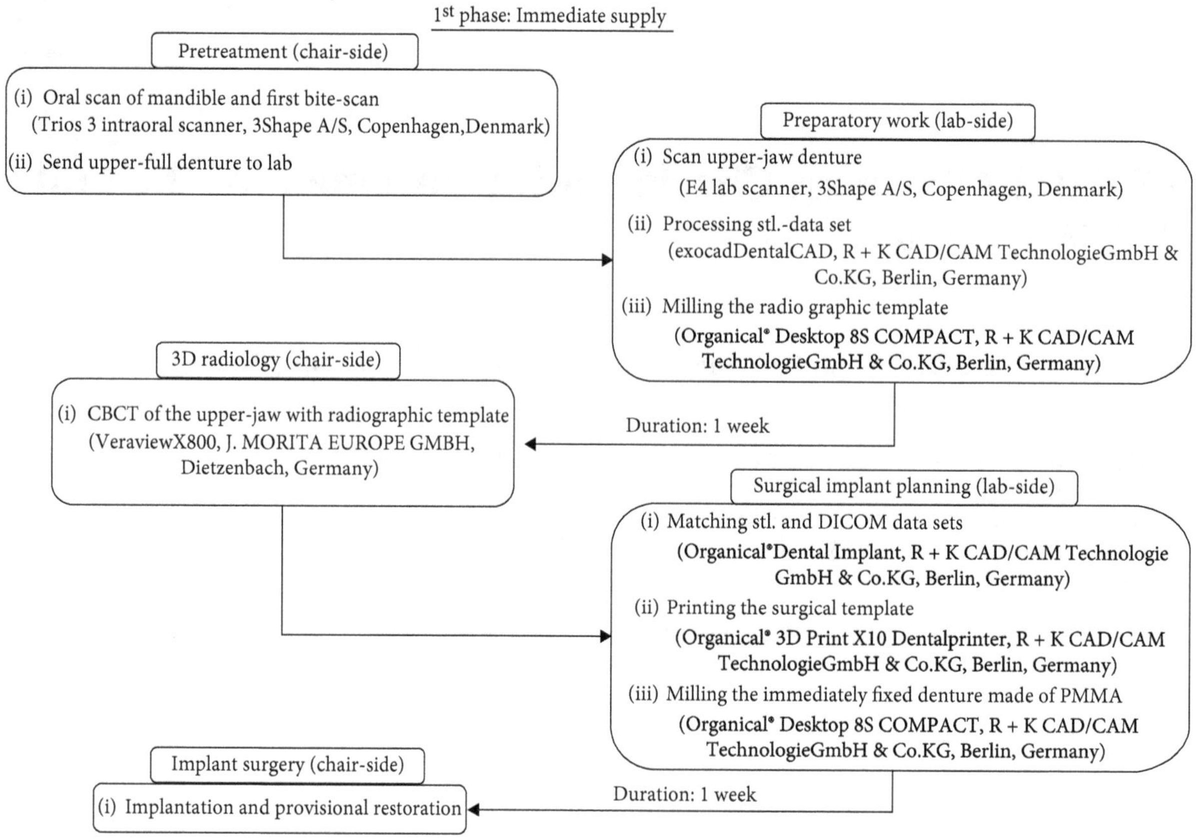

FIGURE 1: Overview of the 1st treatment phase.

posteriorly without compromising relevant anatomical structures and without having to perform extensive bone augmentation measures.

The template used in the present report provided a precise implementation of the digitally determined implant position [5, 9–11, 15, 16]. The navigated procedure offered further advantages by eliminating the need for intraoperative flap formation, thus reducing surgical trauma and reducing the postoperative need for analgesics [8, 17].

However, the main challenge for the prosthetic treatment team (dentist, dental technician) in the implementation of a fully digital All-on-X workflow is to transfer the final implant position to the definitive restoration. The deviations between the virtually planned and the real implant position must be balanced out even with guided implantation [18–25].

Digital impressions represent a reliable impression method for the fabrication of implant-supported full-arch frameworks [26]. Usually, scan-bodies are screwed onto the implants for digital impression making. These can negatively affect the precision of the digital impression [27–29]. However, transmission errors due to the use of scan-bodies must be taken into account. A transfer without the use of scan-bodies could increase the precision of the prosthetic restoration.

In this present case report, we successfully demonstrate the realization of the final prosthodontic restoration while avoiding inaccuracies caused by screwed-in scan-bodies. This was accomplished by the implementation of the digital abutment check without the use of scan-bodies.

2. Initial Situation

The 55-year-old patient first came to the Department of Prosthodontics (Faculty of Medicine, Martin Luther University Halle-Wittenberg) during an outpatient consultation. The patient reported smoking about 10 cigarettes a day but otherwise had an uneventful medical history. The maxilla was edentulous, and the remaining teeth in the mandible were stable from a periodontological and endotontological point of view. The existing prosthetic and conservative restorations were found to be sufficient and restored a continuous dental arch, which extended from the second left to the second right premolar.

According to the patient, the last maxillary teeth had been extracted about one year prior to the initial consultation. Since then, he has been wearing a conventionally made removable complete denture. The patient stated that the stability of the prosthesis was not sufficient to eat properly. He also complained about the extensive coverage of the palate. In the course of weighing up the different therapy options, the patient decided on an implant-supported, fixed full-arch prosthesis without palatal coverage. The mandible shortened dental arch was to be maintained in agreement with the patient.

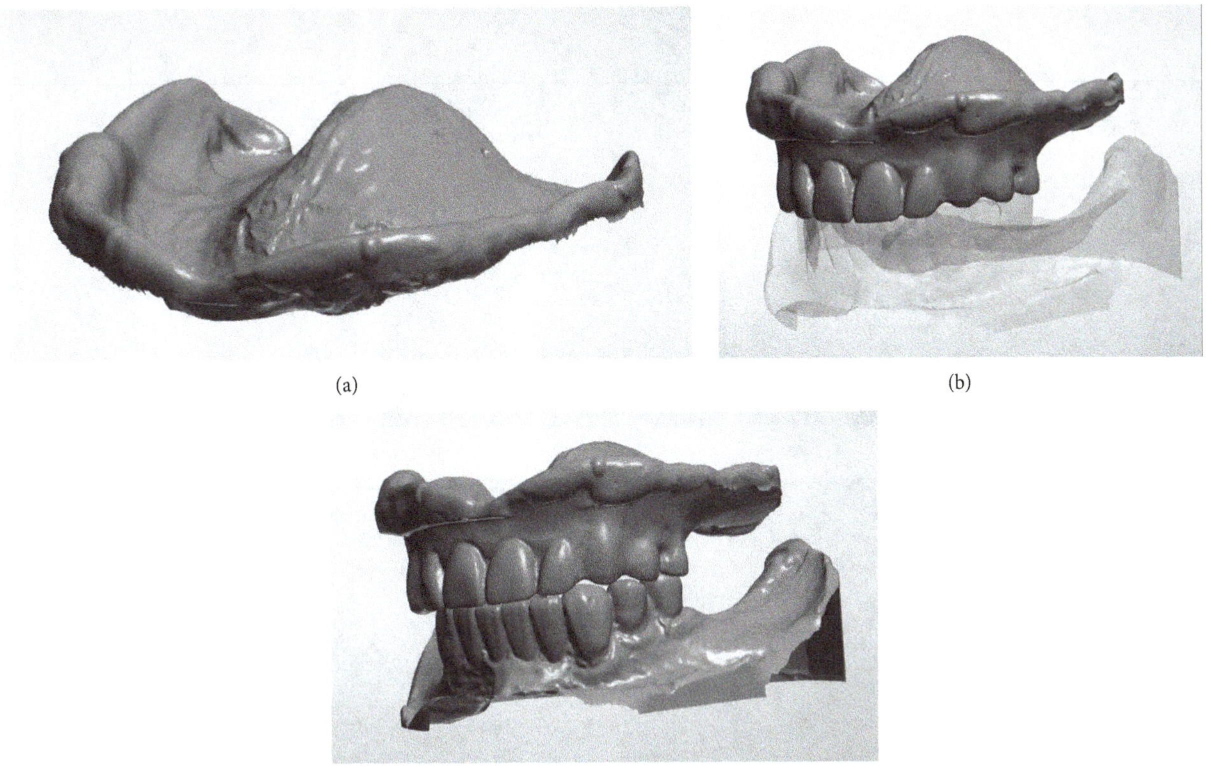

(a) (b) (c)

FIGURE 2: (a) Base area scan of the upper full denture. (b) Scan of the entire upper full denture. (c) Matched scans of the upper full denture and lower jaw.

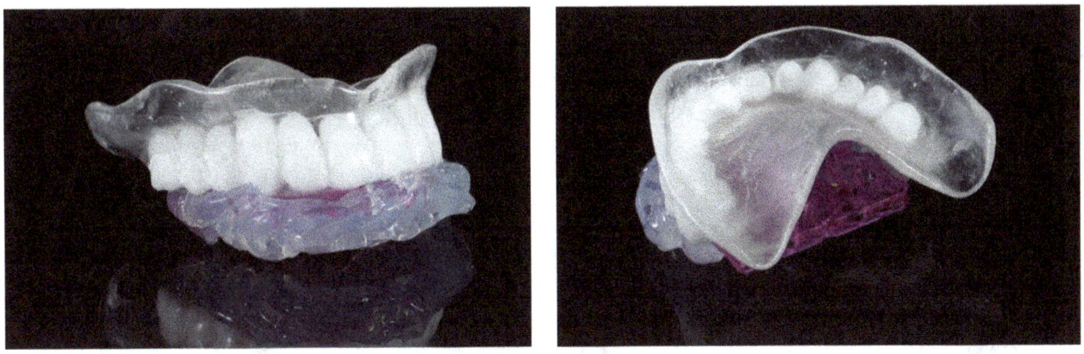

(a) (b)

FIGURE 3: (a) Frontal view of the radiographic template. (b) View on the base area of the radiographic template.

3. Therapy Considerations

The aim of the decided upon therapy was to achieve stable, palate-free care, involving little surgical effort and with as few treatment sessions as possible. We decided to use a gentle, minimally invasive procedure without any additional augmentations. The final planning included the insertion of four implants in the upper jaw and a fixed, provisional immediate restoration, which should be transferred to a definitive fixed partial denture (FPD) after the healing period of six months. The treatment was divided into two independent phases. The first treatment phase involves diagnostics and therapy planning, as well as surgical intervention and the immediate provision of an interim restoration. The second treatment phase consists of the transfer of the interim FPD to the definitive FPD after the successful healing period.

We decided to use the COMFOUR® system (Camlog, Wimsheim, Germany) to maximise patient comfort during the treatment. The advantages of the COMFOUR® system are the possibility of immediate loading with appropriate primary stability of the implants (>35 Ncm) and the targeted avoidance of augmentation by angulation of the posterior implants.

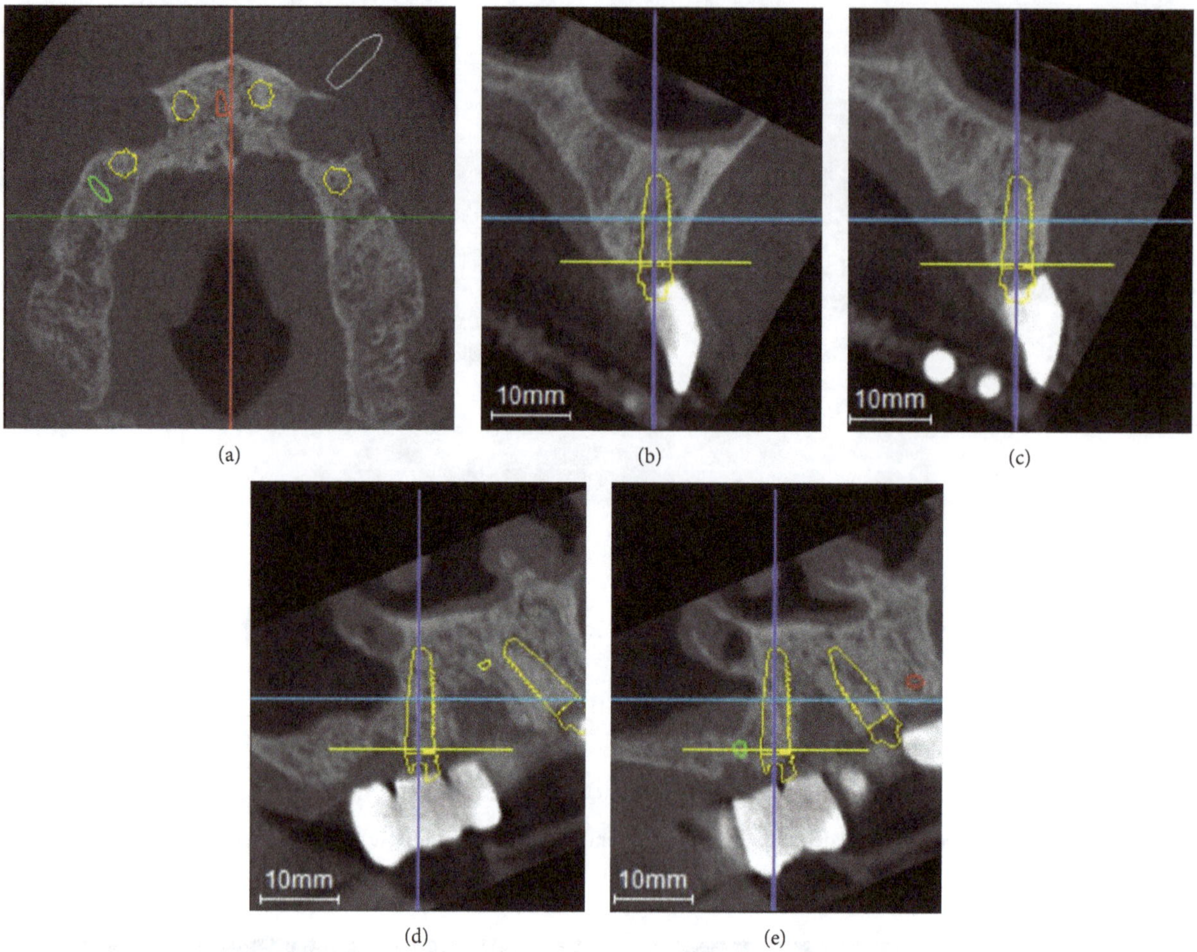

Figure 4: (a) Axial view of all planned implants. (b) Transversal view of planned implant 12. (c) Transversal view of planned implant 22. (d) Transversal view of planned implant 25. (e) Transversal view of planned implant 15.

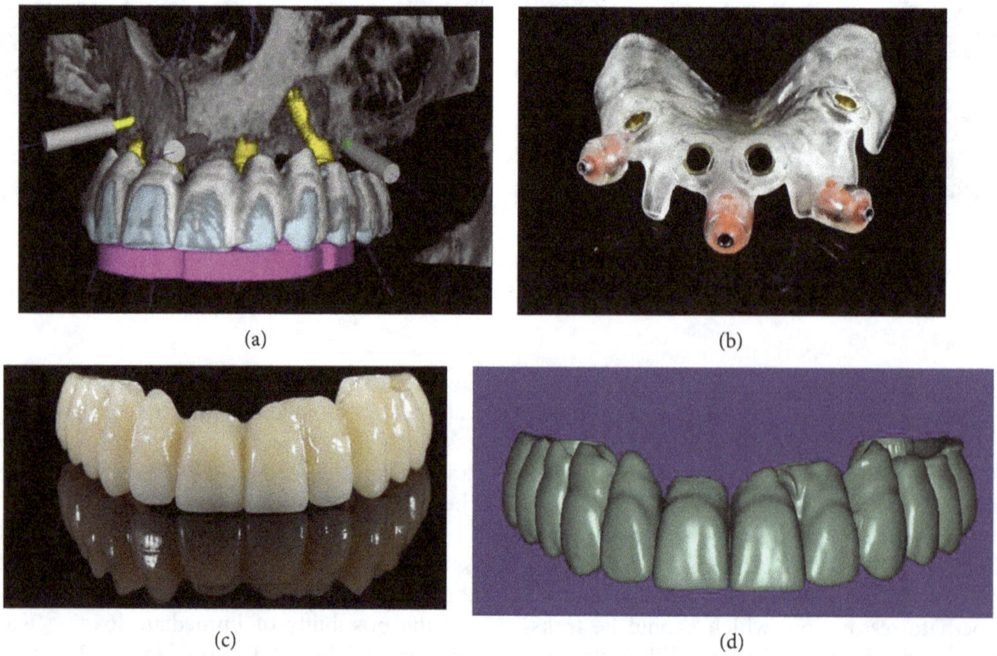

Figure 5: (a) Planning the surgical template. (b) Finished printed surgical template. (c) Design of the provisional FPD. (d) Finished provisional FPD milled from PMMA.

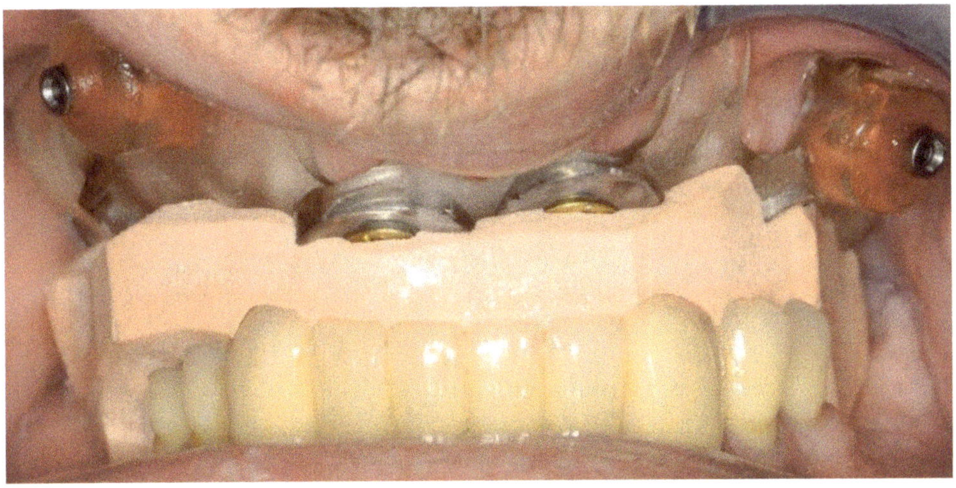

(a)

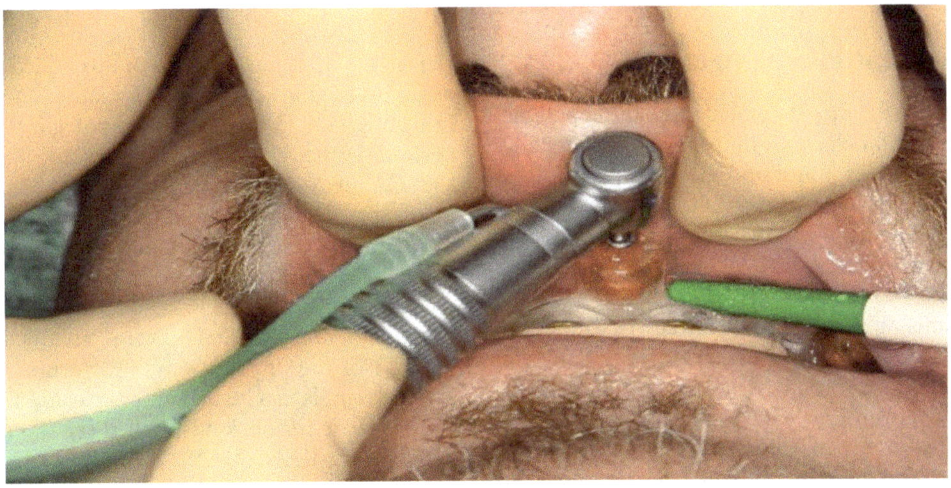

(b)

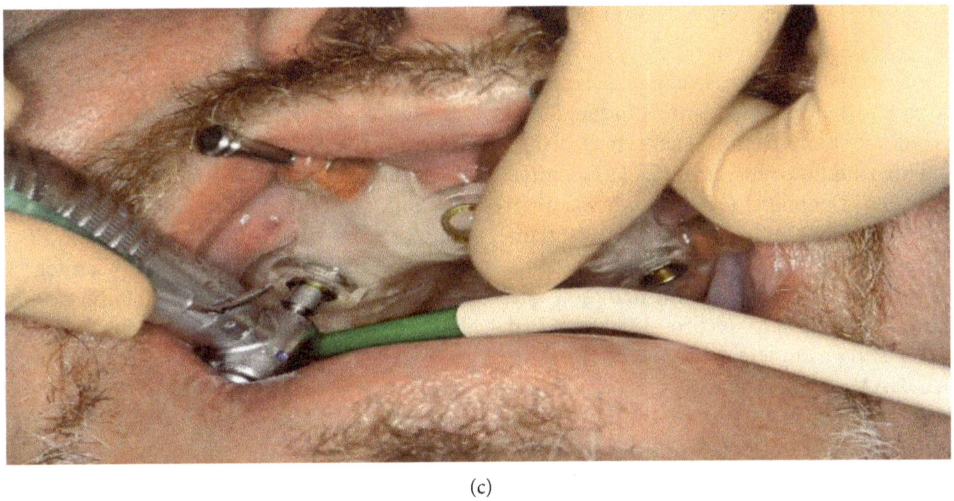

(c)

FIGURE 6: Continued.

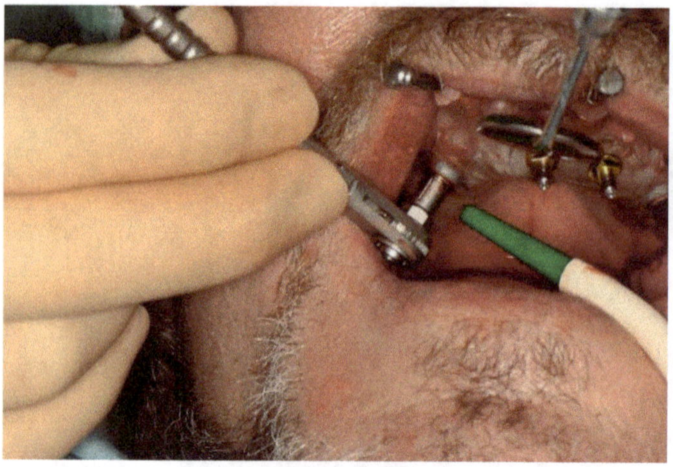

(d)

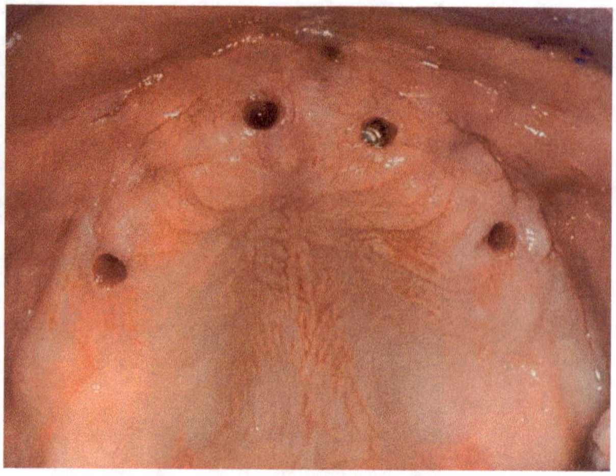

(e)

FIGURE 6: (a) Surgical template with occlusion key. (b) Drilling the holes for the anchor pins. (c) Drilling the implant bearings. (d) Inserting the implants. (e) Upper jaw after implant insertion.

4. The 1st Treatment Phase (Figure 1)

4.1. Pretreatment. As the first treatment step, the mandible and the maxillomandibular relationship were digitally recorded intraorally (Trios 3 intraoral scanner, 3Shape A/S, Copenhagen, Denmark). The correct fit of the maxillary removable complete denture was checked in advance using low viscosity polyvinyl siloxane (GC Fit Checker® Advanced, GC EUROPE N.V., Leuven, Belgium). The correct maxillomandibular relationship was checked clinically based on the resting position of the mandible. If the measured parameters are inadequate, dentures would have to be adjusted in advance. Alternatively, if the patient does not wear any removable dentures or the maxillomandibular relationship has to be changed, the maxillomandibular relationship can be adjusted with digital measurement systems (JMAnalyser +, zebris Medical GmbH, Isny, Germany), due to the fact that these systems offer a digital interface for Computer-Aided Design/Computer-Aided Manufacturing (CAD/CAM).

4.2. Preparatory Work. In the present case, the existing maxillary removable complete denture was scanned in the dental laboratory (Rüberling & Klar Dental Laboratory, Halle (Saale), Germany) with a laboratory scanner (E4 lab scanner, 3Shape A/S, Copenhagen, Denmark) (Figure 2). It was then used as a template for the radiographic and the surgical template and the provisional FPD. The Standard Triangulation/-Tesselation Language (STL) data records of the mandible and the maxillomandibular relationship record were matched with the data of the existing complete denture (exocad DentalCAD, R+K CAD/CAM Technologie GmbH & Co.KG, Berlin, Germany). The soft tissue situation of the edentulous maxilla was picked up using the base area of the complete denture. This procedure resulted in the manufacturing of the radiographic template. The base of the radiographic template was milled from clear polymethylmethacrylate (PMMA; Organic PMMA clear, Organical Dental Implant, R+K CAD/CAM Technologie GmbH & Co.KG, Berlin, Germany), while the dental arch was milled from barium sulphate containing acrylic resin (Organic RO, Organical Dental Implant, R+K CAD/CAM Technologie GmbH & Co.KG, Berlin, Germany) (Organical® Desktop 8S COMPACT, R +K CAD/CAM Technologie GmbH & Co.KG, Berlin, Germany). Finally, both parts of the radiographic template were connected with an autopolymerizing resin (FuturaGen, Schütz Dental, Rosbach, Germany) (Figure 3).

4.3. 3D Radiology. Cone Beam Volumetric Tomography (CBCT) of the upper jaw was performed using the radiographic template. The patient's occlusion was blocked using a silicone occlusion key supplied by the dental laboratory (Transpasil, KANIEDENTA GmbH & Co.KG, Herford, Germany). In this procedure, a Digital Imaging and Communications in Medicine (DICOM®) data record of the upper jaw (Veraview X800, J. MORITA EUROPE GMBH, Dietzenbach, Germany) was created.

4.4. Surgical Implant Planning. 3D planning software (Organical® Dental Implant, R+K CAD/CAM Technologie GmbH & Co.KG, Berlin, Germany) was used for surgical implant planning. In this process, the DICOM® data record and the STL data record were matched. Despite the fact that bony conditions in the anterior maxilla area were reduced, the conditions were sufficient for the insertion of two implants with the size of 3.8×11 mm (Guide Camlog®SL Promote plus, CAMLOG Vertriebs GmbH) at the position of the central incisors. In the posterior, the insertion of two implants of size 3.8×13 mm was planned in the position of the second premolars (Camlog®SL Promote plus, CAMLOG Vertriebs GmbH). The posterior implants were planned with an insertion angle of 30 degrees. In addition, 3 anchor pins measuring 1.5×11 mm at positions 013, 011/021, and 023 were planned for the fixation of the surgical template (Guided Anchor Pin, Nobel Biocare AG, Kloten, Switzerland) (Figure 4). Following the complete surgical implant planning, a corresponding surgical template was printed (VeriGuide™

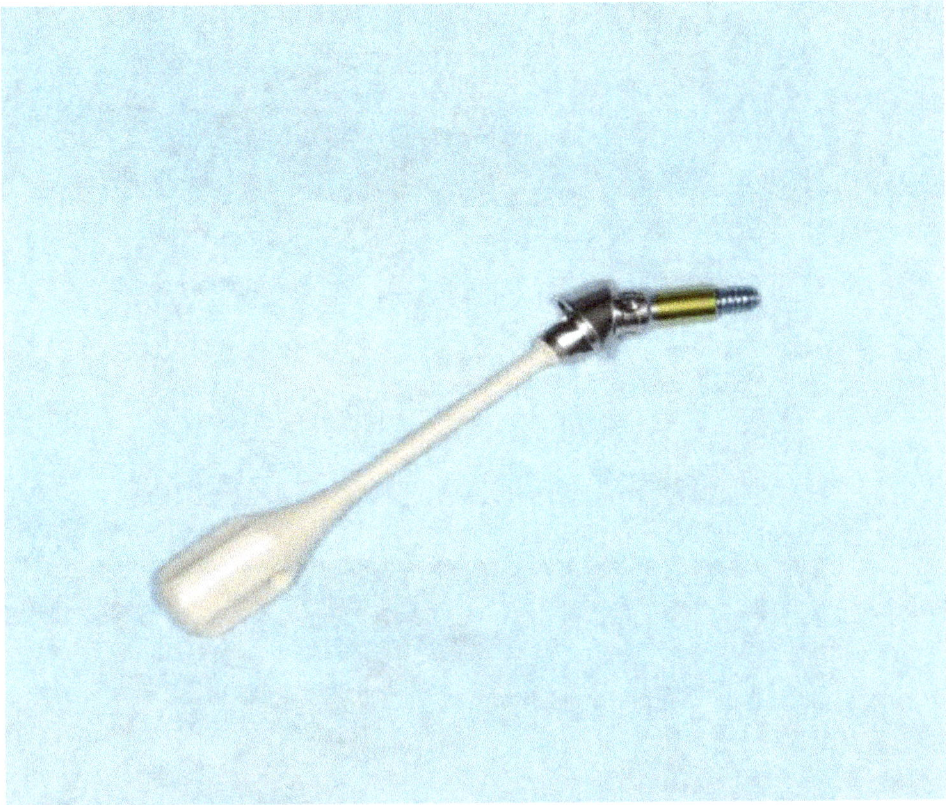

(a)

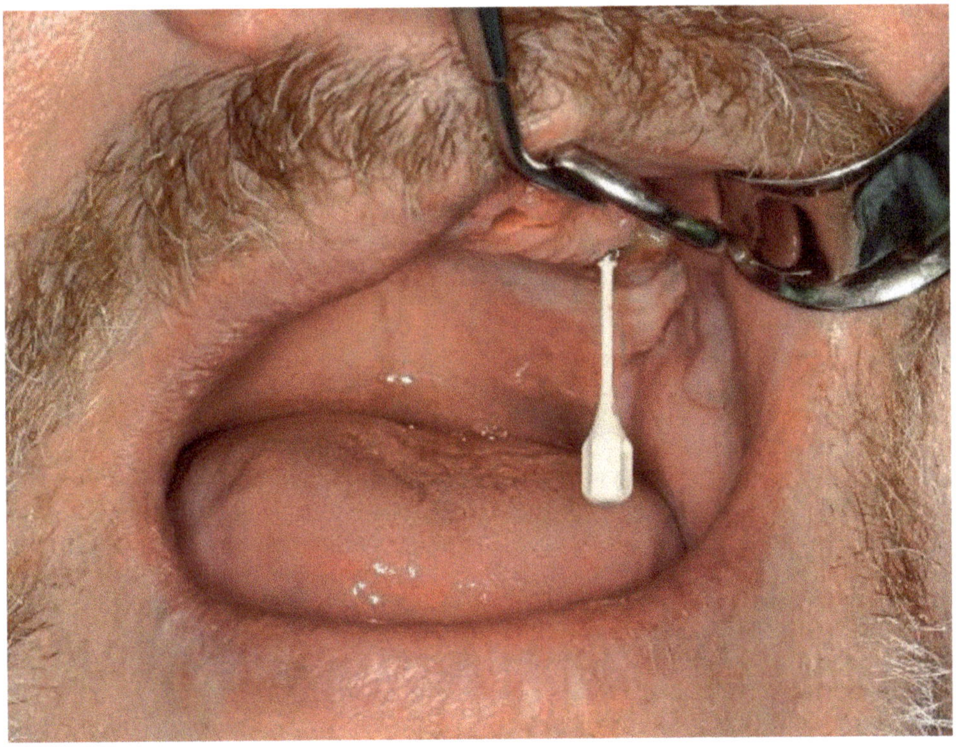

(b)

FIGURE 7: Continued.

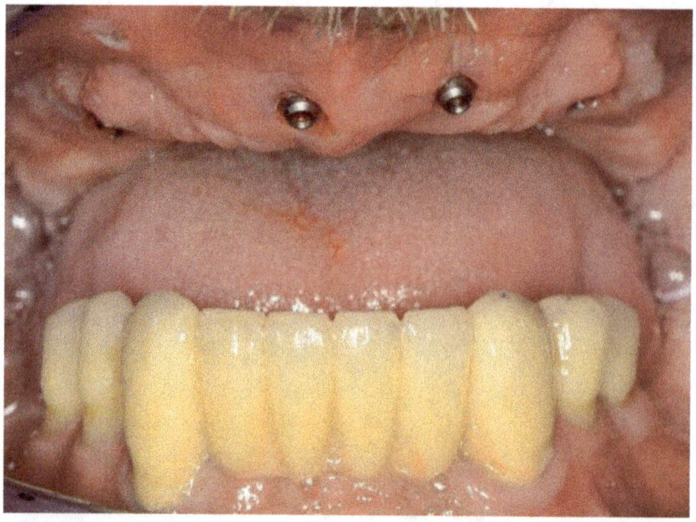

(c)

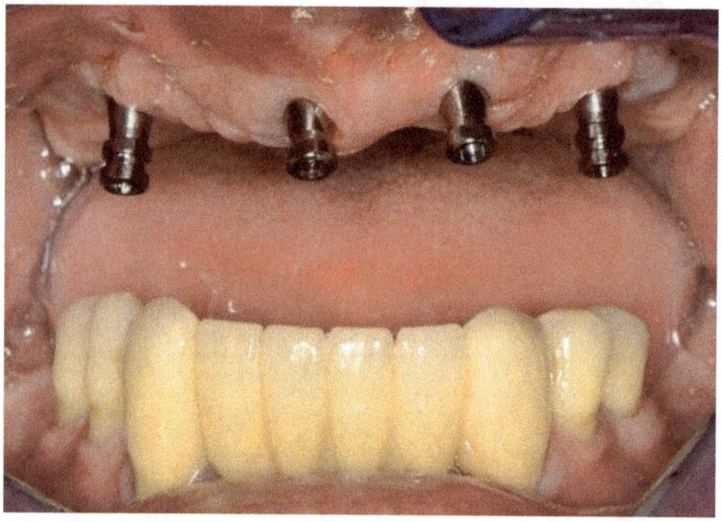

(d)

FIGURE 7: (a) Bar abutment with handle. (b) Inserted bar abutment. (c) Frontal view with inserted bar abutments. (d) Screwed-on adhesive bases.

OS Clear, R+K CAD/CAM Technologie GmbH & Co.KG, Berlin, Germany) (Organical® 3D Print X10 Dentalprinter, R+K CAD/CAM Technologie GmbH & Co.KG, Berlin, Germany) and an interim FPD made of PMMA (Organic PMMA eco A3, Organical Dental Implant, R+K CAD/CAM Technologie GmbH & Co.KG, Berlin, Germany) was milled (Organical® Desktop 8S COMPACT, R+K CAD/CAM Technologie GmbH & Co.KG) (Figure 5).

4.5. Implant Surgery. Using a silicone occlusion key (SHERA-DUETT-SOFT, SHERA Werkstoff-Technologie GmbH & Co.KG, Lemförde, Germany), the surgical template was placed in the patient and fixed in its definite position with anchor pins (Guided Anchor Pin, Nobel Biocare AG). For a flapless surgery, the mucous membrane was punched through the drill sleeves and removed. Afterwards, the implant bearings were reprocessed using 6-13 mm drill bits. For the correct transmission of the planned three-dimensional implant position, the implants (Guide Camlog®SL Promote plus, CAMLOG Vertriebs GmbH) were inserted using the torque wrench up to the marking of the rotation indicator on the drill sleeves. The bone quality corresponded to D2 and the implants performed primary stability (>35 Ncm). Immediate loading was therefore possible (Figure 6).

Abutments compensating for the implant angulation were connected to the implants (bar abutments, CAMLOG Vertriebs GmbH). A flexible handle (COMFOUR®, CAMLOG Vertriebs GmbH) was used to screw in the posterior implants (Figure 7).

4.6. Immediate Restoration. Titanium adhesive bases (titanium adhesive base for bar abutment, passive fit, Camlog, Wimsheim, Germany) were screwed onto the bar abutments. This resulted in an intraoral and tension-free bonding of the provisional FPD. The static and dynamic occlusion was checked and adjusted. The provisional FPD was then drained and cleaned using alcohol. Afterwards, the provisional FPD

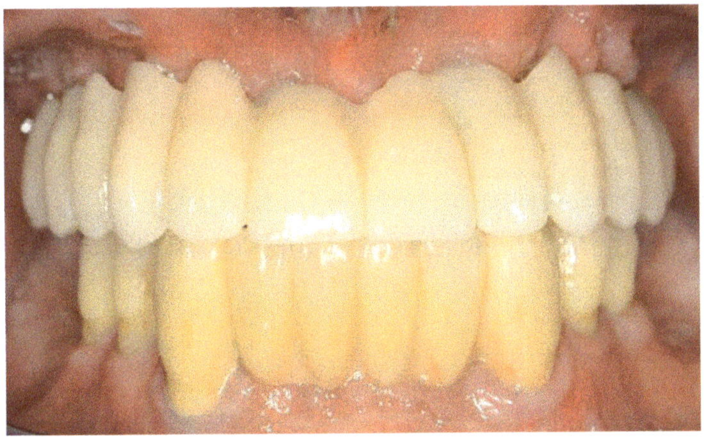

(a)

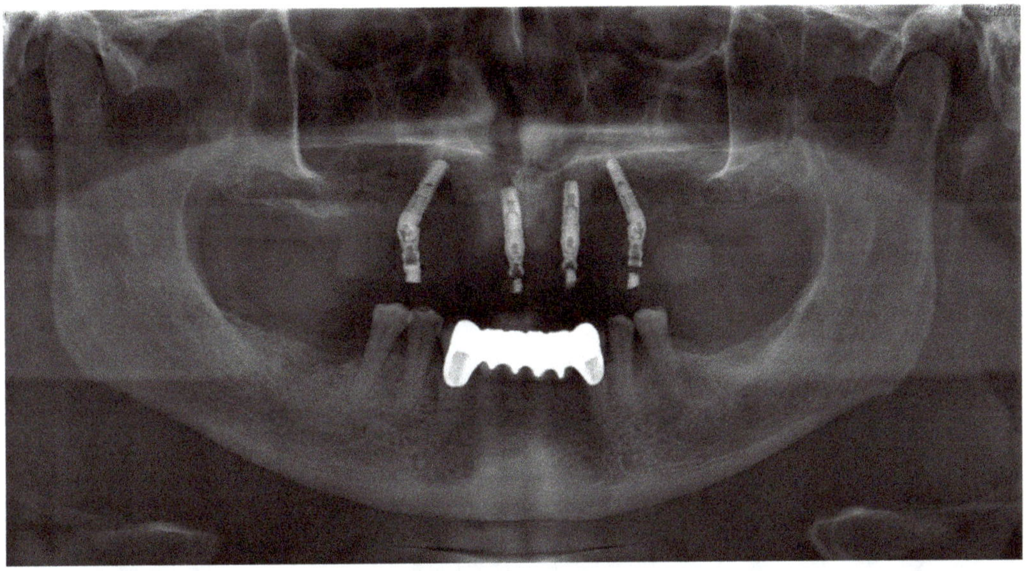

(b)

Figure 8: (a) Frontal view of the final inserted provisional FPD. (b) Orthopantomogram to control the implant position.

was bonded to the titanium adhesive bases (titanium adhesive base for bar abutment, passive fit, camlog) using autopolymerizing prosthesis repair resin (Qu resin, bredent GmbH & Co.KG, Senden, Germany).

The basal surface of the interim FPD was elaborated and polished, and then, the interim FPD was tightened to the implants at 15 Ncm and the occlusion finally checked. The screw channels were closed with foam pellets and a gypsum-based sealing material (Cavit™, 3M Deutschland GmbH, Seefeld, Germany), and a postoperative orthopantomogram was then performed (Figure 8).

5. The 2nd Treatment Phase (Figure 9)

5.1. Abutment Scan. After a six-month implant healing period, the interim FPD had to be replaced by a definitive screw-retained FPD. For this purpose, the occlusion of the existing interim situation and the maxillomandibular relationship were reevaluated.

A digital maxillomandibular relation record was made with the interim restoration in place using an intraoral scanner (Trios 3 intraoral scanner, 3Shape A/S). Then, the interim FPD was unscrewed in order to scan the bar abutments screwed onto the implants and the adjacent soft tissues. After the scan was completed, the provisional FPD was screwed back on.

5.2. Abutment Check. The STL scan data were sent to the dental laboratory for further processing. In the dental laboratory, the existing planning data record is matched with the new maxillomandibular relation record scan and the abutment and soft tissue scan. The incisive papilla, palatine raphe, and palatine rugae served as points of reference for matching the scans. As a result, changes in the jaw relation and soft tissue, as well as minimal positional deviations of the abutments, can be transferred to the definitive FPD (Figure 10).

The cobalt-chromium alloy (CoCrMo) FPD framework (Organic CoCr, Organical Dental Implant, R+K CAD/CAM Technologie GmbH & Co.KG, Berlin, Germany) was designed in accordance with the generated data set (exocad DentalCAD, R+K CAD/CAM Technologie GmbH & Co.KG) and subsequently milled (Organical® 5x dental milling

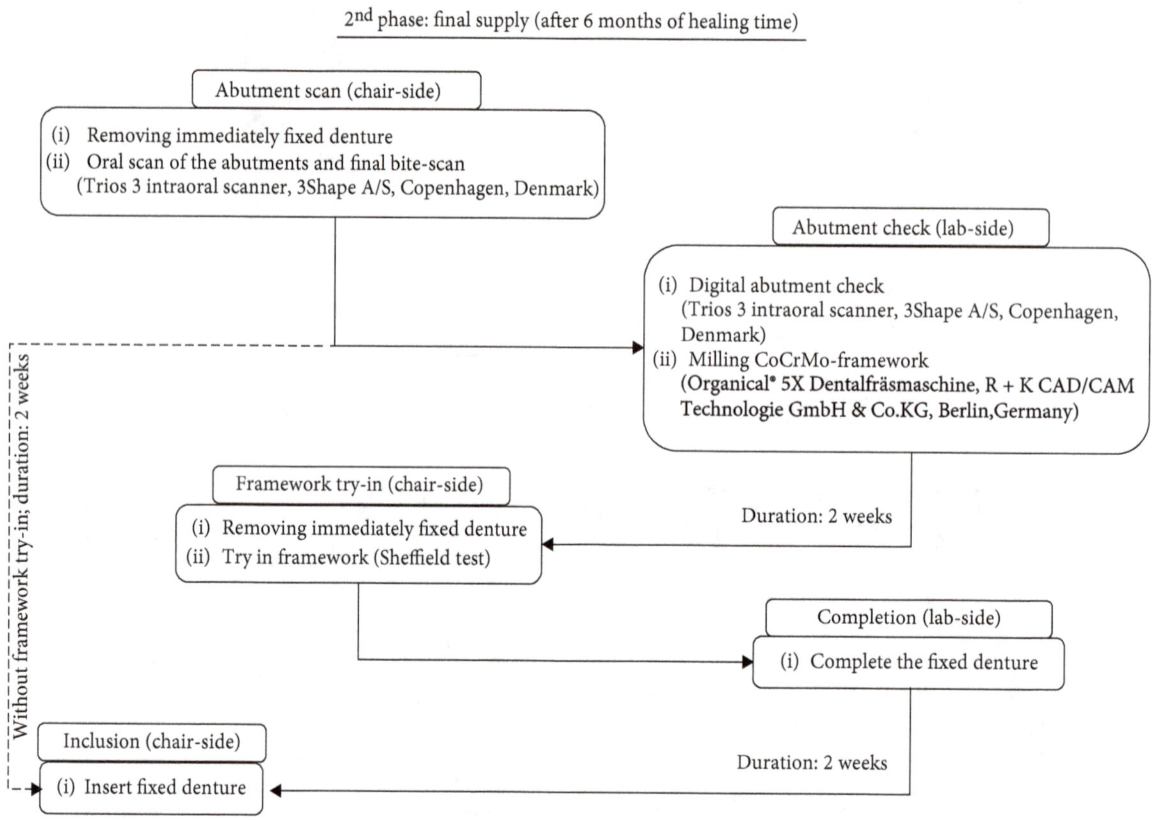

FIGURE 9: Overview of the 2nd treatment phase.

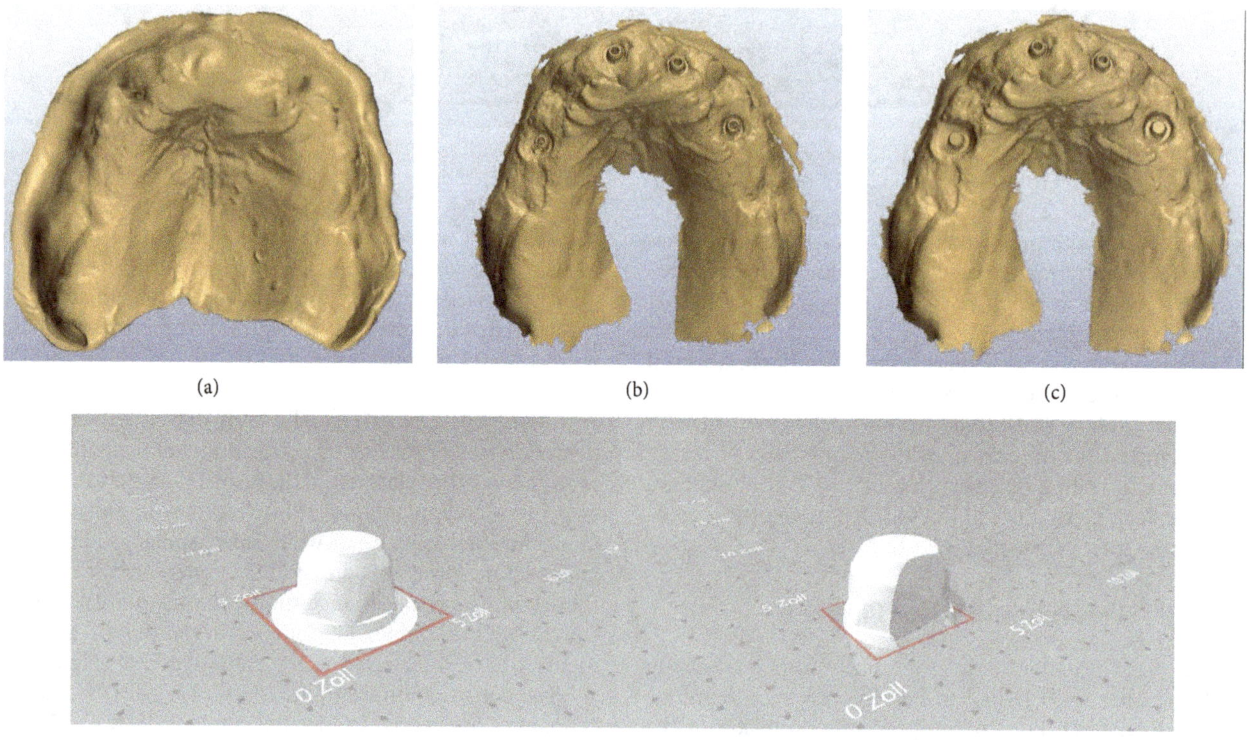

FIGURE 10: (a) Axial view of the modified upper jaw base initial scan. (b) Axial view of the scanned bar abutments. (c) Axial view of the matched scans. (d) For digital abutment check, the shape of the bar abutments stored in CAD software.

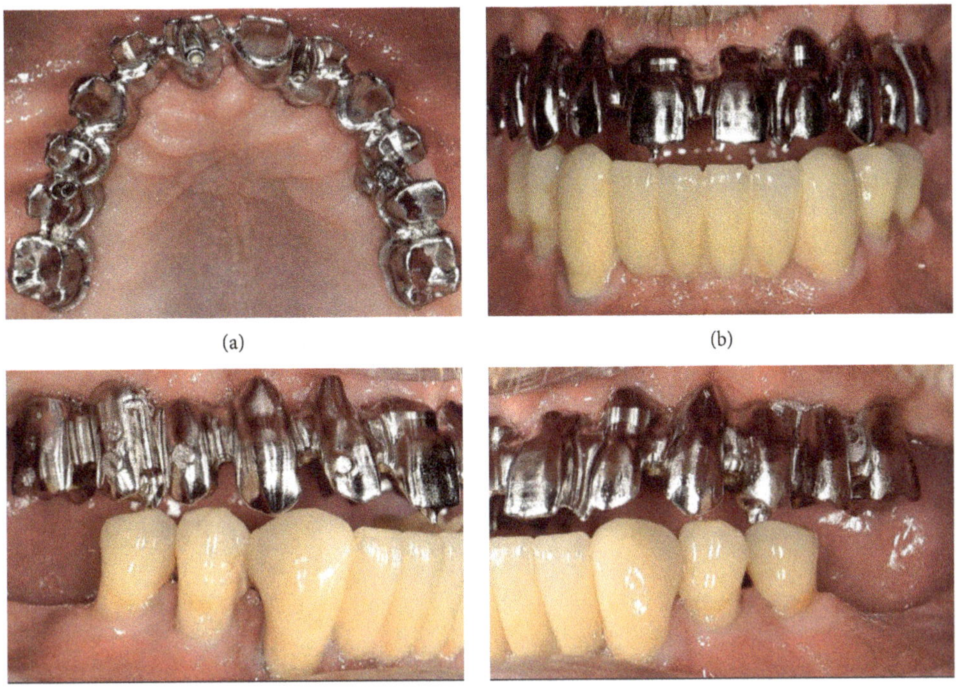

(a) (b) (c) (d)

FIGURE 11: (a) Axial view of the CoCrMo framework. (b) Frontal view of the CoCrMo framework. (c) Right view of the CoCrMo framework. (d) Left view of the CoCrMo framework.

machine, R+K CAD/CAM Technologie GmbH & Co.KG, Berlin, Germany).

5.3. Framework Try-In. The interim FPD was unscrewed in order to try it in the definitive FPD framework and to check the passivity of fit using the Sheffield test [30]. In the present case, the FPD scaffold fitted without the need for any adjustment (Figure 11). The provisional FPD was then screwed back on, and the definitive FPD scaffold was sent to the dental laboratory for final veneering.

5.4. Completion and Inclusion of the FPD. The CoCrMo FPD framework was veneered individually in the laboratory using composite resin material (SR Chromasit, Ivoclar Vivadent, Schaan, Liechtenstein).

In the final treatment session, the provisional FPD was removed and the definitive and veneered FPD was screwed on with 15 Ncm. The fit of the FPD was optimal; the occlusion was checked and optimized with minimal grinding measures. Finally, the screw channels were covered with foam pellets and composite resin (CRB-Bonding, SHOFU INC., Kyoto, Japan; Tetric EvoFlow, Ivoclar Vivadent, Schaan, Liechtenstein) (Figure 12). The final orthopantomogram was performed (Figure 13).

6. Conclusion

The present case report demonstrates the effective use of the available modern digital manufacturing processes in dentistry. The treatment procedure integrated consequent digital backward planning, fully navigated implantation, and completely digital dental prosthesis production. The procedure described here is in contrast to most of the other All-on-X concepts, which do not involve purely digital processes [6, 7, 12–14].

As conventional impressions could be avoided completely in this workflow, the number of individual treatment sessions (session for maxillomandibular relationship record and try-in) and individual session time could be significantly shortened. For example, the entire surgical procedure up to the installation of the provisional FPD could be carried out by an experienced practitioner in about 75 minutes. The relatively short duration of treatment in combination with a minimally invasive procedure lowers the risk of postoperative complaints such as swelling and pain [8, 17].

The key innovation of this case report is the digital abutment check, which is carried out directly using an intraoral scanner without screwed-in scan-bodies. This is possible because the exact geometry of the bar abutments is stored in the CAD software databases (Organical® Dental Implant, R+K CAD/CAM Technologie GmbH & Co.KG). The direct scan of the bar abutments without the use of scan-bodies again offers advantages in terms of digital impression precision. Possible errors due to incorrect positioning of the scan-body on the implants can thus be excluded [27–29]. Ultimately, this in turn influences the exact fit of the final FPD.

In the present case report, an indication-oriented application of both 3D printing methods and CAM milling methods is also demonstrated. Nowadays, surgical templates can be printed with a clinically acceptable fit [31, 32]. If anchor pins have to be used, the 3D printing process is ideal when compared to milling because even with the most

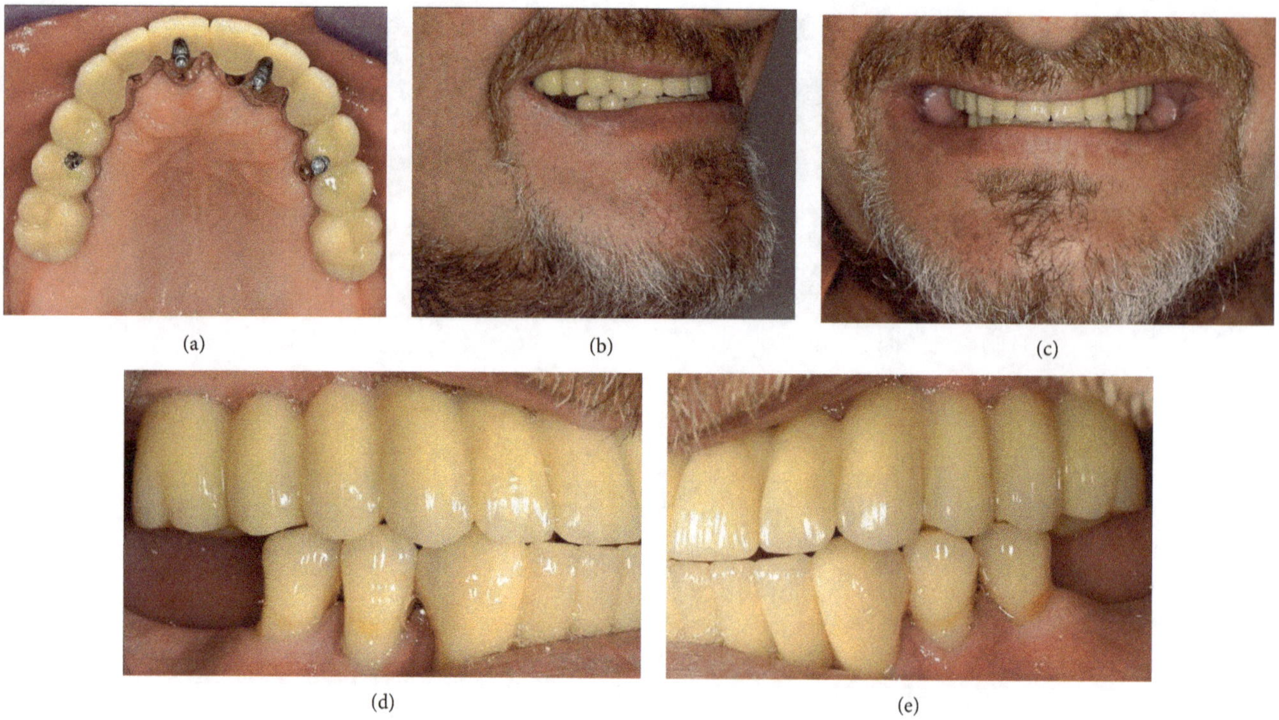

FIGURE 12: (a) Axial view of the definitive FDP. (b) Right view of the patient smile. (c) Frontal view of the patient smile. (d) Right view of the definitive FDP. (e) Left view of the definitive FPD.

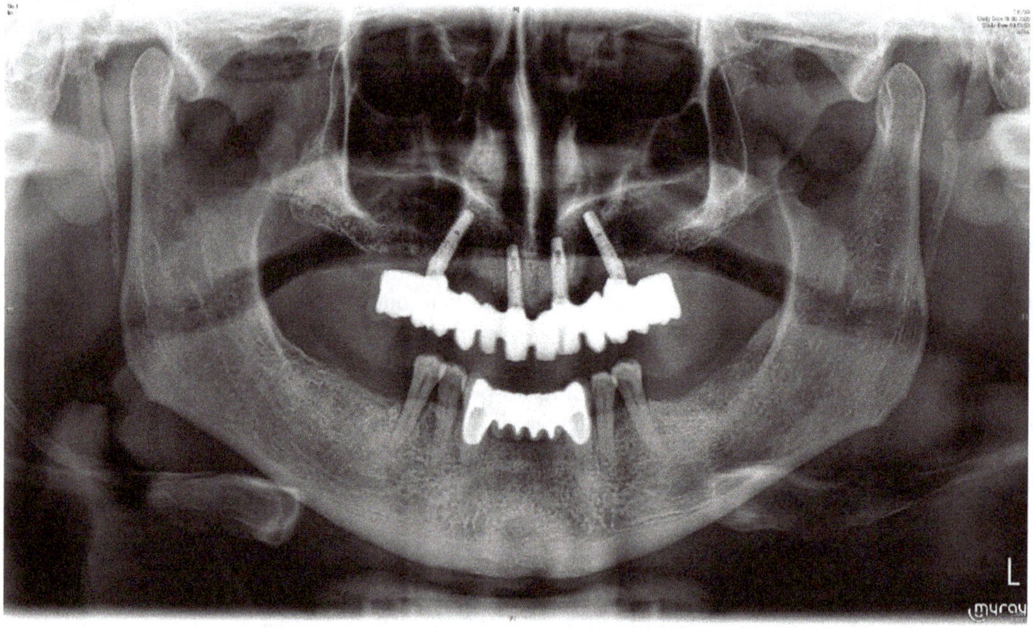

FIGURE 13: Orthopantomogram to control the definitive FDP.

modern 5-axis milling machines, the tool angle is limited. With 3D printing, the drilling channels for the anchor pins, which are often at an angle of 90° to the actual machining axis, can be more easily realized. The printing material, like the milling material, offers the possibility of sterilization before insertion in the patient during the surgery. The ability to sterilize any used dental laboratory materials in order to avoid the chain of infection during the surgical treatment is essential and not just since the beginning of the COVID-19 pandemic situation [33].

The construction of the interim FPD is an additional advantage of the performed digital workflow. The interim FPD was deliberately manufactured using PMMA. In contrast to more stable materials like zirconium dioxide, PMMA offers potential material-specific benefits. These benefits result in the ability to check and adapt the maxillomandibular relationship during the provisional restoration phase. This means that the occlusion of the provisional PMMA-FPD could be either easily reduced by grinding or increased by adding self-curing resin material. The higher abrasiveness of the material offers some protection against overloading the implants during the healing process.

Finally, the definitive FPD may be veneered with ceramic instead of composite resin. In contrast, it is also possible to produce a fully anatomical milled FPD, which can be inserted as the definitive dental restoration. This procedure could avoid the previous scaffold try-in. In this case report, one of the objectives of the treatment procedure was that the denture should be easily repairable. Therefore, the veneering material chosen for the definitive FPD was composite resin. However, compared to ceramic veneering material, composite resin enables easier occlusal adaptation to the opposing jaw.

In contrast to a conventional treatment process, not only are sessions for the maxillomandibular relationship and possibly the scaffold try-in avoided, but the process described here also creates an accurate adjustment of the definitive restoration. The treatment concept shown in this present case report combines a safe and time-saving digital workflow with demanding, predictable therapy results. In addition, the surgical intervention was not a major burden for the patient. The enormous gain in quality of life exceeds the manageable treatment effort for the patient and is clearly in focus.

The patient's wish to switch from a removable complete denture to a fixed, palate-free prosthetic restoration could be fulfilled after three sessions following the end of the first treatment phase. In addition, both the original tooth position and aesthetics could be transferred to the provisional and definitive FPD, producing a harmonious appearance that was familiar to the patient.

References

[1] M. Howashi, Y. Tsukiyama, Y. Ayukawa et al., "Relationship between the CT value and cortical bone thickness at implant recipient sites and primary implant stability with comparison of different implant types," *Clinical Implant Dentistry and Related Research*, vol. 18, no. 1, pp. 107–116, 2016.

[2] P. Smitkarn, K. Subbalekha, N. Mattheos, and A. Pimkhaokham, "The accuracy of single-tooth implants placed using fully digital-guided surgery and freehand implant surgery," *Journal of Clinical Periodontology*, vol. 46, no. 9, pp. 949–957, 2019.

[3] Z. Chen, J. Li, K. Sinjab, G. Mendonca, H. Yu, and H. L. Wang, "Accuracy of flapless immediate implant placement in anterior maxilla using computer-assisted versus freehand surgery: a cadaver study," *Clinical Oral Implants Research*, vol. 29, no. 12, pp. 1186–1194, 2018.

[4] W. Derksen, D. Wismeijer, T. Flügge, B. Hassan, and A. Tahmaseb, "The accuracy of computer-guided implant surgery with tooth-supported, digitally designed drill guides based on CBCT and intraoral scanning. A prospective cohort study," *Clinical Oral Implants Research*, vol. 30, no. 10, pp. 1005–1015, 2019.

[5] J. D'haese, J. Ackhurst, D. Wismeijer, H. De Bruyn, and A. Tahmaseb, "Current state of the art of computer-guided implant surgery," *Periodontology 2000*, vol. 73, no. 1, pp. 121–133, 2017.

[6] P. Maló, M. A. Nobre, A. Lopes, A. Ferro, and M. Nunes, "The All-on-4 concept for full-arch rehabilitation of the edentulous maxillae: a longitudinal study with 5-13 years of follow-up," *Clinical Implant Dentistry and Related Research*, vol. 21, no. 4, pp. 538–549, 2019.

[7] P. Malo, M. de Araujo Nobre, and A. Lopes, "The use of computer-guided flapless implant surgery and four implants placed in immediate function to support a fixed denture: preliminary results after a mean follow-up period of thirteen months," *The Journal of Prosthetic Dentistry*, vol. 97, no. 6, pp. S26–S34, 2007.

[8] I. Laleman, L. Bernard, M. Vercruyssen, R. Jacobs, M. M. Bornstein, and M. Quirynen, "Guided implant surgery in the edentulous maxilla: a systematic review," *International Journal of Oral & Maxillofacial implants*, vol. 31, pp. 103–117, 2016.

[9] K. T. Simpson, M. Bryington, M. Agusto, M. Harper, A. Salman, and G. P. Schincaglia, "Computer-guided surgery using Human Allogenic Bone ring with simultaneous implant placement: a case report," *Clinical Advances in Periodontics*, vol. 10, no. 1, pp. 16–22, 2020.

[10] T. Schelbert, T. Gander, M. Blumer, R. Jung, M. Rücker, and C. Rostetter, "Accuracy of computer-guided template-based implant Surgery," *Implant Dentistry*, vol. 28, no. 6, pp. 556–563, 2019.

[11] M. Colombo, C. Mangano, E. Mijiritsky, M. Krebs, U. Hauschild, and T. Fortin, "Clinical applications and effectiveness of guided implant surgery: a critical review based on randomized controlled trials," *BMC Oral Health*, vol. 17, no. 1, p. 150, 2017.

[12] P. Maló, M. de Araújo Nobre, C. Moura Guedes et al., "Short-term report of an ongoing prospective cohort study evaluating the outcome of full-arch implant-supported fixed hybrid polyetheretherketone-acrylic resin prostheses and the All-on-four concept," *Clinical Implant Dentistry and Related Research*, vol. 20, no. 5, pp. 692–702, 2018.

[13] A. Lopes, P. Maló, M. de Araújo Nobre, E. Sánchez-Fernández, and I. Gravito, "The NobelGuide®All-on-4®treatment concept for rehabilitation of edentulous jaws: a retrospective report on the 7-years clinical and 5-years radiographic outcomes," *Clinical Implant Dentistry and Related Research*, vol. 19, no. 2, pp. 233–244, 2017.

[14] A. Lopes, P. Maló, M. de Araújo Nobre, and E. Sanchez-Fernández, "The NobelGuide® All-on-4® treatment concept for rehabilitation of edentulous jaws: a prospective report on medium-and long-term outcomes," *Clinical Implant Dentistry and Related Research*, vol. 17, pp. e406–e416, 2015.

[15] A. M. Albiero, L. Quartuccio, A. Benato, and R. Benato, "Accuracy of computer-guided flapless implant surgery in fully edentulous arches and in edentulous arches with fresh extraction sockets," *Implant Dentistry*, vol. 28, no. 3, pp. 256–264, 2019.

[16] L. Gillot, B. Cannas, B. Friberg, L. Vrielinck, D. Rohner, and A. Pettersson, "Accuracy of virtually planned and conventionally placed implants in edentulous cadaver maxillae and mandibles: a preliminary report," *The Journal of Prosthetic Dentistry*, vol. 112, no. 4, pp. 798–804, 2014.

[17] T. Joda, W. Derksen, J. G. Wittneben, and S. Kuehl, "Static computer-aided implant surgery (s-CAIS) analysing patient-reported outcome measures (PROMs), economics and surgical

complications: a systematic review," *Clinical Oral Implants Research*, vol. 29, no. S16, pp. 359–373, 2018.

[18] E. Varga, M. Antal, L. Major, R. Kiscsatári, G. Braunitzer, and J. Piffkó, "Guidance means accuracy: a randomized clinical trial on freehand versus guided dental implantation," *Clinical Oral Implants Research*, vol. 31, no. 5, pp. 417–430, 2020.

[19] C. A. Aydemir and V. Arısan, "Accuracy of dental implant placement via dynamic navigation or the freehand method: a split-mouth randomized controlled clinical trial," *Clinical Oral Implants Research*, vol. 31, no. 3, pp. 255–263, 2019.

[20] A. Mediavilla Guzmán, E. Riad Deglow, Á. Zubizarreta-Macho, R. Agustín-Panadero, and S. Hernández Montero, "Accuracy of computer-aided dynamic navigation compared to computer-aided static navigation for dental implant placement: an in vitro study," *Journal of Clinical Medicine*, vol. 8, no. 12, p. 2123, 2019.

[21] K. El Kholy, S. F. M. Janner, M. Schimmel, and D. Buser, "The influence of guided sleeve height, drilling distance, and drilling key length on the accuracy of static computer-assisted implant surgery," *Clinical Implant Dentistry and Related Research*, vol. 21, no. 1, pp. 101–107, 2019.

[22] K. El Kholy, R. Lazarin, S. F. M. Janner, K. Faerber, R. Buser, and D. Buser, "Influence of surgical guide support and implant site location on accuracy of static computer-assisted implant surgery," *Clinical Oral Implants Research*, vol. 30, no. 11, pp. 1067–1075, 2019.

[23] M. Tallarico, Y. J. Kim, F. Cocchi, M. Martinolli, and S. M. Meloni, "Accuracy of newly developed sleeve-designed templates for insertion of dental implants: a prospective multicenters clinical trial," *Clinical Implant Dentistry and Related Research*, vol. 21, no. 1, pp. 108–113, 2019.

[24] M. Tallarico, M. Martinolli, Y.-J. Kim et al., "Accuracy of computer-assisted template-based implant placement using two different surgical templates designed with or without metallic sleeves: a randomized controlled trial," *Dentistry Journal*, vol. 7, no. 2, p. 41, 2019.

[25] S. Kühl, M. Payer, N. U. Zitzmann, J. T. Lambrecht, and A. Filippi, "Technical accuracy of printed surgical templates for guided implant surgery with the coDiagnostiXTMSoftware," *Clinical Implant Dentistry and Related Research*, vol. 17, pp. e177–e182, 2015.

[26] P. Pesce, F. Pera, P. Setti, and M. Menini, "Precision and accuracy of a digital impression scanner in full-arch implant rehabilitation," *The International Journal of Prosthodontics*, vol. 31, no. 2, pp. 171–175, 2018.

[27] H. Skjerven, H. Olsen-Bergem, H. J. Rønold, U. H. Riis, and J. E. Ellingsen, "Comparison of postoperative intraoral scan versus cone beam computerised tomography to measure accuracy of guided implant placement-a prospective clinical study," *Clinical Oral Implants Research*, vol. 30, no. 6, pp. 531–541, 2019.

[28] S. W. Pyo, Y. J. Lim, K. T. Koo, and J. Lee, "Methods used to assess the 3D accuracy of dental implant positions in computer-guided implant placement: a review," *Journal of Clinical Medicine*, vol. 8, no. 1, p. 54, 2019.

[29] M. Stimmelmayr, K. Erdelt, J. F. Güth, A. Happe, and F. Beuer, "Evaluation of impression accuracy for a four-implant mandibular model—a digital approach," *Clinical Oral Investigations*, vol. 16, no. 4, pp. 1137–1142, 2012.

[30] E. Eisenmann, A. Mokabberi, M. H. Walter, and W. B. Freesmeyer, "Improving the fit of implant-supported superstructures using the spark erosion technique," *The International Journal of Oral & Maxillofacial Implants*, vol. 19, no. 6, pp. 810–818, 2004.

[31] L. Herschdorfer, W. M. Negreiros, G. O. Gallucci, and A. Hamilton, "Comparison of the accuracy of implants placed with CAD-CAM surgical templates manufactured with various 3D printers: an in vitro study," *The Journal of Prosthetic Dentistry*, vol. S0022-3913, no. 20, 2020.

[32] R. E. Matta, B. Bergauer, W. Adler, M. Wichmann, and H. J. Nickenig, "The impact of the fabrication method on the three-dimensional accuracy of an implant surgery template," *Journal of Cranio-Maxillo-Facial Surgery*, vol. 45, no. 6, pp. 804–808, 2017.

[33] S. Romano-Bertrand, L.-S. A. Glele, B. Grandbastien, and D. Lepelletier, "Preventing SARS-CoV-2 transmission in rehabilitation pools and therapeutic water environments," *The Journal of Hospital Infection*, vol. 105, no. 4, pp. 625–627, 2020.

28

Florid Cemento-Osseous Dysplasia-Associated Simple Bone Cyst Showing Marked Irregular Border and High Apparent Diffusion Coefficient Value

Ikuho Kojima[1], **Takashi Nishioka**[1], **Maya Sakamoto**[1], **Yuko Sai**[2], **Yushi Ezoe**[2], **Masahiro Iikubo**[1], **Hiroyuki Kumamoto**[3], **and Tetsu Takahashi**[2]

[1]*Division of Oral Diagnosis, Tohoku University Graduate School of Dentistry, 4-1 Seiryo-machi, Aoba-ku, Sendai, Miyagi 980-8575, Japan*
[2]*Division of Oral and Maxillofacial Surgery, Tohoku University Graduate School of Dentistry, 4-1 Seiryo-machi, Aoba-ku, Sendai, Miyagi 980-8575, Japan*
[3]*Division of Oral Pathology, Tohoku University Graduate School of Dentistry, 4-1 Seiryo-machi, Aoba-ku, Sendai, Miyagi 980-8575, Japan*

Correspondence should be addressed to Ikuho Kojima; ikh-koji213@dent.tohoku.ac.jp

Academic Editor: Sukumaran Anil

A simple bone cyst (SBC) is an intrabone cavity without epithelial lining, which occasionally occur with fibrous-osseous lesions. The imaging finding of the scalloped border and conserving the lamina dura, periodontal ligament spaces, or follicular spaces are considered radiographically pathognomonic of SBC. SBC has been reported to occur with fibrous-osseous lesions, including cemento-osseous dysplasia (COD). Computed tomography (CT) imaging findings are sparse, and there are no reports of magnetic resonance imaging (MRI) findings, including apparent diffusion coefficient (ADC) value calculated by diffusion-weighted MRI for the florid COD-associated SBC. We report a case of a 39-year-old woman who was referred to our hospital because a panoramic radiograph of her right mandible showed asymptomatic radiolucency in the apical molar area. CT images showed a low-density lesion in the periapical areas of the right mandible, which accompanied a well-defined, high-density lesion, and a mixed low/high-density lesion with an unusual marked irregular border in the left mandible. The MRI showed cyst-like extremely hyperintense signals on fat-suppressed T2-weighted images at the right mandibular low-density and the left mandibular mixed low/high-density areas. ADC map showed high values (over 2.5×10^{-3} mm^2/s) at the cystic areas in the bilateral mandible. We performed incisional biopsies of the bilateral mandibular lesions and resections of the bilateral maxillary lesions. Surgical and histopathological findings established a diagnosis of florid COD in the bilateral mandible and maxilla, simultaneously complicated by multiple SBCs in the bilateral mandible. The ADC value of cystic component is useful for the diagnosis, if the COD-associated SBC exhibits solitary, nonspecific, or rare imaging findings.

1. Introduction

A simple bone cyst (SBC) is a pseudocyst, which is diagnosed based on the finding of an intrabone cavity without epithelial lining [1]. SBC appears as a well-defined cystic lesion with thin sclerotic borders or an ill-defined cystic lesion on the panoramic radiograph. In the jaws, the imaging appearances of the scalloped border and conserving the lamina dura, periodontal ligament spaces, or follicular spaces are considered radiographically pathognomonic of SBC [2]. SBCs are often found incidentally in young patients and resolve spontaneously after aspiration of the cavity or surgical biopsy without curettage [1, 3]. Interestingly, SBC has been reported to occur with fibrous-osseous lesions, including cemento-osseous dysplasia (COD) [4–8]. Although the radiologic features of SBC or COD, including computed tomography (CT) imaging findings, are well described, those of florid COD-associated SBC are sparse. Moreover, differentiation of SBC from other

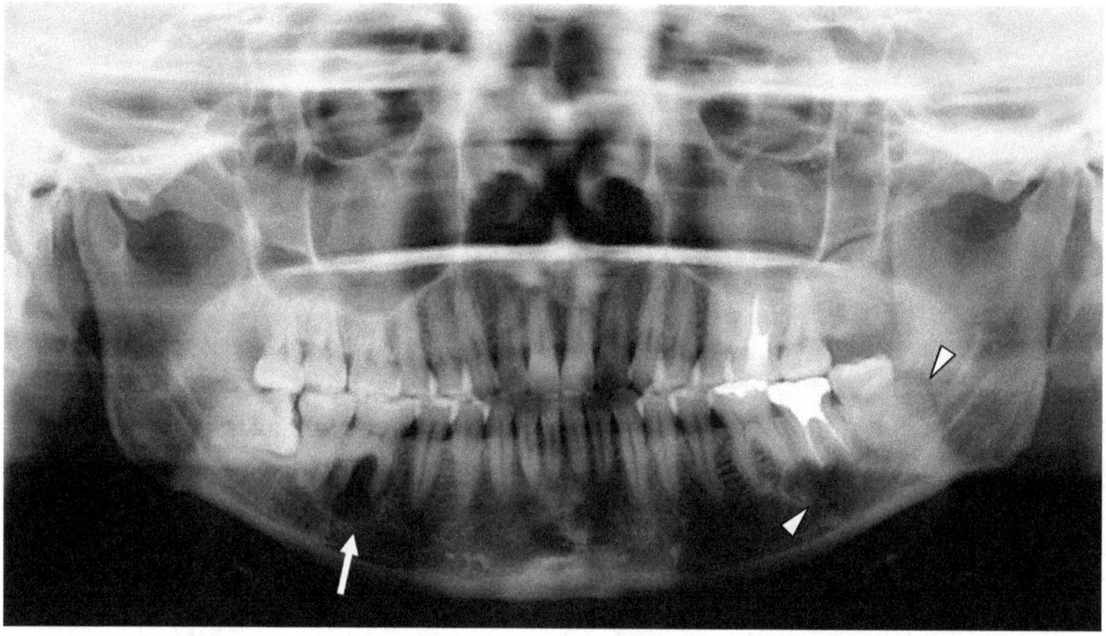

Figure 1: Panoramic X-ray radiogram. Radiolucent lesions are seen in the right mandible (*arrow*). The high-density lesion is complicated by the periapical right mandibular 2nd molar. Additionally, mixed radiolucent/radiopaque lesion was shown in the left molar region (*arrowheads*).

cystic lesions may be difficult when these lesions appear with nonspecific cystic or unusual imaging appearance. Magnetic resonance imaging (MRI) features of SBC are previously reported using apparent diffusion coefficient (ADC) calculated by diffusion-weighted MRI (DW-MRI) [9–11]. However, there are no reports of MRI findings for COD-associated multiple SBCs. The differential diagnosis is difficult, if the COD-associated SBC exhibits solitary, nonspecific, or rare imaging findings. The purpose of this report was to describe the findings of a panoramic radiograph, CT, MRI, and bone scintigram of florid COD-associated SBCs adjacent to radiopaque bone/cementum-density masses in multiquadrant periapical regions.

2. Case Presentation

This case report was approved by our institutional ethics committee (No. 18651). All procedures followed were in accordance with the ethical standards of the responsible committee on human experimentation (institutional and national) and with the Helsinki Declaration of 1975, as revised in 2008. Informed consent was obtained from the patient for being included in the study.

2.1. Patient. A 39-year-old woman had asymptomatic radiolucency of the right mandible on X-ray radiographic examination for caries treatment at a primary dental office. She was referred to our hospital for further radiographic examination and treatment of the lesion. Her medical history revealed postoperative uterine cervical cancer. She had no significant family history. Clinical findings of extra- and intraoral appearances were unremarkable.

2.2. Imaging Findings. Panoramic X-ray radiograph showed radiolucency in the apical region of the vital right lower 1st molar. Mixed radiolucent/radiopaque lesion was shown in the left molar region (Figure 1). CT findings showed multiple low- or high-density lesions in the bilateral mandible and additional high-density lesions in the bilateral maxilla. The right mandibular lesion showed a well-defined low-density lesion with scalloped border in the periapical areas of the right lower 1st molar, which accompanied a well-defined high-density lesion in the adjacent 2nd molar periapical area (Figures 2(a) and 2(b)). The left lesion presented mixed low/-high-density lesion with an unusual, marked irregular border that was more irregular than the scalloped border in the molar region (Figures 2(a) and 2(b)). Both these lesions showed erosion of the cortical bone. Additional high-density lesions were observed in the left 3rd molar and right lateral incisor areas of the maxilla, which were well-defined (Figures 2(c) and 2(d)). No demonstrable finding of root resorption was detected on CT. The MRI showed cyst-like extremely hyperintense signals on fat-suppressed T2-weighted images and thin peripheral enhancement on contrast-enhanced T1-weighted images at the right low-density areas (Figures 3(a) and 3(b)). Hyperintense signals on fat-suppressed T2-weighted image and heterogeneous enhancement on contrast-enhanced T1-weighted image were shown in the adjacent 2nd molar peripheral area of the right high-density lesion (Figures 3(a) and 3(b)). For left mandibular mixed low/high-density lesion on CT finding, MRI showed marked irregular cystic/fluid-collected lesion that was hyperintense signals on fat-suppressed T2-weighted image and thin peripheral enhancement on contrast-enhanced T1-weighted image (Figures 3(a) and 3(b)). No demonstrable findings were found about the high-density

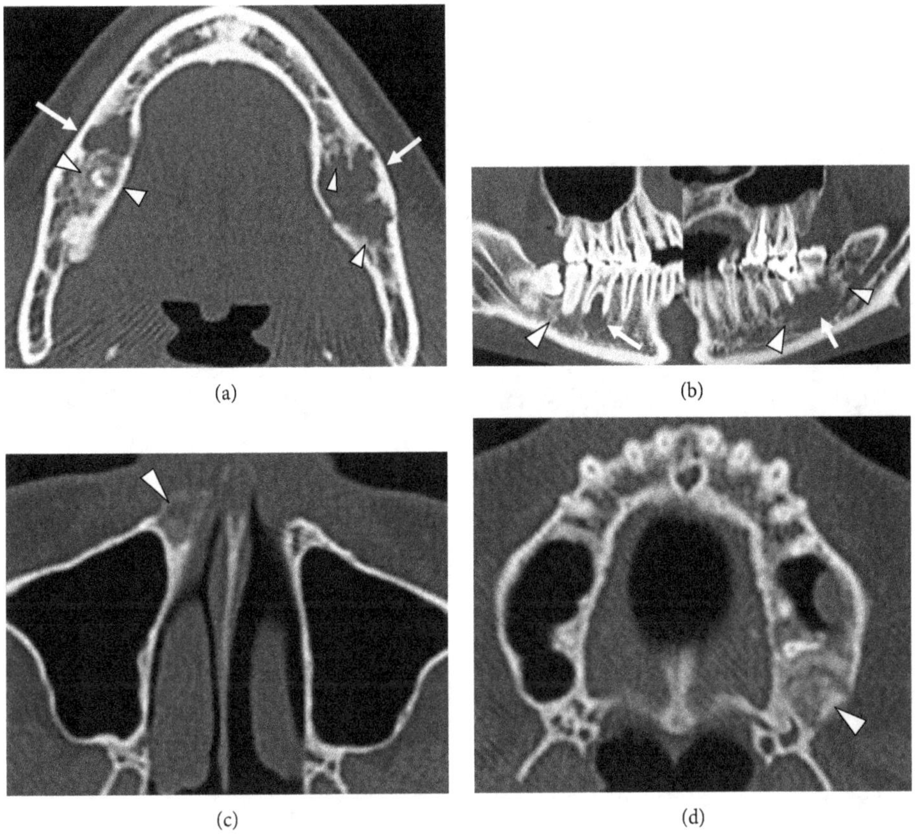

FIGURE 2: CT images. (a, b) Well-defined, low-density lesions (*arrows*) with scalloped border, which accompanies a well-defined high-density appearance (*arrowheads*) are observed in the right mandibular molars on transverse and sagittal images. The left lesion shows mixed main low- (*arrows*) and partial high- (*arrowheads*) density areas with an unusual, marked irregular border in the molar region. The right lesion shows a unilocular, slightly irregular border. (c, d) Transverse CT images show high-density lesions in the right anterior and left posterior maxilla (*arrowheads*). CT: computed tomography.

area in the left mandible, which may be due to metal artifact on MRI. Although no hyperintense signals were found on DW-MRI, ADC showed high values (over 2.5×10^{-3} mm^2/s) at cystic areas in the bilateral mandible (Figure 3(c)). Compared to the CT findings, bone scintigram results showed high tracer uptake in the high-density lesions (Figure 4).

2.3. Clinical Diagnosis. We diagnosed this case as a florid COD-associated SBC based on the plural cystic lesions showing high ADC value with multiquadrant fibrous lesions.

2.4. Treatment and Prognosis. Incisional biopsies of the bilateral mandibular lesions and resection of the bilateral maxillary lesions were performed. Gross examination revealed a mixture of tiny bone-like material within an empty cavity bone in the bilateral mandible. The high-density lesions that resembled bone-like structures were easily removed. Histopathological examination of the tissue specimens was performed. The histopathological findings showed multiple irregular pieces of fibrous connective tissue adjacent to the woven bone trabeculae with an osteoid rim-like border and prominent osteoblasts (Figure 5(a)). Histological examination of the bilateral mandibular specimens of the peripheral low-density lesions showed remnants of a partial bony cavity lined by slightly thin connective tissue. There was no epithelium component in the tissue (Figure 5(b)). Both surgical and histopathological findings matched the diagnosis of a florid COD, which were simultaneously complicated by multiple SBCs.

According to the standard treatment protocol for each of the two lesions, we longitudinally followed up the mandibular lesions after the biopsy by routine imaging examination. A posterior half area in the mixed low/high-density lesion of the left mandible and resected cavities of the bilateral maxilla gradually decreased in size with bone formation. In contrast, twenty-seven months after the biopsy, a follow-up CT showed that an anterior half area in the left mandibular lesion enlarged and changed to multilocular shape. The unilocular, slightly irregular border, low-density lesion of the right mandible, also enlarged with bone expansion (Figure 6). Since then, we have continuously followed up this patient.

3. Discussion

The CT findings of our patient showed low-density lesions next to the high-density lesion of the periapical areas in the right mandibular molars and mixed low/high-density lesion in the left mandibular molars; these lesions had an irregular

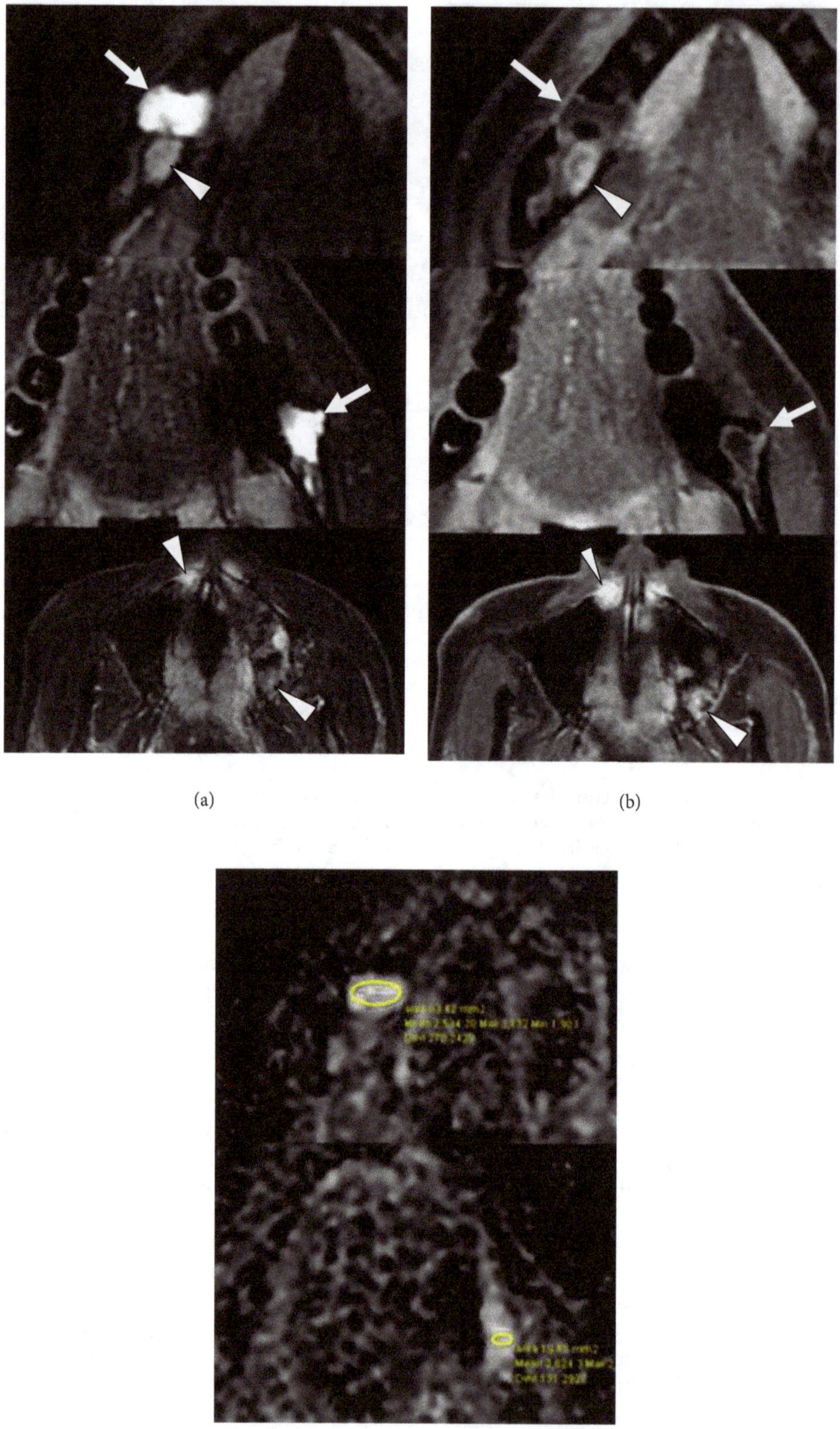

(a) (b) (c)

Figure 3: Magnetic resonance images. (a) Transverse fat-suppressed T2-weighted images show extremely hyperintense signal areas in the bilateral mandible (*arrows*) and hyperintense signal areas in the right mandible and bilateral maxilla (*arrowheads*). (b) Contrast-enhanced T1-weighted images show thin, peripherally enhanced lesions in the bilateral mandible (*arrows*) and heterogeneously enhanced lesions in the right mandible and bilateral maxilla (*arrowheads*). (c) The ADC maps show extremely high ADC values (over 2.5×10^{-3} mm^2/s) at cystic areas in the bilateral mandible. ADC: apparent diffusion coefficient.

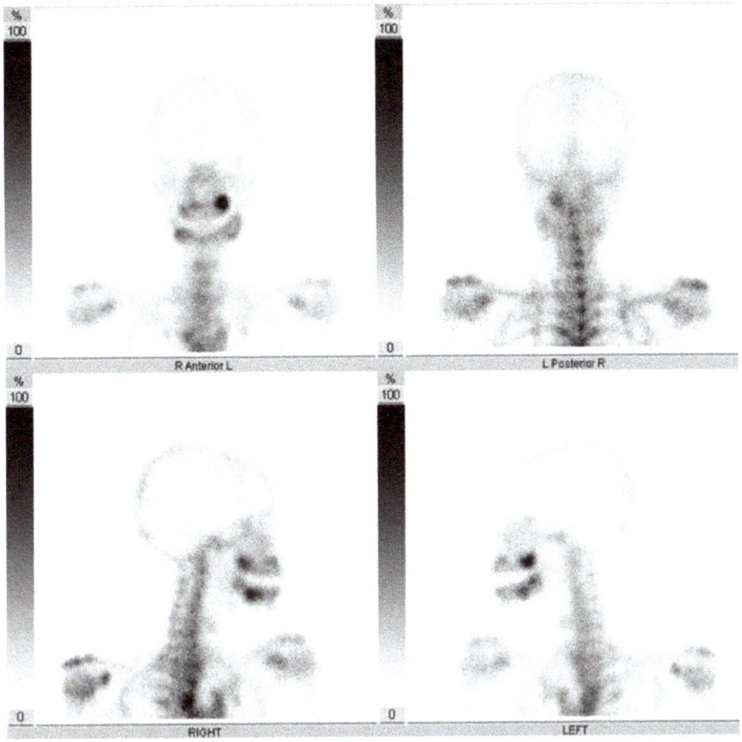

Figure 4: Bone scintigram. Tracer accumulations are observed in the high-density lesion on CT finding of the mandible and maxilla.

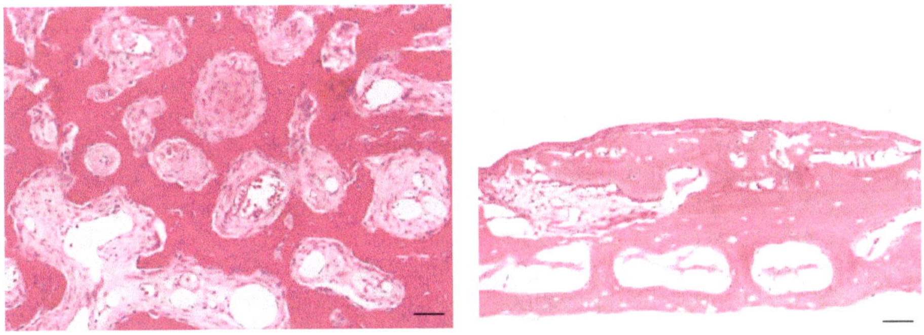

(a) (b)

Figure 5: Histopathological findings (original magnification, ×100). (a) Specimens of the high-density lesions comprised irregular piece of fibrous connective tissue adjacent to the woven bone trabecula, which had an osteoid rim-like border and prominent osteoblasts. Bar: 100 μm. (b) Specimens of the bilateral mandibular low-density lesions exhibited remnants of a partial bony cavity lined by slightly compressed connective tissue. Bar: 100 μm.

border, cortical bone erosion, and loss of the lamina dura. In particular, the appearance of a marked, irregular border in the left mandibular lesion on CT image was rare for the patient with SBC [2, 3]. If the left mandibular lesion presented solitary mixed low/high-density with an irregular border, desmoplastic ameloblastoma should be considered a first differential diagnosis. There are no reports of MRI findings for COD-associated multiple SBCs. We could diagnose this case as a florid COD-associated SBCs based on the plural high ADC cystic lesions, which suggested SBC with multi-quadrant fibrous lesions. Eida et al. [10] reported the efficacy of the ADC value of the cystic component on DW-MRI for differentiation of odontogenic lesion and demonstrated SBC and ameloblastoma had a high ADC value. Desmoplastic ameloblastoma that presented mixed radiolucent-radiopaque appearance with ill-defined borders has been radiographically reported in many cases [12–14]. Although ameloblastoma showed high ADC value in previous reports [10, 11, 15, 16], there is no report on the ADC of the desmoplastic variant. Therefore, desmoplastic ameloblastoma might be considered a differential diagnosis, if a solitary lesion. The imaging finding of bone scintigraphy showed tracer accumulations in the high-density lesion of CT finding of the mandible and maxilla. This finding was nonspecific and consistent with previously published reports [17, 18]. In this report, we have presented the case of a patient with

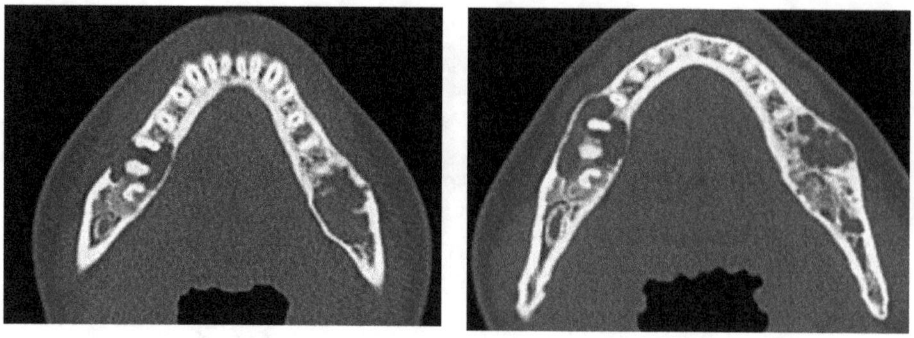

(a) (b)

FIGURE 6: Follow-up CT images. (a) Three months and (b) twenty-seven months after the incisional biopsy; the CT images indicate enlargement of the right and an anterior half area of the left low-density lesions. CT: computed tomography.

florid COD-associated SBCs diagnosed by the imaging finding of plural cystic lesion exhibiting high ADC value with multiquadrant high-density lesions.

Follow-up CT images obtained twenty-seven months after the incisional biopsy indicated that part of the lesions seen previously had gradual regression with bone formation. On the contrary, the bilateral SBCs showed enlargement in size and changed to marked multilocular low-density lesions with bone expansion after the biopsy. Suei et al. [3] retrospectively reviewed 108 cases of solitary SBC from the literature and thirty-one of their cases and demonstrated that the SBCs with multiple, scalloped borders, bone expansion, root resorption, a radiopaque mass including fibrous-osseous lesions, or loss of the lamina dura had a higher recurrence rate (enlargement after surgery including only curettage and exploration of the intrabone cavity wall) than the lesion with smooth borders, no bone expansion, and intact lamina dura. On the other hand, no histopathological analysis has been studied on the recurrence rate of SBCs. Matsumura et al. [19] reviewed the correlation between histopathological and radiological findings of fifty-three cases of SBCs and demonstrated that many SBCs radiographically presenting bone expansion and radiopaque finding had histopthologically thickened wall with dysplastic bone formation. Recurrent SBCs might have a varying degree of osteoblastic change irrespective of the presence or absence of the radiopaque masses. Taking these reports into account, therefore, the marked irregular border on CT images of our case may reflect heterogeneous fibrous-osseous changes in the lesion's peripheral margin. We cannot precisely analyze the histopathological finding, and no other demonstrable finding of MRI was found for the irregular border in the recurrence. In the future, histopathological analysis or MRI finding review of the irregular border might be expected to explain the mechanism of recurrence and contribute to treatment decisions.

Some previous reports assessed the subject population, age distribution, and anatomical distribution of patients with SBC. In one of the previous reports which had the largest number of cases, 87% (20/23) of COD-associated SBCs occurred in women with a mean age in the 40s, and the majority (95.7%) of the cases occurred in the mandibular molar area [8]. In contrast, solitary SBCs were found in equal numbers in both sexes in their second decade of life and typically occurred in the anterior mandible [5–8]. These differences may be related to the pathogenesis of the disease. Chadwick et al. [8] discussed that solitary and COD-associated SBCs might be the same lesion but arising as separate lesions owing to different biological circumstances such as differences in the mean age, sex ratio, and anatomical distribution. They hypothesized that in adolescents, disturbance of normal osteoblast and osteoclast activity may depend on a new and constantly changing biomechanical property of the mandible during growth and development. This indicates that bone cells, especially the osteoblasts, could not satisfy these demands. In contrast, in patients with full skeletal maturity, and especially in women with a significantly higher incidence of COD-associated SBCs, the occurrence of SBCs might indicate differential activity in the normal bone cells because of different underlying reasons. Bones of middle-aged women with possible osteoporosis are more likely to have low or insufficient osteoblast numbers. If this hypothesis is credible, COD-associated SBC caused by osteoporosis in middle-aged women is likely to have a high recurrence rate regardless of imaging findings. The histopathological analysis is expected as evidence.

4. Conclusion

We have reported an interesting case of florid COD-associated multiple SBCs, which showed a rare CT finding of mixed low/high-density with the marked irregular border and high ADC values of cystic components on MRI. The ADC value of cystic component is useful for the diagnosis, if the COD-associated SBC exhibits solitary, nonspecific, or rare imaging findings.

Consent

Informed consent was obtained from the patient for being included in the study.

Acknowledgments

This study was supported in part by the Japan Society for the Promotion of Science (JSPS) Grants-in-Aid for Scientific Research [Grant number 18K09804]. We would like to thank Editage (http://www.editage.com) for English language editing.

References

[1] P. J. Chapman and K. Romaniuk, "Traumatic bone cyst of the mandible; regression following aspiration," *International Journal of Oral Surgery*, vol. 14, no. 3, pp. 290–294, 1985.

[2] M. J. Paroah, "Cysts and cyst-like lesions of the jaws," in *Oral Radiology: Principles and Interpretation*, S. C. White and M. Paroah, Eds., pp. 361–364, Mosby, Philadelphia, PA, 2009.

[3] Y. Suei, A. Taguchi, T. Nagasaki, and K. Tanimoto, "Radiographic findings and prognosis of simple bone cysts of the jaws," *Dento Maxillo Facial Radiology*, vol. 39, no. 2, pp. 65–72, 2010.

[4] R. J. Melrose, A. M. Abrams, and B. G. Mills, "Florid osseous dysplasia," *Oral Surgery, Oral Medicine, and Oral Pathology*, vol. 41, no. 1, pp. 62–82, 1976.

[5] M. Miyauchi, I. Ogawa, T. Takata et al., "Florid cemento-osseous dysplasia with concomitant simple bone cysts: a case in a Japanese woman," *Journal of Oral Pathology & Medicine*, vol. 24, no. 6, pp. 285–287, 1995.

[6] M. Mupparapu, S. R. Singer, M. Milles, and J. Rinaggio, "Simultaneous presentation of focal cemento-osseous dysplasia and simple bone cyst of the mandible masquerading as a multilocular radiolucency," *Dento Maxillo Facial Radiology*, vol. 34, no. 1, pp. 39–43, 2005.

[7] K. A. Rao, S. R. Shetty, S. G. Babu, and R. L. Castelino, "Co-occurrence of florid cemento-osseous dysplasia and simple bone cyst: a case report," *Journal of Oral & Maxillofacial Research: JOMR*, vol. 2, no. 3, article e5, 2011.

[8] J. W. Chadwick, N. A. Alsufyani, and E. W. Lam, "Clinical and radiographic features of solitary and cemento-osseous dysplasia-associated simple bone cysts," *Dento Maxillo Facial Radiology*, vol. 40, no. 4, pp. 230–235, 2011.

[9] Y. Yanagi, J. I. Asaumi, T. Unetsubo et al., "Usefulness of MRI and dynamic contrast-enhanced MRI for differential diagnosis of simple bone cysts from true cysts in the jaw," *Oral Surgery, Oral Medicine, Oral Pathology, Oral Radiology, and Endodontics*, vol. 110, no. 3, pp. 364–369, 2010.

[10] S. Eida, Y. Hotokezaka, I. Katayama et al., "Apparent diffusion coefficient-based differentiation of cystic lesions of the mandible," *Oral Radiology*, vol. 28, no. 2, pp. 109–114, 2012.

[11] K. Srinivasan, A. Seith Bhalla, R. Sharma, A. Kumar, A. Roychoudhury, and O. Bhutia, "Diffusion-weighted imaging in the evaluation of odontogenic cysts and tumours," *The British Journal of Radiology*, vol. 85, no. 1018, pp. e864–e870, 2012.

[12] R. S. Pillai, R. Ongole, A. Ahsan, R. A. Radhakrishnan, and K. M. Pai, "Recurrent desmoplastic ameloblastoma of the maxilla: a case report," *Journal of the Canadian Dental Association*, vol. 70, no. 2, pp. 100–104, 2004.

[13] M. L. Beckley, V. Farhood, L. K. Helfend, and A. Alijanian, "Desmoplastic ameloblastoma of the mandible: a case report and review of the literature," *Journal of Oral and Maxillofacial Surgery*, vol. 60, no. 2, pp. 194–198, 2002.

[14] I. Kaffe, A. Buchner, and S. Taicher, "Radiologic features of desmoplastic variant of ameloblastoma," *Oral Surgery, Oral Medicine, and Oral Pathology*, vol. 76, no. 4, pp. 525–529, 1993.

[15] M. Sumi, Y. Ichikawa, I. Katayama, S. Tashiro, and T. Nakamura, "Diffusion-weighted MR imaging of ameloblastomas and keratocystic odontogenic tumors: differentiation by apparent diffusion coefficients of cystic lesions," *AJNR. American Journal of Neuroradiology*, vol. 29, no. 10, pp. 1897–1901, 2008.

[16] Y. Han, X. Fan, L. Su, and Z. Wang, "Diffusion-weighted mr imaging of unicystic odontogenic tumors for differentiation of unicystic ameloblastomas from keratocystic odontogenic tumors," *Korean Journal of Radiology*, vol. 19, no. 1, pp. 79–84, 2018.

[17] D. D. Yang, A. Ghuman, R. Stratton, M. Hall, and A. Parthipun, "Appearance of florid cemento-osseous dysplasia on SPECT/CT," *Clinical Nuclear Medicine*, vol. 44, no. 5, pp. e357–e359, 2019.

[18] M. A. Lopes, H. S. Kim, F. V. Mariano, M. B. Corrêa, N. T. A. Rabelo, and P. A. Vargas, "Clinico-pathologic conference: case 1. High-grade osteosarcoma (OS) and florid cemento-osseous dysplasia (FCOD)," *Head and Neck Pathology*, vol. 4, no. 4, pp. 329–333, 2010.

[19] S. Matsumura, S. Murakami, N. Kakimoto et al., "Histopathologic and radiographic findings of the simple bone cyst," *Oral Surgery, Oral Medicine, Oral Pathology, Oral Radiology, and Endodontics*, vol. 85, no. 5, pp. 619–625, 1998.

Multiple Dental Inclusion in Monozygotic Twins with Congenital Visual Impairment

G. Galluccio,[1] A. Impellizzeri,[1] A. A. De Stefano,[1,2] E. Serritella,[1] and E. Guercio Monaco[2]

[1]*Department of Oral and Maxillo Facial Sciences, Faculty of Medicine and Dentistry, Sapienza Università di Roma, Italy*
[2]*Department of Orthodontics, Faculty of Dentistry, University Central of Venezuela, Caracas, Venezuela*

Correspondence should be addressed to G. Galluccio; gabriella.galluccio@uniroma1.it

Academic Editor: Rui Amaral Mendes

The study presents two monozygotic twins (MZ) with multiple impacted teeth, affecting the upper canines and lower second molars, as well as congenital aniridia. The clinical aspect of the upper canines is peculiar because of the different positions—palatal in one and buccal in the other twin. Studies reporting different scenarios of impaction in monozygotic twins can contribute more data to the debate on tooth eruption aetiology and more so in this case because of the association with a genetic panocular disease. *Patients' Concerns*. The patients were referred by a general dentist, who diagnosed the presence of multiple inclusions. *Diagnostic Study*. Both patients showed severe malocclusion, classified as grade 5 of the Index of Orthodontic Treatment Need (IOTN). The MZ showed class I malocclusion, upper and lower crowding, and impacted lower right and left second molars. A Dentascan was prescribed for the canine impaction. The impaction of the upper canine was palatal of 2.3 in one of the MZ and buccal of 1.3 in the other one. The same altered pattern of eruption of the lower second molars was identified in both twins. The proposed treatment plan contemplated orthodontic surgical recovery of the impacted elements, followed by orthodontic treatment with multibracket appliance after the extraction of the first four premolars, given the crowding entity. The use of a retraction spring action was chosen for the recovery of the lower second molars. Many aspects of the possible genetic aetiology of tooth impaction are still under discussion. The study of diseases in twins offers decisive information. Finally, the possibility that alterations in the eruptive pattern of the dental elements may be associated with other congenital problems broadens the range of investigations related to the possible aetiological causes of the inclusions in humans.

1. Introduction

Dental anomalies such as hypodontia, supernumerary teeth, enamel defects, and abnormalities of eruption and position are prominent in a large segment of the population.

Although treatment strategies for these conditions are steadily improving, much remains to be understood about their aetiology and pathophysiology [1].

Studies on monozygotic twins may elucidate the genetics underlying the specific aspects of malocclusions and tooth anomalies in the analysis, improving the possibilities of performing a correct treatment plane [2–7].

The presence of concordant or nonconcordant malocclusion traits in monozygotic twins is a special occasion to test the hypothesis in the aetiology of inclusions, which is still nonconcordant in the literature [6, 8].

Special interest is present when specific occlusal alterations are associated with other systemic anomalies and overall when the association is with congenital anomalies.

The case presented, of the monozygotic twins V. P. and L. P., is the concurrent presence of multiple-tooth impaction affecting the upper canines and lower second molars and congenital aniridia. This particular congenital panocular disease is described as the partial or complete absence of the iris and often recognized in association with other diseases [9]. The aetiology of aniridia is recognized as genetic; for example, it was recently identified to be referred to as a deletion in the regulatory region of PAX6 [10, 11].

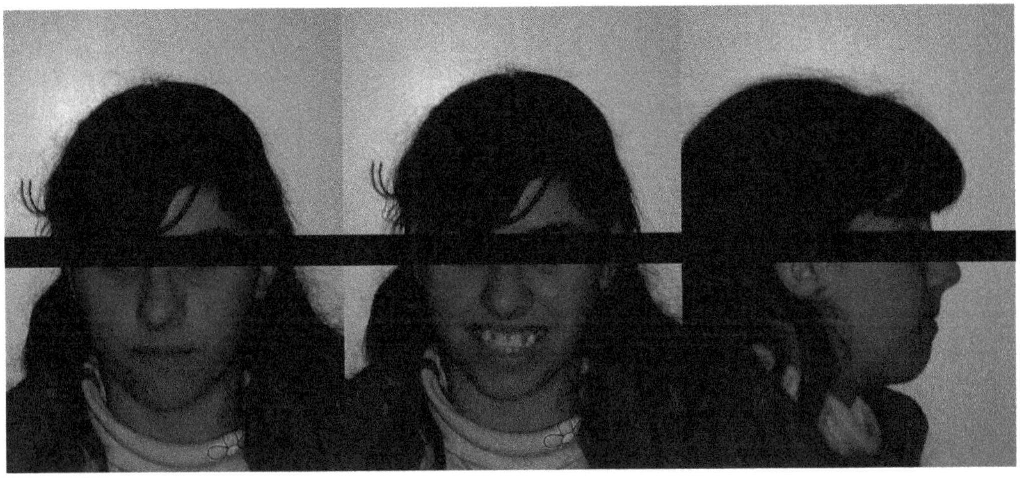

Figure 1: MZ V. P.'s extraoral examination.

1.1. Clinical Findings. The twins came for an orthodontic evaluation accompanied by their parents. The patients (Caucasian, 14 yo) were referred by the general dentistry after their first visit during which the observation of a panorex revealed the presence of an altered pattern of eruption on several dental elements and multiple inclusions. Both the twins had a severe visual impairment with a limitation up to shadow perception due to the presence of congenital aniridia.

The principal concern of the family was related to the misalignment of the teeth and related difficulties in maintaining proper oral hygiene. The parents and the general dentistry considered visual impairment a possible limitation in the compliance, eventually needing restorative dentistry procedures.

From the age of 6 yo, the patients had undergone regular dentistry controls and periodic procedures of oral hygiene with professional deplaquing and instructional reinforcement. The provision of further preventive procedures such as sealants or varnish was not referred.

1.2. Medical History. The parents reported a course of pregnancy without major problems, birth at term by a caesarean section for malposition of the foetuses, and an Apgar score of 8–10. The lactation was mixed (natural/artificial).

The twins were born from the only pregnancy of the couple, and no other sibling was known.

For both the patients, the presence of congenital aniridia was definitively diagnosed at three months of age.

The two patients showed regular somatic development (L. P.'s menarche at the age of 12.3; V. P.'s menarche at the age of 11.9).

The patients had no need for drug treatments for specific conditions.

1.3. Family History. Both parents appeared to be in good health. The anamnesis was negative for the presence of malocclusion and dental impaction in the family.

In medical dental history, the mother reported the need for restorations while the father reported a previous need for restorative and prosthetic dental procedures. Neither had undergone orthodontic treatment.

1.4. Lifestyle and Psychosocial Information. Due to their visual impairment, social interactions, as were for performing physical activity, were limited as much as possible. The schooling was regular as per the age, albeit with the need for devices and supplementary support from teachers due to the visual limitation.

The two sisters showed a strong relationship, evident in their need for each other's presence during the diagnostic and therapeutic procedures.

1.5. Genetic Information. Genetic assessment of the patients was not performed at birth and was refused by the parents after it because it was referred to as insignificant in the medical treatment choices of the disease and for economic reasons.

1.5.1. Case # 1: Twin V. P. The medical history of the patient reported that she was diagnosed with bilateral aniridia with congenital bilateral polar cataracts, highlighted at the age of three months, later surgically treated by removing it and by placing cosmetic intraocular implants in both eyes.

Visus was equal to 2/30 in the right eye and 1/10 in the left eye, without any possibility of improvement.

Any kind of dental or orthodontic treatment was previously performed.

(1) Physical Examination. The extraoral examination showed an increased lower facial height (dolichofacial), slight convex profile, lines of symmetry respected, and lip incompetence at rest (Figure 1).

The intraoral examination presented that the patient had late mixed dentition; it was noticeable in the presence of the arches of deciduous teeth, not consistent with the age: upper left canine and lower left second molar. Both lower second permanent molars showed a semi-inclusion with only the distal cusps visible in the mouth (Table 1).

Table 1: V. P. twin dental formulae (*semi-inclusion). Monozygotic twin V. P.'s dental formula as in ISO (International Organization for Standardization) 5 with the mesiodistal (MD) crown diameters of permanent teeth (in mm to the nearest 0.5 mm). Bold numbers report the mesiodistal dimension of a deciduous tooth, and italic numbers report the mesiodistal dimension of an unerupted tooth, evaluated on the panorex and calculated based on the magnification coefficient.

Twin V. P.: tooth number (ISO two-digit system)														
Maxillary teeth														
Upper arch		16	15	14	13	12	11	21	22	63	24	25	26	
MD diameter (mm)		11	8	7.5	8	7	9	9	7	**6** *8*	7.5	8	11	
Dentoalveolar discrepancy = −13 mm														
Mandibular teeth														
Lower arch	47*	46	45	44	43	42	41	31	32	33	34	75	36	37*
MD diameter (mm)		11	8	7.5	7.5	6.5	6	6	6.5	7.5	7.5	**9.5** *8*	11	
Dentoalveolar discrepancy = −14 mm														

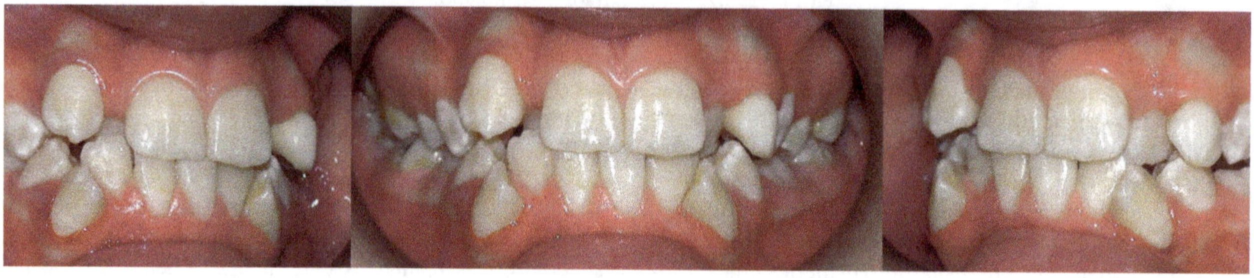

Figure 2: MZ V. P.'s intraoral examination.

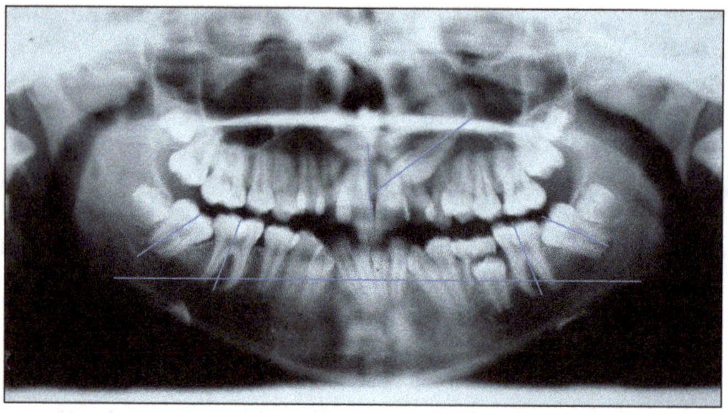

Figure 3: MZ V. P.'s panorex. The upper left canine α angle is 57°, and the vertical distance from the occlusal plane is 9.5 mm. The inclination of the second molar axis is 38° for 4.7 and 40° for 3.7.

The occlusal molar relationships were of class I on the right and the left side, while the canine relationship was undetectable because of the ectopic position of the upper right canine and the absence in the arch of the left one. There was deviation of the lower midline (Figure 2).

Overjet and overbite were increased; a severe dentoalveolar discrepancy, with evident upper and lower crowding, was evident. The oral hygiene was poor, with bacterial plaque, probably due to the limited visual capacity. Decays were present on elements 3.6 and 3.7. An amalgam restoration was present on the vestibular surface of 4.6.

(2) Radiographic Examination. The orthopantomography of the dental arches reveals the presence of all permanent teeth, with the upper left canine impacted; mesial inclination of the lower second molars is seen, with the mesial cusps impacted under the crown of the first molars.

The inclination of the second molar axis related to the first molar axis was analysed for the prognostic value of this measurement [12] and was 38° for 4.7 and 40° for 3.7 (Figure 3).

The inclination of the upper left canine was 57° as evaluated with the α angle, and the vertical distance from the occlusal plane was 9.5 mm. The evaluation of the alpha angle and the D-distance has a prognostic value in relation to the success of surgical orthodontic treatment. The angle is formed from the canine axis and the midline between the

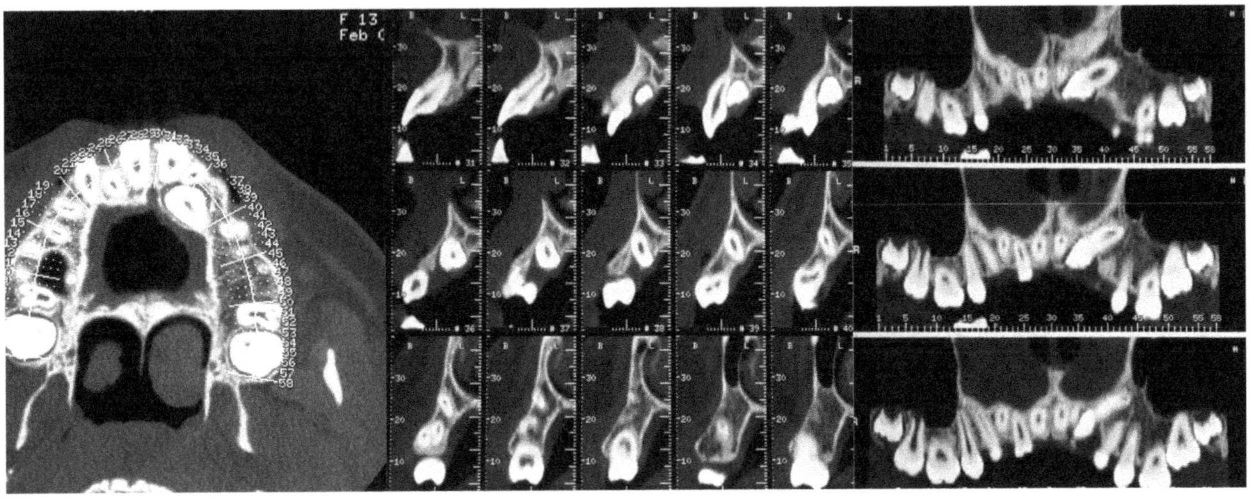

FIGURE 4: MZ V. P.'s upper arch Dentascan: upper left canine palatal impaction.

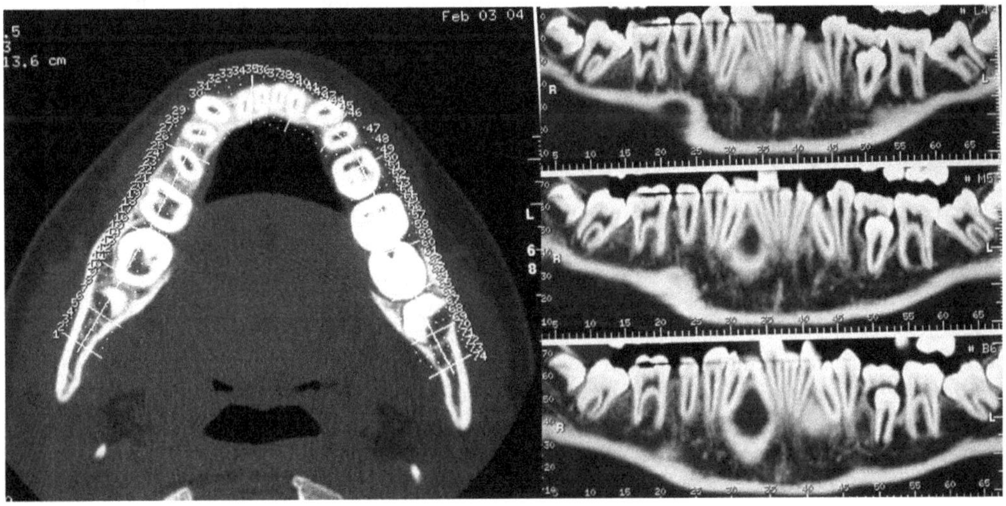

FIGURE 5: MZ V. P.'s lower arch Dentascan: mesial impaction of both the lower second molars.

central incisors. The D-distance is measured from the canine cusp to the occlusal plane [13]. The evaluation of these parameters can be also read, in an early stage of dentition, as an indication of progressive canine impaction. However, these radiographic variables take on a diagnostic and prognostic significance of canine dislocation at a later age group, i.e., only after 10–11 years [14].

The presence of severe eruptive disturbances suggested the prescription of further radiographic evaluation with a TC Dentascan of the upper and lower arch.

The observation revealed an inclusion of 2.3 in the palatal position. A tight contact was evident between the palatal surface of the central and lateral left incisors' roots and the crown of the impacted canine. However, no signs of root resorption were evident for the incisors. An eruptive delay of 1.4, 1.5, and 4.5 was detectable with altered axial inclination (Figure 4).

The evaluation of the two lower molars showed an H stage of maturity (Demirjian dental age assessment) [15], acceptable for the age of the patient; the vestibulooral position of both the molars was centred with limited contact with the lingual cortical bone for 3.7 (Figure 5).

For both the second molars, the mesial cusps were positioned under the crown equator of the respective molars.

The cephalometric analysis of the latero-lateral X-ray is summarised in Table 2. The results show a class II malocclusion, an increase in the vertical dimension of the lower third, and the vestibularisation of the upper incisors.

(3) Cast Analysis. A severe dentoalveolar discrepancy was present in the upper arch, equal to −13, and the lower arch, equal to −14 (Table 1).

1.5.2. Case # 2: Twin L. P. The medical history of the patient reports that at the age of three months, she was diagnosed with bilateral aniridia with congenital bilateral polar cataracts, which was treated surgically by removing it and by placing cosmetic intraocular implants to both eyes. Secondary retinal detachment resulted in corneal opacity in the right eye.

Visus was equal to light perception in the right eye and 2/30 in the left eye, without any possibility of improvement.

Any kind of dental or orthodontic treatment was previously performed.

TABLE 2: MZ V. P.'s cephalometric analysis.

MZ V. P.	
Maxilla to cranial base	
SNA (°)	80.4
Mandible to cranial base	
SNB (°)	76.2
SN-GoGn (°)	45.2
FMA (MP-FH) (°)	32.1
Maxillo-mandibular	
ANB (°)	4.2
Maxillary dentition	
U1-NA (mm)	4.7
U1-SN (°)	103.1
Mandibular dentition	
L1-NB (mm)	9.2
L1-MP (°)	88.6
Soft tissue	
Lower lip to E-plane (mm)	0.9
Upper lip to E-plane (mm)	-10.5

(1) Physical Examination. The extraoral examination showed an increased lower facial height (dolichofacial), slight convex profile, lines of symmetry respected, and lip incompetence at rest (Figure 6).

The intraoral examination showed that the patient was in a late mixed dentition stage. The relative formula is reported in Table 3. It was noticeable in the presence of arches in deciduous teeth: upper left canine and upper and lower left second molars. This was not consistent with the age, and both lower second permanent molars showed only the distal cusps visible in the mouth.

The occlusal molar relationships were of class I on the right and the left side, while the canine relationship was undetectable because of the absence of the arch in the right upper canine and the contemporary presence of the permanent and the deciduous upper left canine. Therefore, the ectopic position was of a permanent one. A unilateral crossbite was present on the right side (Figure 7).

Overjet and overbite were increased; a severe dentoalveolar discrepancy with upper and lower crowding was evident. Oral hygiene was poor, with the presence of bacterial plaque, probably due to the heavily limited visual capacity. Decays were also present on elements 1.6, 6.5, 2.6, 3.6, and 3.7.

(2) Radiographic Examination. The orthopantomography of the dental arches revealed the presence of all the permanent teeth, the impacted upper right canine, persistence of the upper left deciduous canine, the second molar, the lower left deciduous second molar, and the eruptive delay of 3.5 with alteration of the axial inclination, mesial inclination of the lower second molars, and horizontal impaction under the crown of the first molars.

The inclination of the second molar axis related to the first molar axis was 68° for 4.7 and 69° for 3.7 [12]. The inclination of the upper left canine was 58°, as evaluated with the α angle, and the vertical distance from the occlusal plane was 16 mm (Figure 8).

In this case, the presence of severe eruptive disturbances also suggested the prescription of a further radiographic evaluation with a TC Dentascan of the upper and lower arches.

The X-ray observation revealed a high vestibular inclusion of 2.3. A tight contact was evident between the crown of the impacted canine and the apical third of the central and lateral left incisor roots. Slight signs of root resorption in the point of contact were advisable for the right lateral incisor. The crown of the upper left canine was superimposed on the gingival third of the lateral incisor root. An eruptive delay of 1.4 and 1.5 was detectable with a palatal axial inclination of 1.5 (Figure 9).

The evaluation of the two lower molars showed an H stage of maturity (Demirjian dental age assessment), acceptable for the age of the patient; the position of both the molars was horizontal with a tight contact with the lingual cortical bone.

Most of the occlusal surfaces of 4.7 and 3.7 were positioned under the crown equator of the respective first molar (Figure 10).

The cephalometric analysis of the latero-lateral radiography is summarised in Table 4. The results showed a skeletal class II malocclusion and an increase in the vertical dimension of the lower third. The maxillary and mandibular incisors were proclined.

1.6. Diagnostic Focus and Assessment. Both the twins showed a class I dental malocclusion with severe dentoalveolar discrepancy.

In the cast analysis of twin V. P., the lack of space was of -13 mm maxilla and -14 mm lower jaw (Table 1). In twin L. P., the discrepancy between the size of the teeth and those of the arches was equal to -11.5 mm in the upper arch and -13 mm in the lower arch (Table 3).

The latero-lateral radiography examination showed skeletal hyperdivergent class II but with signs of mandibular length and therefore a tendency of a class II skeletal pattern of growth; an excessive vestibular inclination of the upper and lower teeth was detected in both the cases.

A protrusive lower lip characterised the profile of both twins.

1.6.1. Treatment Options. The study of clinical and radiographic data of the two sisters indicates the immediate need for orthodontic treatment, which must not be delayed in time (Index of Orthodontic Treatment Need- (IOTN-) 5) [16].

The most evident need of therapy is the presence of multiple inclusions, namely, for the upper canine, right in one sister and left in the other, and of both second molars in the lower arch for both sisters.

The prognosis of a possible surgical orthodontic approach for the impacted teeth, although some similarities were present in the sisters, was significantly different because of the localisation of the upper canine, vestibular or palatal,

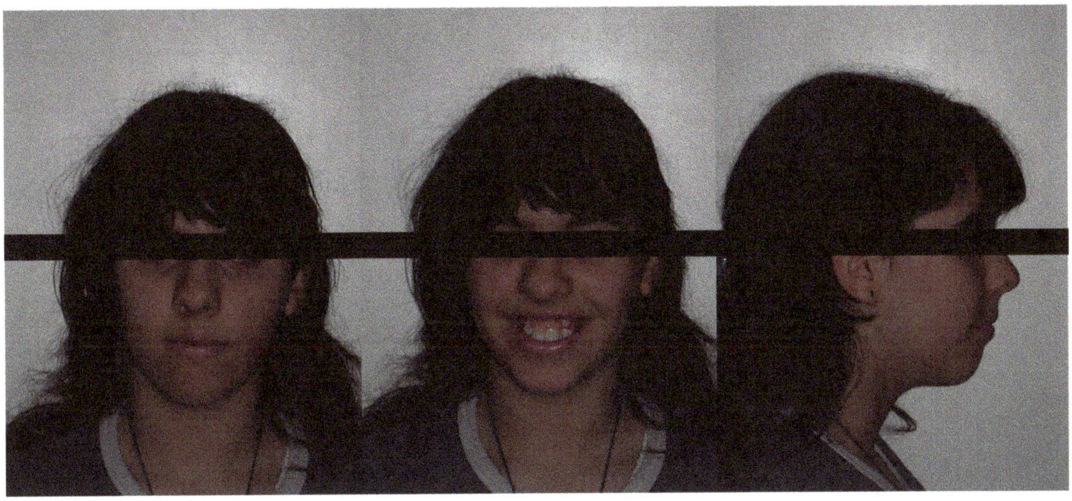

FIGURE 6: MZ L. P.'s extraoral examination.

TABLE 3: L. P. twin dental formulae (*semi-inclusion). Monozygotic twin L. P.'s dental formula as in ISO (International Organization for Standardization) 5 with the mesiodistal (MD) crown diameters of permanent teeth (in mm to the nearest 0.5 mm). Bold numbers report the mesiodistal dimension of a deciduous tooth, and italic numbers report the mesiodistal dimension of an unerupted tooth, evaluated on the panorex and calculated based on the magnification coefficient.

Twin L. P.: tooth number (ISO two-digit system)														
Maxillary teeth														
Upper arch		16	15	14	/	12	11	21	22	23/63	/	65	26	
MD diameter (mm)		11	7.5	7.5	8	7	9	9	7	**8.5** *6*	8.5	**9** *7.5*	11	
Dentoalveolar discrepancy = −11.5 mm														
Mandibular teeth														
Lower arch	47*	46	45	44	43	42	41	31	32	33	34	75	36	37*
MD diameter (mm)		11	8	7.5	7.5	6.5	6	6	6.5	7.5	7.5	**9.5** *8*	11	
Dentoalveolar discrepancy = −13 mm														

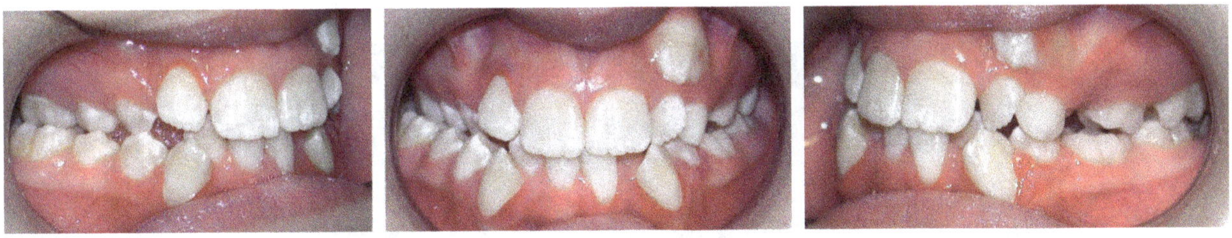

FIGURE 7: MZ L. P.'s intraoral examination.

and the distance of the canine from the occlusal plane, which was far accentuated for the vestibular inclusion. The bilateral inclusion of the lower second molars showed a different degree of mesial inclination, more severe for L. P., in which the deep of the molars' crown was also heightened.

A serious dentoalveolar discrepancy was present in both the patients, leading to a consideration of a fixed multibracket treatment with extraction of four premolars; this is also acceptable for the presence of a protrusive profile.

A possible orthognathic surgery for the correction of the skeletal malocclusion was not considered because of the mild level of the discrepancy and global clinical, medical, and social consideration for which the family refuses to evaluate for this approach.

The treatment plan is therefore different for the two sisters.

For V. P., a surgical orthodontic approach was planned for upper left canine disimpaction, using a transpalatal arch with a cantilever spring soldered to the palatal bar [17]. The aim of the first step is to extrude the canine by a closed eruption technique. Only after the first radiographic evaluation of the effective movement of the canine can a subsequent fixed

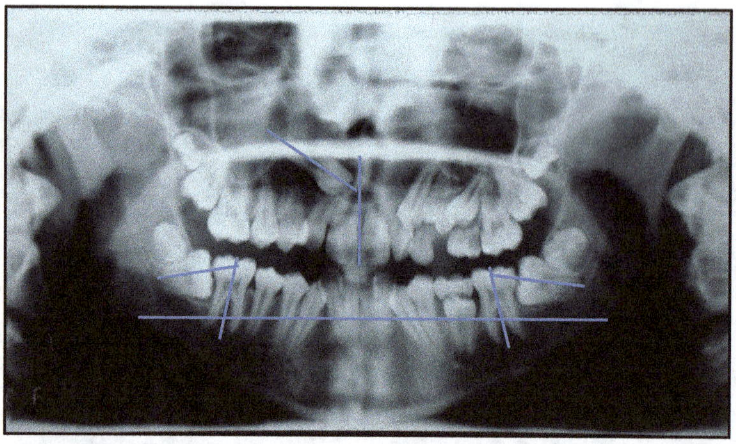

Figure 8: MZ L. P.'s panorex. The right canine α angle is 58°, and the vertical distance from the occlusal plane is 16 mm. The inclination of the second molar axis is 68° for 4.7 and 69° for 3.7.

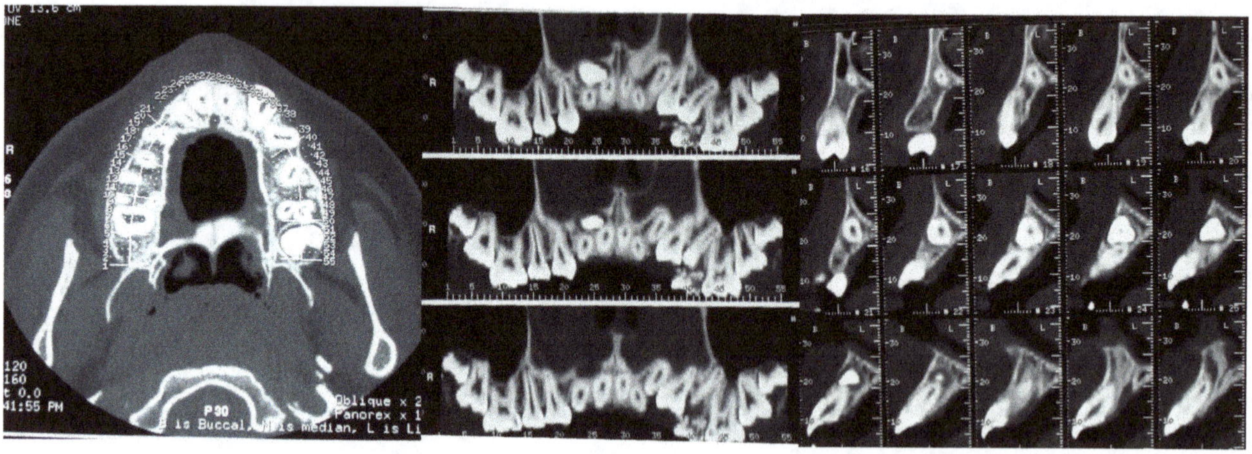

Figure 9: MZ L. P.'s upper arch Dentascan: upper right canine buccal impaction.

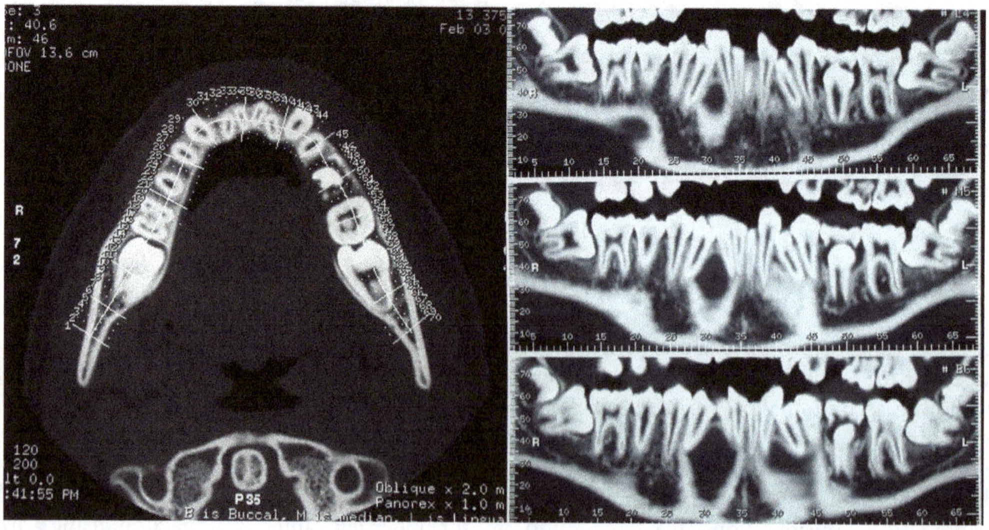

Figure 10: MZ L. P.'s lower arch Dentascan: deep mesial impaction of both the lower second molars.

Table 4: MZ L. P.'s cephalometric analysis.

MZ L. P.	
Maxilla to cranial base	
SNA (°)	83.1
Mandible to cranial base	
SNB (°)	78.4
SN-GoGn (°)	41.3
FMA (MP-FH) (°)	28.9
Maxillo-mandibular	
ANB (°)	4.7
Maxillary dentition	
U1-NA (mm)	6.5
U1-SN (°)	106.9
Mandibular dentition	
L1-NB (mm)	13.9
L1-MP (°)	93.2
Soft tissue	
Lower lip to E-plane (mm)	-0.5
Upper lip to E-plane (mm)	-9.0

multibracket treatment, with extraction of four first premolars, take place. In the lower arch, the second molar disimpaction was considered with the aid of a De-Impactor spring (Dentamate Co.), positioned under the contact point between the first and second molars bilaterally [18]. Once free in the mesial part of the second molars, a complete bonding of the lower arch will take place.

For patient L. P., the surgical orthodontic approach was planned, considering the upper canine disimpaction, using the VISTA technique [19], which entails a closed subperiosteal traction, anchored to a transpalatal bar with a vertical arm vestibular to the upper first right molar. For this patient too, only after the first radiographic evaluation of the effective movement of the canine can a subsequent fixed multibracket treatment, with extraction of four first premolars, take place. The presence of an inclination of over 68° for both the second lower molars indicates the need for a different procedure for the recovery, using a cantilever spring, as described by Doshi et al. [20].

1.6.2. Treatment Alternatives. Only if the canines are not responsive to the orthodontic traction, a possible surgical extraction will take place, planning the substitution of it with the first premolar and, therefore, treating the patients with three premolar extractions.

For L. P., a possible alternative treatment plan should be considered: the extraction of the second lower molars and the mesialization of the third molars.

For V. P., in case the orthodontic uprighting is not achieved, surgical repositioning of the second molars should be considered [21].

2. Discussion

Twin studies in medicine are an important source of information to understand the relative importance of the genetic

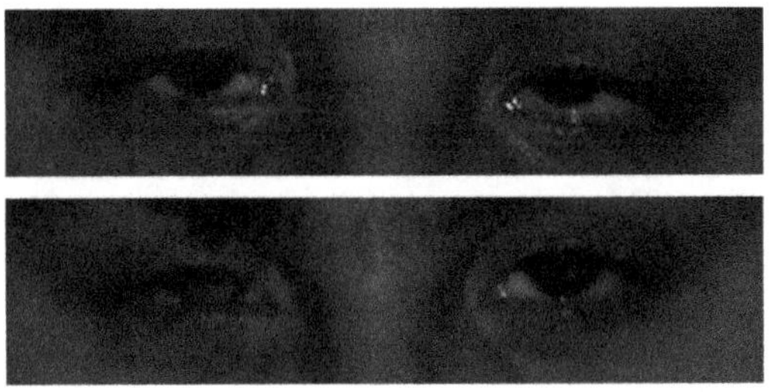

Figure 11: Detail of the clinical aspect of aniridia.

or environmental origin of specific disorders. In monozygotic twins, the gene is equal to 100%, so if a character appears more frequently in monozygotic twins than the expected rate in siblings or dizygotic twins, the genetic factor is important. If not, it must consider greater environmental importance in the aetiology of problems found [22].

The case reported is peculiar under several aspects. A similar but specular canine impaction, both for the side and for the localisation of the tooth, is present in both monozygotic twins.

In the lower arch, however, the same alteration of the eruptive pattern is evident for the same teeth, although with a different degree of severity. The lower second molars showed the same direction of impaction, with mesial inclination, and the same clinical evidence of osteomucosal semi-inclusion.

Moreover, the twins were also characterised for the presence of a congenital ocular malformation because the presence of aniridia was diagnosed early for both (Figure 11). Therefore, the case is interesting due to the simultaneous presence of occlusal and ocular abnormalities, especially in patients with a negative family history for both diseases.

Aniridia is defined as a rare clinical condition in which there is a partial or complete absence of the iris. The prevalence reaches 0.018% and is equally distributed among males and females. This condition is usually congenital; however, its aetiology is still uncertain. The congenital aniridia can be classified as autosomal dominant, autosomal recessive congenital, or sporadic congenital.

Sporadic aniridia can be detected between symptoms in certain clinical conditions, as it happens in WAGR syndrome, a rare genetic disorder characterised by Wilms' tumour, aniridia, genitourinary anomalies, and mental retardation, or in Gillespie syndrome, where it is present in the autosomal recessive congenital aniridia.

Aniridia can be associated with several other anomalies, including sensory deficiency such as abnormal olfaction or hearing loss, absent or hypoplastic patella, and the AGR triad (aniridia, genitourinary abnormalities, mental retardation) [23]. However, to the best of our knowledge, congenital aniridia has not been associated with dental anomalies.

While aniridia is a rare condition, the canine inclusion, particularly in the palatal side, is a frequent abnormality in the Caucasian population, being most common in females. If it is assumed that the prevalence of the upper canine inclusion is equal to 2% in the general population, the probability of finding the same palatal inclusion in monozygotic twins, as a sporadic event, would be questionable

[24]. The frequent association of canine impaction with other dental anomalies, such as tooth number or size anomalies both in the same subject and in families, strongly suggests a genetic origin, and research progressively supports this hypothesis. It, therefore, seems likely that the inclusion is linked to genetic causes [25, 26].

The presence of palatal inclusion of the canine in monozygotic twins has already been reported in the literature. Leonardi et al. [6] report the case of monozygotic twins with palatal inclusion of the canine but in a specular position. In the cases described by the authors, the two lateral incisors were of normal size. From the study of these cases, the authors derive evidence to support the genetic aetiology of palatal inclusion of canine, rather an aetiology connected to the lack of guidance for lateral incisor anomaly [27, 28]. In this study, the twins also showed abnormalities of the position of the lower second molars, showing a mesial inclination. The presence of multiple abnormalities in the same subjects has been variously reported in the literature; the concomitant presence of the most various anomalies, including alterations of the eruptive pattern of the molars, was considered further proof of the genetic cause of these alterations.

In our reported cases, both patients presented with the inclusion of the upper canine and retention of the lower second molars, which showed an altered mesial inclination. This then presents great similarity with Leonardi et al.'s study, but the inclusion is specular not only in the side but also at the position, which is present in one patient in a palatal position and in a buccal position in another one. Moreover, in both patients, there was a considerable dentoalveolar discrepancy with significant space deficit.

While the literature has found significant evidence of the genetic aetiology of palatal canine inclusion, only a few studies report an association between dental anomalies and buccal inclusion [29]. Recently, some authors developed a different theory to explain the possible aetiology of both canine impactions from the vestibular side and on the palatal side: according to this theory, both the canines included in the palatal and buccal position have a genetic origin, but local factors can lead to displacement in the palatal or vestibular direction [30].

The "sequential theory," developed on the basis of a large retrospective study, affirms that genetic and environmental factors act at different times, and therefore, both the palatal and buccal impacted canines have an initial genetic cause while the specific clinical picture is realised according to environmental influences, predominantly referred to as excess of space, as it happens in microdontia. However, previous studies still consider the lack of space a possible local cause for vestibular inclusion. In the monozygotic twins, the lack of space was evident.

The detection of the presence, however, is of very similar alterations in both patients, which shows a correlation in the elements involved in abnormalities—upper canines and lower second molars—and the correlation of dental size detected and the presence of similar values of dentoalveolar discrepancy, which seems to indicate a genetic basis for these characteristics.

The observation, in the same subjects, of ocular congenital anomalies is not easy to analyse, given that research has only recently identified several genes involved in the pathogenesis of aniridia, such as the regulatory region deletions in PAX6 and PITX2 and, in cases of anterior segment dysgenesis (ASD) disorders, mutations in the alpha-1 collagen type IV (COL4A1) and beta-1,3-galactosyltransferase-like (B3GALTL) [11, 31, 32].

These conditions are not, however, related to concurrent dental alterations.

In the genesis of ocular development, alterations then reconnect with genetic alterations in which the transcription factors have an important role, in particular some DNA-binding transcription factors such as PAX6, FOXC1, SOX2, FOXE3, OTX2, PITX2, and PAX2 [33].

Alterations in the same PITX2, FOXC1, and PAX6 genes, linked to important dental abnormalities, were identified in other clinical conditions such as Rieger syndrome [34, 35].

Therefore, only on a speculative level, it could be imagined as an alteration, intervened in the gestational period and capable of inducing alterations in the same embryological derivation areas.

In the cases presented, the parents did not refer to genetic analysis at birth or in the moment of congenital aniridia diagnosis. A possible deepening of the diagnosis of the underlying causes of aniridia was refused by the parents in that moment because the ocular pathology treatment possibilities were not influenced from a more accurate genetic knowledge and for economic reasons. Alike, the parents refused the genetic analysis also when the multiple dental impaction became evident.

Some clinical considerations influenced this decision; several conditions involving the presence of multiple impactions are known to be related to a genetic mutation that also involves the failure of all the orthodontic strategies of recovery of the impacted teeth. Nevertheless, some clinical observations can lead to substantially excluding these conditions for the MZ, as it happens for the primary failure of eruption (PFE). In the PFE cases, in fact, the teeth involved are mostly located on only one side, in the posterior area, and showing a progressive worsening of the impaction from the first tooth to the last one of the areas affected. This condition is clinically evident with a posterior open bite. Similarly, a differential diagnosis is possible on a clinical base also for the anchyloses, clinically characterised for a single tooth involved and with a vertical alteration of its position [36]. The treatment choices in the other cases of impaction always comprehend a treatment with an orthodontic-surgical approach.

For the MZ, therefore, a deepening of the diagnostic procedures adding a genetic mapping would not change in the treatment plane and was therefore refused by the patients and their parents.

However, not having subjected our patients to a genetic investigation, the data of the present study is limited to a simple hypothesis that suggests a possible diagnostic genetic study in cases with similar dental and ocular abnormalities.

3. Conclusions

The debate about the aetiology of inclusions sees many points that are still under discussion, especially the different genetic bases of the inclusions in the front or rear area or different importance of the genetic factor in the inclusion of the upper canines. Finally, the possibility that alterations in the path and of the dental element eruptive potential may be associated with other congenital problems broadens the range of possibilities of aetiological causes of the inclusions.

The present case study of the monozygotic twins provides information on the possible genetic basis of dental inclusions. The potential link between inclusions and abnormalities of eruption and other genetic alterations can push towards finding genetic factors involved in the anomalies. This then affects both the possibilities of early diagnosis of clinical conditions that require treatment with chances of therapy success. It particularly affects the determination of the aetiology of malocclusion's tractability. The possible genetic aetiology can improve the chances of early interception but does not allow preventive treatments solely based on changing environmental conditions.

Additional Points

Guidelines. The authors used appropriate guidelines (CARE for case reports).

Consent

All patients signed an informed consent form and gave the necessary approval for the use of the clinical documentation.

References

[1] T. J. Pemberton, G. Mendoza, J. Gee, and P. I. Patel, "Inherited dental anomalies: a review and prospects for the future role of clinicians," *Journal of the California Dental Association*, vol. 35, no. 5, pp. 324–326, 2007.

[2] J. Cohen-Levy, A. S. Kamoun-Goldrat, Y. Simon, and A. Lautrou, "Jumeaux et héritabilité des phénotypes dento-faciaux," *L'Orthodontie Française*, vol. 78, no. 1, pp. 69–77, 2007.

[3] M. Markovic, "Hypodontia in twins," *Swedish Dental Journal. Supplement*, vol. 15, pp. 153–162, 1982.

[4] K. Ulrich, "Isolated canine aplasia in monozygotic twins," *Fortschritte der Kieferorthopädie*, vol. 50, no. 5, pp. 415–422, 1989.

[5] S. Peck, L. Peck, and G. Hirsh, "Mandibular lateral incisor-canine transposition in monozygotic twins," *ASDC Journal of Dentistry for Children*, vol. 64, no. 6, pp. 409–413, 1997.

[6] R. Leonardi, S. Peck, M. Caltabiano, and E. Barbato, "Palatally displaced canine anomaly in monozygotic twins," *The Angle Orthodontist*, vol. 73, no. 4, pp. 466–470, 2003.

[7] F. B. Naini and J. P. Moss, "Three-dimensional assessment of the relative contribution of genetics and environment to various facial parameters with the twin method," *American Journal of Orthodontics and Dentofacial Orthopedics*, vol. 126, no. 6, pp. 655–665, 2004.

[8] S. Camilleri, C. M. Lewis, and F. McDonald, "Ectopic maxillary canines: segregation analysis and a twin study," *Journal of Dental Research*, vol. 87, no. 6, pp. 580–583, 2008.

[9] K. Tripathy and B. Salini, "Aniridia," in *StatPearls*, StatPearls Publishing, Treasure Island (FL), 2020.

[10] L. Hyun Taeka, K. Dae Heeb, and K. Hyunaa, "*PAX6* aniridia syndrome clinics, genetics, and therapeutics," *Current Opinion in Ophthalmology*, vol. 28, no. 5, pp. 436–447, 2017.

[11] L. M. Reis and E. V. Semina, "Genetics of anterior segment dysgenesis disorders," *Current Opinion in Ophthalmology*, vol. 22, no. 5, pp. 314–324, 2011.

[12] A. Alligri, A. Putrino, M. Cassetta, A. Silvestri, E. Barbato, and G. Galluccio, "The mandibular permanent second molars and their risk of impaction: a retrospective study," *European Journal of Paediatric Dentistry*, vol. 16, no. 3, pp. 246–250, 2015.

[13] S. Ericson and J. Kurol, "Early treatment of palatally erupting maxillary canines by extraction of the primary canines," *European Journal of Orthodontics*, vol. 10, no. 1, pp. 283–295, 1988.

[14] S. J. Lindauer, L. K. Rubenstein, W. M. Hang, W. C. Andersen, and R. J. Isaacson, "Canine impaction identified early with panoramic radiographs," *The Journal of the American Dental Association*, vol. 123, no. 3, pp. 91–97, 1992.

[15] A. Demirjian, H. Goldstein, and J. M. Tanner, "A new system of dental age assessment," *Human Biology*, vol. 45, no. 2, pp. 211–227, 1973.

[16] P. H. Brook and W. C. Shaw, "The development of an index of orthodontic treatment priority," *European Journal of Orthodontics*, vol. 11, no. 3, pp. 309–320, 1989.

[17] R. Nanda, *Biomechanics in Clinical Orthodontics*, WB Saunders, 1997.

[18] S. Calasso, M. Cassetta, G. Galluccio, and E. Barbato, "Impacted lower second molars [Aspetti clinici del secondo molare inferiore incluso]," *Dental Cadmos*, vol. 76, no. 2, pp. 41–54, 2008.

[19] R. C. Bariani, R. Milani, C. H. Guimaraes Junior, W. S. Moura, and C. L. Ortolani, "Orthodontic traction of impacted upper canines using the VISTA technique," *Journal of Clinical Orthodontics*, vol. 51, no. 2, pp. 76–85, 2017.

[20] J. Doshi, K. Trivedi, and S. Traulatha, "Management of partially impacted mandibular second molars with an Australian uprighting spring," *The Orthodontic Ciber Journal*, vol. 9, pp. 1–22, 2009.

[21] G. La Monaca, M. P. Cristalli, N. Pranno, G. Galluccio, S. Annibali, and R. Pippi, "First and second permanent molars with failed or delayed eruption: clinical and statistical analyses," *American Journal of Orthodontics and Dentofacial Orthopedics*, vol. 156, no. 3, pp. 355–364, 2019.

[22] S. A. Burt and K. L. Klump, "The Michigan State University Twin Registry (MSUTR): 15 years of twin and family research," *Twin Research and Human Genetics*, vol. 22, no. 6, pp. 741–745, 2019.

[23] M. Hingorani, I. Hanson, and V. van Heyningen, "Aniridia," *European Journal of Human Genetics*, vol. 20, no. 10, pp. 1011–1017, 2012.

[24] S. Peck, L. Peck, and M. Kataja, "The palatally displaced canine as a dental anomaly of genetic origin," *The Angle Orthodontist*, vol. 64, no. 4, pp. 249–256, 1994.

[25] S. Pirinen, S. Arte, and S. Apajalahti, "Palatal displacement of canine is genetic and related to congenital absence of teeth," *Journal of Dental Research*, vol. 75, pp. 1742–1746, 1996.

[26] S. Peck and L. Peck, "Letter to the editor," *Journal of Dental Research*, vol. 76, no. 3, pp. 728-729, 2016.

[27] A. Becker and S. Chaushu, "Etiology of maxillary canine impaction: a review," *American Journal of Orthodontics and Dentofacial Orthopedics*, vol. 148, no. 4, pp. 557–567, 2015.

[28] S. Peck, "Misleading article on palatally displaced canines," *American Journal of Orthodontics and Dentofacial Orthopedics*, vol. 149, no. 2, pp. 149-150, 2016.

[29] A. Nagpal, K. M. Pal, and G. Sharma, "Palatal and labially impacted maxillary canine e associated dental anomalies: a comparative study," *The Journal of Contemporary Dental Practice*, vol. 10, pp. 67–74, 2009.

[30] A. K. Sajnani and N. M. King, "The sequential hypothesis of impaction of maxillary canine - a hypothesis based on clinical and radiographic findings," *Journal of Cranio-Maxillo-Facial Surgery*, vol. 40, no. 8, pp. e375–e385, 2012.

[31] M. Moosajee, M. Hingorani, and A. T. Moore, "PAX6-related aniridia," in *Gene Reviews®*, M. P. Adam, H. H. Ardinger, and R. A. Pagon, Eds., pp. 1993–2020, Seattle (WA), University of Washington, Seattle, 2003.

[32] R. E. Ferrell, A. Chakravarti, H. M. Hittner, and V. M. Riccardi, "Autosomal dominant aniridia: probable linkage to acid phosphatase-1 locus on chromosome 2," *Proceedings of the National Academy of Sciences of the United States of America*, vol. 77, no. 3, pp. 1580–1582, 1980.

[33] B. Käsmann-Kellner, K. Moslemani, and B. Seitz, "Clinical and genetic characteristics of ocular developmental disorders: MAC-spectrum, anterior segment dysgenesis," *Klinische Monatsblätter für Augenheilkunde*, vol. 236, no. 3, pp. 269–285, 2019.

[34] Y. Wang, H. Zhao, X. Zhang, and H. Feng, "Novel identification of a four-base-pair deletion mutation in PITX2 in a Rieger syndrome family," *Journal of Dental Research*, vol. 82, no. 12, pp. 1008–1012, 2016.

[35] C. R. Haldeman-Englert, A. Biser, E. H. Zackai, and J. E. Ming, "A 223-kb de novo deletion of *PAX9* in a patient with oligodontia," *The Journal of Craniofacial Surgery*, vol. 21, no. 3, pp. 837–839, 2010.

[36] S. G. Rhoads, H. M. Hendricks, and S. A. Frazier-Bowers, "Establishing the diagnostic criteria for eruption disorders based on genetic and clinical data," *American Journal of Orthodontics and Dentofacial Orthopedics*, vol. 144, no. 2, pp. 194–202, 2013.

Permissions

All chapters in this book were first published by Frontiers; hereby published with permission under the Creative Commons Attribution License or equivalent. Every chapter published in this book has been scrutinized by our experts. Their significance has been extensively debated. The topics covered herein carry significant findings which will fuel the growth of the discipline. They may even be implemented as practical applications or may be referred to as a beginning point for another development.

The contributors of this book come from diverse backgrounds, making this book a truly international effort. This book will bring forth new frontiers with its revolutionizing research information and detailed analysis of the nascent developments around the world.

We would like to thank all the contributing authors for lending their expertise to make the book truly unique. They have played a crucial role in the development of this book. Without their invaluable contributions this book wouldn't have been possible. They have made vital efforts to compile up to date information on the varied aspects of this subject to make this book a valuable addition to the collection of many professionals and students.

This book was conceptualized with the vision of imparting up-to-date information and advanced data in this field. To ensure the same, a matchless editorial board was set up. Every individual on the board went through rigorous rounds of assessment to prove their worth. After which they invested a large part of their time researching and compiling the most relevant data for our readers.

The editorial board has been involved in producing this book since its inception. They have spent rigorous hours researching and exploring the diverse topics which have resulted in the successful publishing of this book. They have passed on their knowledge of decades through this book. To expedite this challenging task, the publisher supported the team at every step. A small team of assistant editors was also appointed to further simplify the editing procedure and attain best results for the readers.

Apart from the editorial board, the designing team has also invested a significant amount of their time in understanding the subject and creating the most relevant covers. They scrutinized every image to scout for the most suitable representation of the subject and create an appropriate cover for the book.

The publishing team has been an ardent support to the editorial, designing and production team. Their endless efforts to recruit the best for this project, has resulted in the accomplishment of this book. They are a veteran in the field of academics and their pool of knowledge is as vast as their experience in printing. Their expertise and guidance has proved useful at every step. Their uncompromising quality standards have made this book an exceptional effort. Their encouragement from time to time has been an inspiration for everyone.

The publisher and the editorial board hope that this book will prove to be a valuable piece of knowledge for researchers, students, practitioners and scholars across the globe.

List of Contributors

Nada Fathalla Abdelbagi, Ibrahim Ahmed Ismail and Fadia Awadalkreem
Department of Oral Rehabilitation, Faculty of Dentistry, University of Khartoum, Khartoum, Sudan

Mohammed Nasser Alhajj
Department of Prosthodontics, Faculty of Dentistry, Thamar University, Dhamar, Yemen

V. Keerthi Narayan
Department of Oral Pathology and Microbiology, Thai Moogambigai Dental College and Hospital, Dr. MGR Educational and Research Institute, 600107, Chennai, Tamil Nadu, India

Anand deep Shukla, G. Srikanth, A. Chitra, Anupam Singh and Sunil Nayak
Department of Oral and Maxillofacial Surgery, MCODS, Manipal, India

Aya Mtiri, Ghada Bouslama, Nour-sayda Ben Messouad, Iyadh Abidi and Souha Ben Youssef
Department of Oral Surgery, University Hospital Farhat Hached Sousse, University of Monastir, Tunisia

Badreddine Sriha
Department of Histopathology, University Hospital Farhat Hached, Sousse, Tunisia
Cytology and Pathological Anatomy Department, Farhat Hached Hospital (Sousse), University of Sousse, Tunisia
Faculty of Medicine, University of Sousse, Farhat Hached Hospital of Sousse, Department of Pathology, Sousse, Tunisia

Farnoush Mohammadi and Nariman Nikparto
Department of Oral and Maxillofacial Surgery, School of Dentistry, Tehran University of Medical Sciences, 1439955991, Kargar North St., Tehran, Iran

Abbas Azari
Department of Prosthodontics, School of Dentistry, Tehran University of Medical Sciences, 1439955991, Kargar North St., Tehran, Iran

Heliya Ziaei
School of Dentistry, Tehran University of Medical Sciences, 1439955991, Kargar North St., Tehran, Iran

Noura A. Alsufyani
Oral & Maxillofacial Radiology, Oral Medicine and Diagnostic Sciences Department, College of Dentistry, King Saud University, Riyadh, Saudi Arabia
School of Dentistry, Department of Medicine and Dentistry, University of Alberta, Canada

Mohammed A. Alsufyani
Cosmetic and Dermatologic Surgery, Department of Dermatology and Dermatologic Surgery, Prince Sultan Military Medical City, Riyadh, Saudi Arabia

Ramtin Dastgir
Faculty of Dentistry, Tehran Medical Sciences, Islamic Azad University, Tehran, Iran

Maryam Sohrabi
Department of Oral and Maxillofacial Surgery, School of Dentistry, Tehran University of Medical Sciences, Tehran, Iran

Christian Boliere and Henry Fung
Division of Oral & Maxillofacial Surgery, John H. Stroger Hospital of Cook County, Chicago, IL, USA

James Murphy
Division of Oral & Maxillofacial Surgery, John H. Stroger Hospital of Cook County, Chicago, IL, USA
Division of Plastic and Reconstructive Surgery, Rush University Medical Center, Chicago, IL, USA

Mohammed Qaisi
Division of Oral & Maxillofacial Surgery, John H. Stroger Hospital of Cook County, Chicago, IL, USA
Division of Otolaryngology, John H. Stroger Hospital of Cook County, Chicago, IL, USA

Frances Manosca
Department of Pathology, John H. Stroger Hospital of Cook County, Chicago, IL, USA

Aryen Kaushik
Department of Prosthodontics, ITS Dental College, Greater Noida, India

HarshVardhan Sinha
Department of Prosthodontics, Saraswati Dental College, Lucknow, India

M. N. Hombesh and Taranjeet Kaur
Department of Prosthodontics, College of Dental Sciences, Davangere, India

Pooja Rani
Department of Prosthodontics, Buddha Institute of Dental Sciences and Hospital, Patna, India

Mahamadou Konate, Dounia Sarfi, Mounia El Bouhairi and Ihsane Benyahya
Department of Oral Surgery, Universitè Hassan II, Casablanca, Morocco

Taylor Ellingsen
School of Dentistry, University of Washington, 1959 NE Pacific St, Seattle, WA 98195, USA

Andrew Nalley
Clinical Instructor, Division of Radiology, Department of Oral Medicine, School of Dentistry, University of Washington, 1959 NE Pacific St, Seattle, WA 98195, USA

Dolphine Oda and Thomas B. Dodson
Department of Oral and Maxillofacial Surgery, School of Dentistry, University of Washington, 1959 NE Pacific St, Seattle, WA 98195, USA

Peggy P. Lee
Department of Oral Medicine, School of Dentistry, University of Washington, 1959 NE Pacific St, Seattle, WA 98195, USA

Mohammed A. AlZayer and Ali Matouq AlMarzouq
Dammam Medical Complex, Saudi Arabia

Zahrah Hasan Al-Faraj
Qatif Central Hospital, Saudi Arabia

Eman F. Al-Saleh
Dammam regional lab and blood bank, Saudi Arabia

Eya Moussaoui, Yassine Oueslati, Lamia Oualha and Nabiha Douki
Department of Dental Medicine, Sahloul Hospital (Sousse), Dental Faculty of Monastir, University of Monastir, Tunisia
Laboratory of Oral Health and Maxillofacial Rehabilitation (LR12ES11), University of Monastir, Tunisia

Mohamed Denguezli
Dermatology Department, Farhat Hached Hospital (Sousse), University of Sousse, Tunisia

Min A. Kwon, Jaegyok Song and Seokkon Kim
Department of Anaesthesiology and Pain Medicine, Dankook University College of Medicine, Cheonan, Republic of Korea

Pyeung-wha Oh and Minji Kang
Department of Anaesthesiology and Pain Medicine, Dankook University Hospital, Cheonan, Republic of Korea

Xu Wei, X. F. Meng, Xiaoping Luo and Wei Han
Department of Prosthodontics, Nanjing Stomatological Hospital, Medical School of Nanjing University, Nanjing, China

Lang Guo
Department of Otolaryngology, Nanjing Stomatological Hospital, Medical School of Nanjing University, Nanjing, China

Shamimul Hasan and Mandeep Kaur
Department of Oral Medicine and Radiology, Faculty of Dentistry, Jamia Millia Islamia, New Delhi, India

Syed Ansar Ahmad
Department of Oral and Maxillofacial Surgery, Faculty of Dentistry, Jamia Millia Islamia, New Delhi, India

Rajat Panigrahi
Department of Oral Medicine and Radiology, Institute of Dental Sciences, Siksha 'O' Anusandhan University, Bhubaneswar, Odisha, India

Swagatika Panda
Department of Oral and Maxillofacial Pathology, Institute of Dental Sciences, Siksha 'O' Anusandhan University, Bhubaneswar, Odisha, India

Saeed Shirafkan, Mehdi Gholamian, Ali Rohani, Sadaf Sadat Mahmoudinezhad and Kooshan Moradi
Department of Oral and Maxillofacial Surgery, School of Dentistry, Ahvaz Jundishapur University of Medical Sciences, Ahvaz, Iran

Mahshid Razavi
Department of Oral and Maxillofacial Radiology, School of Dentistry, Ahvaz Jundishapur University of Medical Sciences, Ahvaz, Iran

Ratna Meidyawati, Endang Suprastiwi and Hasti Dwi Setiati
Department of Conservative Dentistry, Faculty of Dentistry, Universitas Indonesia, Indonesia

Metab Algeffari
Department of Family and Community Medicine, College of Medicine, Qassim University, Saudi Arabia

Mansour Alsharidah
Department of Physiology, College of Medicine, Qassim University, Saudi Arabia

Zanab Malik
Registrar Special Needs Dentistry, Department of Oral Medicine, Oral Pathology and Special Needs Dentistry, Level 3 Westmead Centre for Oral Health, Westmead, NSW, Australia

Takashi Ito, Satoshi Fukuzawa, Kenji Yamagata, Shohei Takaoka, Makiko Ohkubo-Sato, Fumihiko Uchida, Naomi Ishibashi-Kanno and Hiroki Bukawa
Department of Oral and Maxillofacial Surgery, Faculty of Medicine, University of Tsukuba, Tennodai 1-1-1, Tsukuba, Ibaraki 305-8575, Japan

Zhaoguo Yue, Haidong Zhang, Lili Miao and Jianxia Hou
Department of Periodontology, Peking University School and Hospital of Stomatology, National Engineering Laboratory for Digital and Material Technology of Stomatology, Research Center of Engineering and Technology for Digital Dentistry of Ministry of Health, Beijing Key Laboratory of Digital Stomatology, Beijing, China

Qi Liu
BYBO Dental Hospital, Beijing, China

Jingwen Yang
Department of Prosthodontics, Peking University School and Hospital of Stomatology & National Clinical Research Center for Oral Diseases & National Engineering Laboratory for Digital and Material Technology of Stomatology & Beijing Key Laboratory of Digital Stomatology, Beijing, China

Maya Fedhila, Raouaa Belkacem Chebil, Lamia Oualha and Nabiha Douki
Department of Oral Medicine and Oral Surgery, SAHLOUL Hospital (Sousse), Dental Faculty of Monastir, University of Monastir, Tunisia
Laboratory of Oral Health and Maxillofacial Rehabilitation (LR12ES11), University of Monastir, Tunisia

Sonia Karray
National Center of Medicine in Schools and Universities, Tunisia

Ivan Pedro Taffarel
School of Life Sciences, Pontifícia Universidade Católica do Paraná, Curitiba, Brazil
Brazilian Board of Orthodontics and Dentofacial Orthopedics, Brazil

Thiago Martins Meira
School of Life Sciences, Pontifícia Universidade Católica do Paraná, Curitiba, Brazil
Bahia State University (UNEB), Guanambi, Bahia, Brazil

Lara Karolina Guimarães
School of Life Sciences, Pontifícia Universidade Católica do Paraná, Curitiba, Brazil

Oscar Mario Antelo
School of Life Sciences, Pontifícia Universidade Católica do Paraná, Curitiba, Brazil
Universidad Intercontinental, Cidade de Mexico, Mexico

Orlando Motohiro Tanaka
School of Life Sciences, Pontifícia Universidade Católica do Paraná, Curitiba, Brazil
Brazilian Board of Orthodontics and Dentofacial Orthopedics, Brazil
The Center for Advanced Dental Education, Saint Louis University, USA

Hossein Behnia
Department of Oral and Maxillofacial Surgery, Dental School, Shahid Beheshti University of Medical Sciences, Tehran, Iran

Hossein Mohammad-Rahimi
Dental Research Center, Dental Research Institute, Dental School, Shahid Beheshti University of Medical Sciences, Tehran, Iran

Mohammad Behnaz
Department of Orthodontics, Dental School, Shahid Beheshti University of Medical Sciences, Tehran, Iran

Ibrahem Amro and Lyana Shawar
Lebanon Dental Clinic, State of Palestine

Raed abu Hantash, Basem Abuquba and Akram Amro
Al-Quds University, State of Palestine

Sebastian Hinz, Christian Wegner and Tobias Bensel
Department of Prosthodontics, Faculty of Medicine, Martin Luther University Halle-Wittenberg, Magdeburger Straße 16, 06112 Halle (Saale), Germany

Daniel Ellmann
R+K CAD/CAM Technologie GmbH & Co.KG, Ruwerstieg 43, 12681 Berlin, Germany

Wolfgang Bömicke
Department of Oral, Dental and Maxillofacial Diseases, Heidelberg University Hospital, Im Neuenheimer Feld 400, Heidelberg 69120, Germany

Ikuho Kojima, Takashi Nishioka, Maya Sakamoto and Masahiro Iikubo
Division of Oral Diagnosis, Tohoku University Graduate School of Dentistry, 4-1 Seiryo-machi, Aoba-ku, Sendai, Miyagi 980-8575, Japan

Yuko Sai, Yushi Ezoe and Tetsu Takahashi
Division of Oral and Maxillofacial Surgery, Tohoku University Graduate School of Dentistry, 4-1 Seiryo-machi, Aoba-ku, Sendai, Miyagi 980-8575, Japan

Hiroyuki Kumamoto
Division of Oral Pathology, Tohoku University Graduate School of Dentistry, 4-1 Seiryo-machi, Aoba-ku, Sendai, Miyagi 980-8575, Japan

G. Galluccio, A. Impellizzeri and E. Serritella
Department of Oral and Maxillo Facial Sciences, Faculty of Medicine and Dentistry, Sapienza Università di Roma, Italy

A. A. De Stefano
Department of Oral and Maxillo Facial Sciences, Faculty of Medicine and Dentistry, Sapienza Università di Roma, Italy
Department of Orthodontics, Faculty of Dentistry, University Central of Venezuela, Caracas, Venezuela

E. Guercio Monaco
Department of Orthodontics, Faculty of Dentistry, University Central of Venezuela, Caracas, Venezuela

Index